Diabetes in pregnancy

management of diabetes and its complications from preconception to the postnatal period

National Collaborating Centre for Women's and Children's Health

Commissioned by the National Institute for Health and Clinical Excellence

March 2008

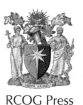

RCOG Press

Published by the **RCOG Press** at the Royal College of Obstetricians and Gynaecologists, 27 Sussex Place, Regent's Park, London NW1 4RG

www.rcog.org.uk

Registered charity no. 213280

First published 2008

ISBN 978-1-904752-47-9

NCC-WCH Editor: Andrew Welsh
Original design: FiSH Books, London
Typesetting: Andrew Welsh
Proofreading: Elisabeth Rees Evans
Index: Jan Ross (Merrall-Ross (Wales) Ltd)
Printed by Henry Ling Ltd, The Dorset Press, Dorchester DT1 1HD

Contents

Guideline Development Group membership and acknowledgements

Guideline Development Group

GDG member	Job title and affiliation	Area of expertise
Dominique Acolet (until October 2007)	Clinical Director (Perinatal Epidemiology), Confidential Enquiry into Maternal and Child Health (CEMACH), London	Neonatal paediatrician
Lynne Carney	Development Officer, Fair Share Trust, Community Foundation for Shropshire and Telford	Patient/carer representative
Anne Dornhorst	Consultant Physician and Honorary Senior Lecturer in Metabolic Medicine, Hammersmith Hospital, London	Diabetes physician
Robert Fraser	Reader in Obstetrics and Gynaecology, University of Sheffield	Obstetrician (GDG chair)
Roger Gadsby	General Practitioner, Nuneaton, and Senior Lecturer in Primary Care, University of Warwick	General practitioner
Jane Hawdon (from October 2007)	Consultant Neonatologist, University College Hospitals London NHS Foundation Trust	Neonatal paediatrician
Richard Holt	Reader of Endocrinology and Metabolism, University of Southampton	Diabetes physician
Ann Parker	Diabetes Advisory Midwife, Royal Shrewsbury Hospital	Diabetes specialist midwife
Nickey Tomkins	Advanced Nurse Practitioner in Diabetes/Diabetes Specialist Midwife, Medway Primary Care Trust, Kent	Diabetes nurse practitioner
Stephen Walkinshaw	Consultant in Maternal and Fetal Medicine, Liverpool Women's Hospital	Obstetrician
Jackie Webb	Diabetes Specialist Nurse Manager, Heart of England NHS Foundation Trust, Birmingham	Diabetes specialist nurse
Saiyyidah Zaidi	Programme Manager, Building Schools for the Future, London	Patient/carer representative

NCC-WCH staff	Job title and affiliation	Area of expertise
Paula Broughton-Palmer	Senior Work Programme Coordinator, NCC-WCH	Guideline methodologist
Michael Corkett	Senior Information Specialist, NCC-WCH	Guideline methodologist
Anthony Danso-Appiah	Research Fellow, NCC-WCH	Guideline methodologist
Paul Jacklin	Senior Health Economist, NCC-WCH	Guideline methodologist
Lorelei Jones	Research Fellow, London School of Hygiene & Tropical Medicine (formerly Research Fellow, NCC-WCH)	Guideline methodologist
Moira Mugglestone	Deputy Director, NCC-WCH	Guideline methodologist (NCC-WCH project director)
Jeffrey Round	Health Economist, NCC-WCH	Guideline methodologist
Anuradha Sekhri	Research Fellow, NCC-WCH	Guideline methodologist

External advisers

External adviser	Job title and affiliation	Area of expertise
Anita Holdcroft	Reader in Anaesthesia, Imperial College London, and Honorary Consultant Anaesthetist at Chelsea and Westminster Hospital, London	Obstetric analgesia and anaesthesia
Jo Modder	Clinical Director (Obstetrics), CEMACH, London and Consultant Obstetrician, University College London Hospitals NHS Trust	CEMACH Diabetes in Pregnancy programme
Peter Scanlon	National Co-ordinator, Diabetic Retinopathy Screening Programme (England), Consultant Ophthalmologist, Gloucestershire Eye Unit and Oxford Eye Hospital	Ophthalmologist with an interest in diabetic retinopathy
Roy Taylor	Professor of Medicine and Metabolism, University of Newcastle, and Honorary Consultant Physician, Newcastle Acute Hospitals NHS Trust and Newcastle Primary Care Trust	Diabetes physician with an interest in diabetic retinopathy

Guideline Review Panel

GRP member	Job title and affiliation
Mike Drummond	Director, Centre for Health Economics, University of York (GRP Chair)
Graham Archard	General Practitioner, Dorset
Catherine Arkley	Lay Member
Karen Cowley	Practice Development Nurse, York
David Gillen	Medical Director, Wyeth Pharmaceuticals
Barry Stables	Lay Member

Acknowledgements

Additional support was received from: Anna Burt, Jiri Chard, Sjokvist Garcia-Stewart, Anita Fitzgerald, Alyson Huntley, Debbie Pledge and Jane Tuckerman at the NCC-WCH. We also thank the Patient and Public Involvement Programme (PPIP) of the National Institute for Health and Clinical Excellence (NICE) whose glossary was adapted for use in this guideline. Finally, we thank CEMACH for allowing us to reproduce in our glossary terms from the glossary published in *Confidential Enquiry into Maternal and Child Health. Diabetes in pregnancy: are we providing the best care? Findings of a national enquiry: England, Wales and Northern Ireland*. London: CEMACH; 2007.

Stakeholder organisations

Action on Pre-eclampsia
Addenbrooke's NHS Trust
Adur Arun and Worthing PCT
Afiya Trust
Airedale General Hospital
All Wales Dietetic Advisory Committee
Anglesey Local Health Board
Ashfield and Mansfield District PCT
Association for Improvements in Maternity Services (AIMS)
Association of British Clinical Diabetologists
Association of British Health-Care Industries
Association of Clinical Biochemists
Association of Radical Midwives
Association of the British Pharmaceuticals Industry (ABPI)
AstraZeneca UK
Baby Lifeline
Barnsley Acute Trust
Barnsley PCT
Bedfordshire PCT

Birmingham Women's Healthcare Trust
Blaenau Gwent Local Health Board
BLISS – the premature baby charity
Bournemouth and Poole PCT
Bradford & Airdale PCT
Bradford Hospitals NHS Trust
Brighton & Sussex University Hospitals Trust
Bristol Health Services Plan
British Association for Counselling and Psychotherapy
British Association of Perinatal Medicine
British Dietetic Association
British Maternal and Fetal Medicine Society
British National Formulary (BNF)
British Psychological Society
Buckinghamshire Hospitals NHS Trust
Calderdale PCT
CASPE
CEMACH
City and Hackney PCT
City Hospitals Sunderland NHS Trust
Cochrane Pregnancy & Childbirth Group
Commission for Social Care Inspection
Connecting for Health
Conwy & Denbighshire NHS Trust
Co-operative Pharmacy Association
County Durham and Darlington Acute Hospital Trust
Coventry and Warwickshire Cardiac Network
Craven Harrogate & Rural District PCT
Croydon PCT
Cytyc UK
Daiichi Sankyo UK
Department of Health
Department of Health, Social Security and Public Safety of Northern Ireland
Derbyshire Mental Health Services NHS Trust
Det Norske Veritas – NHSLA Schemes
Diabetes UK
Doncaster PCT
East and North Herts PCT
East Sussex Hospitals NHS Trust
Echo UK (the tiny tickers charity)
Eli Lilly and Company
English National Forum of LSA Midwifery Officers
Evidence Based Midwifery Network
Faculty of Public Health
Fibroid Network Charity
Gloucestershire Hospitals NHS Trust
Guy's and St Thomas' NHS Foundation Trust
Healthcare Commission
Heart of England NHS Foundation Trust
HemoCue Ltd
Independent Midwives Association
Institute of Biomedical Science
Institute of Health and Society
Insulin Dependent Diabetes Trust
JBOL
King's College Acute Trust
La Leche League GB
Leeds PCT
Leeds Teaching Hospitals NHS Trust
Liverpool PCT
Liverpool Women's Hospital NHS Trust

Long Term Medical Conditions Alliance
Luton and Dunstable Hospital NHS Trust
Maidstone and Tunbridge Wells NHS Trust
Maidstone Hospital
Medicines and Healthcare products Regulatory Agency (MHRA)
Medtronic
Medway NHS Trust
Menarini Diagnostics
Merck Pharmaceuticals
Mid and West Regional MSLC
Mid Staffordshire General Hospitals NHS Trust
MIDIRS (Midwives Information & Resource Service)
Milton Keynes PCT
National Audit Office
National Childbirth Trust
National Council for Disabled People and Carers from Black & Minority Ethnic Communities
National Diabetes Consultant Nurse Group
National Kidney Research Fund
National Perinatal Epidemiology Unit
National Public Health Service – Wales
National Screening Committee
Newcastle PCT
NHS Clinical Knowledge Summaries Service
NHS Direct
NHS Quality Improvement Scotland
Norfolk, Suffolk & Cambridgeshire Strategic Health Authority
North Eastern Derbyshire PCT
North Middlesex Hospital University Trust
North Sheffield PCT
North Tees and Hartlepool NHS Trust
North Yorkshire and York PCT
Northumbria Diabetes Service
Northumbria Healthcare NHS Foundation Trust
Northwest London Hospitals NHS Trust
Nottingham City PCT
Novo Nordisk
Nutrition Society
Obstetric Anaesthetists Association
Pennine Acute Hospitals NHS Trust
PERIGON (formerly the NHS Modernisation Agency)
Pfizer
Powys Local Health Board
Primary Care Diabetes Society
Primary Care Pharmacists Association
PRIMIS+
Princess Alexandra Hospital NHS Trust
Prodigy
Queen Elizabeth Hospital NHS Trust
Queen Mary's Hospital NHS Trust (Sidcup)
RCM Consultant Midwives Forum
Regional Maternity Survey Office
Roche Diagnostics
Rotherham PCT
Royal Bolton Hospitals NHS Trust
Royal College of Anaesthetists
Royal College of General Practitioners
Royal College of General Practitioners Wales
Royal College of Midwives
Royal College of Nursing (RCN)
Royal College of Obstetricians and Gynaecologists
Royal College of Ophthalmologists

Royal College of Paediatrics and Child Health
Royal College of Pathologists
Royal College of Physicians of Edinburgh
Royal College of Physicians of London
Royal College of Radiologists
Royal Cornwall Hospitals NHS Trust and Peninsula Medical School
Royal Society of Medicine
Royal United Hospital Bath NHS Trust
Royal West Sussex Trust
Salford PCT
Salford Royal Hospitals Foundation NHS Trust
Sandwell and West Birmingham NHS Trust
Sandwell PCT
Sanofi-Aventis
Scarborough and North Yorkshire Healthcare NHS Trust
School of Midwifery
Scottish Executive Health Department
Scottish Intercollegiate Guidelines Network (SIGN)
Scottish Nutrition & Diet Resources Initiative
Sheffield PCT
Sheffield Teaching Hospitals NHS Trust
Society & College of Radiographers
South Asian Health Foundation
South Staffordshire PCT
South Tees Hospitals NHS Trust
Southend Hospitals NHS Trust
Staffordshire Moorlands PCT
Stockport PCT
Sunderland Royal Hospital NHS Trust
Sure Start Tamworth
Syner-Med Pharmaceutical Products
Takeda UK
Tameside Acute Trust
Tameside and Glossop Acute Services NHS Trust
Trafford PCT
UK Anaemia
UK Clinical Pharmacy Association
UK National Screening Committee
UK Specialised Services Public Health Network
University College London Hospitals NHS Trust
University Hospital Lewisham
University Hospital of North Staffordshire Acute Trust
University Hospitals of Leicester
University of Leicester (The Infant Mortality & Morbidity Studies)
Welsh Assembly Government (formerly National Assembly for Wales)
Welsh Endocrine and Diabetes Society
Welsh Scientific Advisory Committee (WSAC)
West Hertfordshire Hospitals Trust
West Herts PCT
West Middlesex University Hospital NHS Trust
West Midlands Antenatal Diabetes Association
Western Cheshire Primary Care Trust
Whittington Hospital Trust
Wiltshire PCT
Wirral Hospital NHS Trust
Worcestershire Acute Trust
Worthing Hospital
York NHS Trust
Yorkshire and the Humber LSA

Abbreviations

AC	abdominal circumference
ACE	angiotensin-converting enzyme
ACHOIS	Australian Carbohydrate Intolerance Study in Pregnant Women
ADA	American Diabetes Association
AFP	alpha fetoprotein
AGA	appropriate for gestational age
ARB	angiotensin-II receptor blocker (also known as angiotensin-II receptor antagonist)
BMI	body mass index
BP	blood pressure
CBG	capillary blood glucose
CEMACH	Confidential Enquiry into Maternal and Child Health
CI	confidence interval
CINAHL	Cumulative Index to Nursing and Allied Health Literature
CSII	continuous subcutaneous insulin infusion
DAFNE	Dose Adjustment for Normal Eating
DCCT	Diabetes Control and Complications Trial
DESMOND	Diabetes Education and Self Management for Ongoing and Newly Diagnosed
DKA	diabetic ketoacidosis
DPP	Diabetes Prevention Program
DVLA	Driver and Vehicle Licensing Agency
EFW	estimated fetal weight
eGFR	estimated glomerular filtration rate
EL	evidence level
EPO	erythropoietin
ETDRS	Early Treatment Diabetic Retinopathy Study
EUROCAT	European Surveillance of Congenital Anomalies
FBG	fasting blood glucose
FCG	fasting capillary glucose
FPG	fasting plasma glucose
GCT	glucose challenge test
GDG	guideline development group
GI	glycaemic index
GP	general practitioner
HAPO	Hyperglycemia and Adverse Pregnancy Outcome
HbA_{1c}	glycosylated haemoglobin
hCG	human chorionic gonadotropin
HTA	health technology assessment
ICER	incremental cost-effectiveness ratio
IGT	impaired glucose tolerance
IUGR	intrauterine growth restriction
LGA	large for gestational age
LR	likelihood ratio
MIG	Metformin in Gestational Diabetes
MDI	multiple daily injection
MODY	maturity-onset diabetes of the young
MoM	multiple-of-median
NCC-WCH	National Collaborating Centre for Women's and Children's Health
NDDG	National Diabetes Data Group
NHS	National Health Service
NHS EED	NHS Economic Evaluation Database
NHSLA	National Health Service Litigation Authority
NICE	National Institute for Health and Clinical Excellence

NICU	neonatal intensive care unit
NNH	number needed to harm
NNT	number needed to treat
NPDR	non-proliferative diabetic retinopathy
NPV	negative predictive value
NSF	National Service Framework
NT	nuchal translucency
OGTT	oral glucose tolerance test
ONS	Office for National Statistics
OR	odds ratio
PAPP-A	pregnancy-associated plasma protein-A
PDR	proliferative diabetic retinopathy
PPIP	Patient and Public Involvement Programme
PPV	positive predictive value
QALY	quality-adjusted life year
RBG	random blood glucose
RCT	randomised controlled trial
ROC	receiver operating characteristic
RR	relative risk
SD	standard deviation
SE	standard error
SGA	small for gestational age
TA	technology appraisal
TGA	transposition of the great arteries
uE3	unconjugated estriol
VBAC	vaginal birth after previous caesarean section
WHO	World Health Organization

Glossary of terms

ACE inhibitor	Angiotensin-converting enzyme inhibitor; a class of drugs that reduce peripheral arterial resistance by inactivating an enzyme that converts angiotensin-I to the vasoconstrictor angiotensin-II.
Albuminuria	The presence of albumin in the urine, indicating renal dysfunction.
Antenatal	The period of time in pregnancy preceding birth.
Applicability	The extent to which the results of a study or review can be applied to the **target population** for a clinical guideline.
Appraisal of evidence	Formal assessment of the quality of research evidence and its relevance to the clinical question or guideline under consideration, according to predetermined criteria.
Best available evidence	The strongest research evidence available to support a particular guideline recommendation.
Bias	Influences on a study that can lead to invalid conclusions about a treatment or intervention. Bias in research can make a treatment look better or worse than it really is. Bias can even make it look as if the treatment works when it actually does not. Bias can occur by chance or as a result of **systematic errors** in the design and execution of a study. Bias can occur at different stages in the research process, e.g. in the collection, analysis, interpretation, publication or review of research data. For examples see **selection bias, performance bias, information bias, confounding factor, publication bias.**
Blinding or masking	The practice of keeping the investigators or subjects of a study ignorant of the group to which a subject has been assigned. For example, a clinical trial in which the participating patients or their doctors are unaware of whether they (the patients) are taking the experimental drug or a **placebo** (dummy treatment). The purpose of 'blinding' or 'masking' is to protect against **bias**. See also **double-blind study, single-blind study, triple-blind study.**
Body mass index (BMI)	The body's weight in kilograms divided by the square of the height in metres, used in the assessment of obesity.
Cardiomegaly	Enlargement of the heart.
Cardiotocograph	Graphical representation of electronic monitoring of the fetal heart rate and of uterine contractions. The fetal heart rate is recorded by means of either an external ultrasonic abdominal transducer or a fetal scalp electrode. Uterine contractions are recorded by means of an abdominal pressure transducer.
Case report (or case study)	Detailed report on one patient (or case), usually covering the course of that person's disease and their response to treatment.
Case series	Description of several cases of a given disease, usually covering the course of the disease and the response to treatment. There is no comparison (**control**) group of patients.
Case–control study	A study that compares exposure in subjects who have a particular outcome with those who do not. The study starts with the identification of a group of individuals sharing the same characteristics (e.g. people with a particular disease) and a suitable comparison (**control**) group (e.g. people without the disease). All subjects are then assessed with respect to things that happened to them in the past, e.g. things that might be related to getting the disease under investigation. Such studies are also called **retrospective** as they look back in time from the outcome to the possible causes.
Causal relationship	Describes the relationship between two **variables** whenever it can be established that one causes the other. For example, there is a causal relationship between a treatment and a disease if it can be shown that the treatment changes the course or outcome of the disease. Usually **randomised controlled trials** are needed to ascertain causality. Proving cause and effect is much more difficult than just showing an association between two variables. For example, if it happened that everyone who had eaten a particular food became sick, and everyone who avoided that food remained well, then the food would clearly be associated with the sickness. However, even if leftovers were found to be contaminated, it could not be proved that the food caused the sickness – unless all other possible causes (e.g. environmental factors) had been ruled out.

Centile	Any of the 99 numbered points that divide an ordered set of scores into 100 parts each of which contains one-hundredth of the total.
Checklist	See **study checklist**.
Clinical audit	A **systematic** process for setting and monitoring standards of clinical care. Whereas 'guidelines' define what the best clinical practice should be, 'audit' investigates whether best practice is being carried out. Clinical audit can be described as a cycle or spiral. Within the cycle there are stages that follow a systematic process of establishing best practice, measuring care against specific criteria, taking action to improve care, and monitoring to sustain improvement. The spiral suggests that as the process continues, each cycle aspires to a higher level of quality.
Clinical effectiveness	The extent to which a specific treatment or intervention, when used under *usual* or *everyday conditions*, has a beneficial effect on the course or outcome of disease compared with no treatment or other routine care. (Clinical trials that assess effectiveness are sometimes called management trials.) Clinical 'effectiveness' is not the same as **efficacy**.
Clinical impact	The effect that a guideline recommendation is likely to have on the treatment, or treatment outcomes, of the **target population**.
Clinical importance	The importance of a particular guideline recommendation to the clinical management of the **target population**.
Clinical question	This term is sometimes used in guideline development work to refer to the questions about treatment and care that are formulated in order to guide the search for research evidence. When a clinical question is formulated in a precise way, it is called a **focused question**.
Clinical trial	A research study conducted with patients which tests out a drug or other intervention to assess its effectiveness and safety. Each trial is designed to answer scientific questions and to find better ways to treat individuals with a specific disease. This general term encompasses **controlled clinical trials** and **randomised controlled trials**.
Clinician	A qualified healthcare professional providing patient care, e.g. doctor, nurse, physiotherapist.
Cochrane Collaboration	An international organisation in which people find, appraise and review specific types of studies called **randomised controlled trials**. The Cochrane Database of Systematic Reviews contains regularly updated reviews on a variety of health issues and is available electronically as part of the **Cochrane Library**.
Cochrane Library	The Cochrane Library consists of a regularly updated collection of evidence-based medicine databases including the Cochrane Database of Systematic Reviews (reviews of **randomised controlled trials** prepared by the **Cochrane Collaboration**). The Cochrane Library is available on CD-ROM and the internet.
Cohort	A group of people sharing some common characteristic (e.g. patients with the same disease), followed up in a research study for a specified period of time.
Cohort study	An **observational study** that takes a group (cohort) of patients and follows their progress over time in order to measure outcomes such as disease or mortality rates and make comparisons according to the treatments or interventions that patients received. Thus within the study group, subgroups of patients are identified (from information collected about patients) and these groups are compared with respect to outcome, e.g. comparing mortality between one group that received a specific treatment and one group which did not (or between two groups that received different levels of treatment). Cohorts can be assembled in the present and followed into the future (a 'concurrent' or '**prospective**' cohort study) or identified from past records and followed forward from that time up to the present (a 'historical' or '**retrospective**' cohort study). Because patients are not randomly allocated to subgroups, these subgroups may be quite different in their characteristics and some adjustment must be made when analysing the results to ensure that the comparison between groups is as fair as possible.
Comorbidity	Coexistence of a disease or diseases in the people being studied in addition to the health problem that is the subject of the study.
Confidence interval (CI)	A way of expressing certainty about the findings from a study or group of studies, using statistical techniques. A confidence interval describes a range of possible effects (of a treatment or intervention) that are consistent with the results of a study or group of studies. A wide confidence interval indicates a lack of certainty or precision about the true size of the clinical effect and is seen in studies with too few patients. Where confidence intervals are narrow they indicate more precise estimates of effects and a larger sample of patients studied. It is usual to interpret a '95%' confidence interval as the range of effects within which we are 95% confident that the true effect lies.

Confounder or confounding factor	A factor that can bring an alternative explanation to an association observed between an exposure and the outcome of interest. It influences a study and can contribute to misleading findings if it is not understood or appropriately dealt with. For example, if a group of people exercising regularly and a group of people who do not exercise have an important age difference then any difference found in outcomes about heart disease could well be due to one group being older than the other rather than due to the exercising. Age is the confounding factor here and the effect of exercising on heart disease cannot be assessed without adjusting for age differences in some way.
Congenital anomaly	A physical or biochemical malformation which is present at birth
Consensus development conference	A technique used for the purpose of reaching an agreement on a particular issue. It involves bringing together a group of about ten people who are presented with evidence by various interest groups or experts who are not part of the decision-making group. The group then retires to consider the questions in the light of the evidence presented and attempts to reach a consensus. See also **consensus methods**.
Consensus methods	A variety of techniques that aim to reach an agreement on a particular issue. Formal consensus methods include **Delphi** and **nominal group techniques** and consensus development conferences. In the development of clinical guidelines, consensus methods may be used where there is a lack of strong research evidence on a particular topic.
Consensus statement	A statement of the advised course of action in relation to a particular clinical topic, based on the collective views of a body of experts.
Considered judgement	The application of the collective knowledge of a guideline development group to a body of evidence, to assess its **applicability** to the **target population** and the strength of any recommendation that it would support.
Consistency	The extent to which the conclusions of a collection of studies used to support a guideline recommendation are in agreement with each other. See also **homogeneity**.
Control group	A group of patients recruited into a study that receives no treatment, a treatment of known effect or a **placebo** (dummy treatment) in order to provide a comparison for a group receiving an experimental treatment, such as a new drug.
Controlled clinical trial (CCT)	A study testing a specific drug or other treatment involving two (or more) groups of patients with the same disease. One (the experimental group) receives the treatment that is being tested, and the other (the comparison or **control group**) receives an alternative treatment, a **placebo** (dummy treatment) or no treatment. The two groups are followed up to compare differences in outcomes to see how effective the experimental treatment was. A CCT where patients are randomly allocated to treatment and comparison groups is called a **randomised controlled trial**.
Cost–benefit analysis	A type of **economic evaluation** where both costs and benefits of healthcare treatment are measured in the same monetary units. If benefits exceed costs, the evaluation would recommend providing the treatment.
Cost-effectiveness	Value for money. A specific healthcare treatment is said to be 'cost-effective' if it gives a greater health gain than could be achieved by using the resources in other ways.
Cost-effectiveness analysis	A type of **economic evaluation** comparing the costs and the effects on health of different treatments. Health effects are measured in 'health-related units', for example, the cost of preventing one additional heart attack.
Cost–utility analysis	A special form of **cost-effectiveness analysis** where health effects are measured in **quality-adjusted life years**. A treatment is assessed in terms of its ability to both extend life and to improve the quality of life.
Crossover study design	A study comparing two or more interventions in which the participants, upon completion of the course of one treatment, are switched to another. For example, for a comparison of treatments A and B, half the participants are randomly allocated to receive them in the order A, B and half to receive them in the order B, A. A problem with this study design is that the effects of the first treatment may carry over into the period when the second is given. Therefore a crossover study should include an adequate 'wash-out' period, which means allowing sufficient time between stopping one treatment and starting another so that the first treatment has time to wash out of the patient's system.
Cross-sectional study	The observation of a defined set of people at a single point in time or time period – a snapshot. This type of study contrasts with a **longitudinal study**, which follows a set of people over a period of time.
Data set	A list of required information relating to a specific disease.

Decision analysis	The study of how people make decisions or how they *should* make decisions. There are several methods that decision analysts use to help people to make better decisions, including **decision trees**.
Decision tree	A method for helping people to make better decisions in situations of uncertainty. It illustrates the decision as a succession of possible actions and outcomes. It consists of the probabilities, costs and health consequences associated with each option. The overall effectiveness or overall cost-effectiveness of different actions can then be compared.
Declaration of interest	A process by which members of a working group or committee 'declare' any personal or professional involvement with a company (or related to a technology) that might affect their objectivity, for example if their position or department is funded by a pharmaceutical company.
Delphi method	A technique used for the purpose of reaching an agreement on a particular issue, without the participants meeting or interacting directly. It involves sending participants a series of postal questionnaires asking them to record their views. After the first questionnaire, participants are asked to give further views in the light of the group feedback. The judgements of the participants are statistically aggregated, sometimes after weighting for expertise. See also **consensus methods**.
Diabetic ketoacidosis (DKA)	A state of absolute or relative insulin deficiency characterised by hyperglycaemia, dehydration, acidosis and ketosis.
Diabetic nephropathy	Kidney dysfunction or disease occurring as a result of diabetes.
Diabetic retinopathy	A complication of diabetes affecting the blood vessels in the retina at the back of the eye, which can affect vision. There may be bleeding from retinal vessels (non-proliferative retinopathy) or the development of new abnormal vessels (proliferative retinopathy).
Diagnostic study	A study to assess the effectiveness of a test or measurement in terms of its ability to accurately detect or exclude a specific disease.
Dominance	A term used in **health economics** describing when an option for treatment is both less clinically effective and more costly than an alternative option. The less effective and more costly option is said to be 'dominated'.
Double-blind study	A study in which neither the subject (patient) nor the observer (investigator/clinician) is aware of which treatment or intervention the subject is receiving. The purpose of **blinding** is to protect against **bias**.
Economic evaluation	A comparison of alternative courses of action in terms of both their costs and consequences. In **health economic** evaluations the consequences should include health outcomes.
Effectiveness	See **clinical effectiveness**.
Efficacy	The extent to which a specific treatment or intervention, under *ideally controlled conditions* (e.g. in a laboratory) has a beneficial effect on the course or outcome of disease compared with no treatment or other routine care.
Elective	Clinical procedures that are regarded as advantageous to the patient but not urgent.
Empirical	Based directly on experience (observation or experiment) rather than on reasoning alone.
Epidemiology	Study of diseases within a population, covering the causes and means of prevention.
Erb palsy	Injury to the nerve roots of the brachial plexus of an arm mainly related to birth trauma and leading to various degrees of weakness of the affected arm which may resolve during the first year of life.
Evidence based	The process of systematically finding, appraising and using research findings as the basis for clinical decisions.
Evidence level	A code (e.g. 1++, 1+) linked to an individual study, indicating where it fits into the **hierarchy of evidence** and how well it has adhered to recognised research principles. Also called level of evidence.
Evidence table	A table summarising the results of a collection of studies which, taken together, represent the evidence supporting a particular recommendation or series of recommendations in a guideline.
Evidence-based clinical practice	Evidence-based clinical practice involves making decisions about the care of individual patients based on the best research evidence available rather than basing decisions on personal opinions or common practice (which may not always be evidence based). Evidence-based clinical practice therefore involves integrating individual clinical expertise and patient preferences with the best available evidence from research.

Exclusion criteria	See **selection criteria**.
Experimental study	A research study designed to test if a treatment or intervention has an effect on the course or outcome of a condition or disease – where the conditions of testing are to some extent under the control of the investigator. **Controlled clinical trial** and **randomised controlled trial** are examples of experimental studies.
Experimental treatment	A treatment or intervention (e.g. a new drug) being studied to see if it has an effect on the course or outcome of a condition or disease.
Extrapolation	The application of research evidence based on studies of a specific population to another population with similar characteristics.
Fetal growth restriction	Evidence of abnormally slow growth of the fetus within the uterus; either estimated weight or abdominal circumference below the 10th percentile, or slowing growth velocity of the abdominal circumference as measured at a subsequent ultrasound scan.
Fetal surveillance	The process of performing fetal wellbeing tests. These may include ultrasound scans, fetal and placental Doppler ultrasounds, biophysical profiles and fetal heart monitoring.
Focused question	A study question that clearly identifies all aspects of the topic that are to be considered while seeking an answer. Questions are normally expected to identify the patients or population involved, the treatment or intervention to be investigated, what outcomes are to be considered, and any comparisons that are to be made. For example, do insulin pumps (intervention) improve blood sugar control (outcome) in adolescents with type 1 diabetes (population) compared with multiple insulin injections (comparison)? See also **clinical question**.
Folic acid	A water-soluble vitamin in the B-complex group which helps to prevent fetal neural tube defect when commenced by the mother before conception.
Funnel plot	Funnel plots are simple scatter plots on a graph. They show the treatment effects estimated from separate studies on the horizontal axis against a measure of sample size on the vertical axis. **Publication bias** may lead to asymmetry in funnel plots.
Gestation	The time from conception to birth. The duration of gestation is measured from the first day of the last normal menstrual period.
Gestational diabetes	Carbohydrate intolerance of varying severity which is diagnosed in pregnancy and may or may not resolve after pregnancy.
Glucose electrode	Blood glucose measurement using electrochemical biosensors.
Glycaemic control targets	Recommended levels of blood glucose.
Glycosylated haemoglobin (HbA_{1c})	A test which measures the amount of glucose-bound haemoglobin and reflects how well the blood glucose level has been controlled over the previous 2–3 months.
Gold standard	A method, procedure or measurement that is widely accepted as being the best available.
Grey literature	Reports that are unpublished or have limited distribution and are not included in bibliographic retrieval systems.
Guideline	A systematically developed tool that describes aspects of a patient's condition and the care to be given. A good guideline makes recommendations about treatment and care based on the best research available, rather than opinion. It is used to assist clinician and patient decision making about appropriate health care for specific clinical conditions.
Guideline recommendation	Course of action advised by the guideline development group on the basis of their assessment of the supporting evidence.
Health economics	A branch of economics that studies decisions about the use and distribution of healthcare resources.
Health technology	Health technologies include medicines, medical devices such as artificial hip joints, diagnostic techniques, surgical procedures, health promotion activities (e.g. the role of diet versus medicines in disease management) and other therapeutic interventions.
Heterogeneity	Or lack of **homogeneity**. The term is used in **meta-analyses** and **systematic reviews** when the results or estimates of effects of treatment from separate studies seem to be very different in terms of the size of treatment effects or even to the extent that some indicate beneficial and others suggest adverse treatment effects. Such results may occur as a result of differences between studies in terms of the patient populations, outcome measures, definition of **variables** or duration of follow-up.

Hierarchy of evidence	An established hierarchy of study types, based on the degree of certainty that can be attributed to the conclusions that can be drawn from a well-conducted study. Well-conducted **randomised controlled trials** (RCTs) are at the top of this hierarchy (for example, several large statistically significant RCTs which are in agreement represent stronger evidence than one small RCT). Well-conducted studies of patients' views and experiences would appear at a lower level in the hierarchy of evidence.
Homogeneity	This means that the results of studies included in a **systematic review** or **meta-analysis** are similar and there is no evidence of **heterogeneity**. Results are usually regarded as homogeneous when differences between studies could reasonably be expected to occur by chance. See also **consistency**
Hypertension	High blood pressure.
Hypoglycaemia	Low blood glucose level.
Inclusion criteria	See **selection criteria**.
Information bias	Pertinent to all types of study and can be caused by inadequate questionnaires (e.g. difficult or biased questions), observer or interviewer errors (e.g. lack of **blinding**), response errors (e.g. lack of blinding if patients are aware of the treatment they receive) and measurement error (e.g. a faulty machine).
Interquartile range (IQR)	The spread of a set of values between which 25% (25th centile) and 75% (75th centile) of these values lie.
Intervention	Healthcare action intended to benefit the patient, e.g. drug treatment, surgical procedure, psychological therapy, etc.
Level of evidence	See **evidence level**.
Literature review	A process of collecting, reading and assessing the quality of published (and unpublished) articles on a given topic.
Longitudinal study	A study of the same group of people at more than one point in time. This type of study contrasts with a **cross-sectional study**, which observes a defined set of people at a single point in time.
Macrosomia	Oversized baby as seen, for example as a consequence of the effect of diabetes during pregnancy. Often defined as having a birthweight above the 90th centile for gestation or a birthweight of 4000 g or more.
Masking	See **blinding**.
Median	The value of the middle item of a series when the items are arranged in numerical order.
Meta-analysis	Results from a collection of independent studies (investigating the same treatment) are pooled, using statistical techniques to synthesise their findings into a single estimate of a treatment effect. Where studies are not compatible e.g. because of differences in the study populations or in the outcomes measured, it may be inappropriate or even misleading to statistically pool results in this way. See also **systematic review** and **heterogeneity**.
Metformin	An oral antidiabetic agent that decreases glucose production by the liver and lowers plasma glucose levels.
Methodological quality	The extent to which a study has conformed to recognised good practice in the design and execution of its research methods.
Methodology	The overall approach of a research project; for example, that the study will be a **randomised controlled trial** of 200 people over 1 year.
Microalbuminuria	A very small increase in urinary albumin.
Miscarriage	Spontaneous ending of a pregnancy before viability (currently taken as 24 weeks of gestation).
Maturity-onset diabetes of the young (MODY)	A group of autosomal dominant disorders in young people each caused by a single gene defect, associated with decreased insulin production and varying degrees of clinical severity.
Multicentre study	A study where subjects were selected from different locations or populations, e.g. a cooperative study between different hospitals or an international collaboration involving patients from more than one country.
Multidisciplinary clinic	A clinic with access to care from health professionals in more than one discipline. For diabetes, the disciplines recommended are obstetrics, diabetology, nursing, midwifery and dietetics.

Multiparous	A woman who has had at least one previous birth (from 24 weeks onwards).
Negative predictive value (NPV)	The proportion of people with a negative test result who do not have the disease (where not having the disease is indicated by the 'gold standard' test being negative).
Neonatal death	Death of a liveborn baby before 28 completed days after birth.
Neonatal unit	A unit which provides additional care for babies over and above that which can be offered on a postnatal ward or transitional care unit. There are different levels of complexity of care which can be offered by an individual neonatal unit.
Neural tube defect	A major birth defect caused by abnormal development of the neural tube, the structure present during embryonic life which later gives rise to the central nervous system (brain and spinal cord).
Nominal group technique	A technique used for the purpose of reaching an agreement on a particular issue. It uses a variety of postal and direct contact techniques, with individual judgements being aggregated statistically to derive the group judgement. See also **consensus methods**.
Non-experimental study	A study based on subjects selected on the basis of their availability, with no attempt having been made to avoid problems of **bias**.
Non-systematic review	See **review**.
Number needed to treat (NNT)	This measures the impact of a treatment or intervention. It states how many patients need to be treated with the treatment in question in order to prevent an event which would otherwise occur, e.g. if the NNT = 4, then four patients would have to be treated to prevent one bad outcome. The closer the NNT is to 1, the better the treatment is. Analogous to the NNT is the number needed to harm (NNH), which is the number of patients that would need to receive a treatment to cause one additional adverse event, e.g. if the NNH = 4, then four patients would have to be treated for one bad outcome to occur.
Obesity	Increased body weight, defined as a body mass index of 30 kg/m^2 or greater.
Observation	A research technique used to help understand complex situations. It involves watching, listening to and recording behaviours, actions, activities and interactions. The settings are usually natural, but they can be laboratory settings, as in psychological research.
Observational study	In research about diseases or treatments, this refers to a study in which nature is allowed to take its course. Changes or differences in one characteristic (e.g. whether or not people received a specific treatment or intervention) are studied in relation to changes or differences in other(s) (e.g. whether or not they died), without the intervention of the investigator. There is a greater risk of **selection bias** than in **experimental studies**.
Odds ratio (OR)	Odds are a way of representing probability, especially familiar for betting. In recent years odds ratios have become widely used in reports of clinical studies. They are a measure of the excess risk or degree of protection given by exposure to a certain factor. They provide an estimate (usually with a **confidence interval**) for the effect of a treatment. Odds are used to convey the idea of 'risk' and an odds ratio of 1 between two treatment groups would imply that the risks of an adverse outcome were the same in each group. An odds ratio of greater than 1 shows an increased risk and less than 1 shows a protective effect. For rare events the odds ratio and the **relative risk** (which uses actual risks and not odds) will be very similar. See also **relative risk, risk ratio**.
Outcome	The end result of care and treatment and/or rehabilitation. In other words, the change in health, functional ability, symptoms or situation of a person, which can be used to measure the effectiveness of care/treatment/rehabilitation. Researchers should decide what outcomes to measure before a study begins; outcomes are then assessed at the end of the study.
P **value**	If a study is done to compare two treatments then the *P* value is the probability of obtaining the results of that study or something more extreme if there really was no difference between treatments. (The assumption that there really is no difference between treatments is called the 'null hypothesis'.) Suppose the *P* value was $P = 0.03$. What this means is that if there really was no difference between treatments then there would only be a 3% chance of getting the kind of results obtained. Since this chance seems quite low we should question the validity of the assumption that there really is no difference between treatments. We would conclude that there probably is a difference between treatments. By convention, where the value of *P* is below 0.05 (i.e. less than 5%) the result is seen as statistically significant. Where the value of *P* is 0.001 or less, the result is seen as highly significant. *P* values just tell us whether an effect can be regarded as statistically significant or not. In no way do they relate to how big the effect might be, for which we need the **confidence interval**.

Peer review	Review of a study, service or recommendations by those with similar interests and expertise to the people who produced the study findings or recommendations. Peer reviewers can include professional and/or patient/carer representatives.
Performance bias	Systematic differences in care provided apart from the intervention being evaluated. For example, if study participants know they are in the **control group** they may be more likely to use other forms of care; people who know they are in the experimental group may experience **placebo effects**, and care providers may treat patients differently according to what group they are in. Masking (**blinding**) of both the recipients and providers of care is used to protect against performance bias.
Pilot study	A small scale 'test' of the research instrument, for example testing out (piloting) a new questionnaire with people who are similar to the population of the study in order to highlight any problems or areas of concern, which can then be addressed before the full-scale study begins.
Placebo	Fake or inactive treatments received by participants allocated to the **control group** in a clinical trial that are indistinguishable from the active treatments being given in the experimental group. They are used so that participants are ignorant of their treatment allocation in order to be able to quantify the effect of the experimental treatment over and above any **placebo effect** due to receiving care or attention.
Placebo effect	A beneficial (or adverse) effect produced by a **placebo** and not due to any property of the placebo itself.
Positive predictive value (PPV)	The proportion of people with a positive test result who have the disease (where having the disease is indicated by the 'gold standard' test being positive).
Postnatal	The period of time occurring after birth.
Power	See **statistical power**.
Preterm birth	Birth before 37 weeks and 0 days of gestation.
Prevalence	The proportion of individuals in a population having a disease.
Probability	How likely an event is to occur, e.g. how likely a treatment or intervention will alleviate a symptom.
Prospective study	A study in which people are entered into the research and then followed up over a period of time with future events recorded as they happen. This contrasts with studies that are **retrospective**.
Protocol	A plan or set of steps that defines appropriate action. A research protocol sets out, in advance of carrying out the study, what question is to be answered and how information will be collected and analysed. Guideline implementation protocols set out how guideline recommendations will be used in practice by the NHS, both at national and local levels.
Publication bias	Studies with statistically significant results are more likely to get published than those with non-significant results. **Meta-analyses** that are exclusively based on published literature may therefore produce biased results. This type of bias can be assessed by a **funnel plot**.
Quality-adjusted life years (QALYs)	A measure of health outcome that looks at both length of life and quality of life. QALYs are calculated by estimating the years of life remaining for a patient following a particular care pathway and weighting each year with a quality of life score (on a zero to one scale). One QALY is equal to 1 year of life in perfect health or 2 years at 50% health, and so on.
Quantitative research	Research that generates numerical data or data that can be converted into numbers, for example clinical trials or the national Census that counts people and households.
Quintile	The portion of a frequency distribution containing one-fifth of the total sample.
Random allocation or randomisation	A method that uses the play of chance to assign participants to comparison groups in a research study, for example, by using a random numbers table or a computer-generated random sequence. Random allocation implies that each individual (or each unit in the case of **cluster randomisation**) being entered into a study has the same chance of receiving each of the possible interventions.

Randomised controlled trial (RCT)	A study to test a specific drug or other treatment in which people are randomly assigned to two (or more) groups: one (the experimental group) receiving the treatment that is being tested, and the other (the comparison or **control group**) receiving an alternative treatment, a **placebo** (dummy treatment) or no treatment. The two groups are followed up to compare differences in outcomes to see how effective the experimental treatment was. Through randomisation, the groups should be similar in all aspects apart from the treatment they receive during the study.
Range	The difference or interval between the smallest and largest values in a frequency distribution.
Relative risk (RR)	A summary measure which represents the ratio of the risk of a given event or outcome (e.g. an adverse reaction to the drug being tested) in one group of subjects compared with another group. When the 'risk' of the event is the same in the two groups the relative risk is 1. In a study comparing two treatments, a relative risk of 2 would indicate that patients receiving one of the treatments had twice the risk of an undesirable outcome than those receiving the other treatment. Relative risk is sometimes used as a synonym for **risk ratio**.
Reliability	Reliability refers to a method of measurement that consistently gives the same results. For example, someone who has a high score on one occasion tends to have a high score if measured on another occasion very soon afterwards. With physical assessments it is possible for different clinicians to make independent assessments in quick succession and if their assessments tend to agree then the method of assessment is said to be reliable.
Retinal assessment	Examining the fundi through pupils which have been dilated with eye drops.
Retrospective study	A study that deals with the present/past and does not involve studying future events. This contrasts with studies that are **prospective**.
Review	Summary of the main points and trends in the research literature on a specified topic. A review is considered non-systematic unless an extensive literature search has been carried out to ensure that all aspects of the topic are covered and an objective appraisal made of the quality of the studies.
Risk ratio	Ratio of the risk of an undesirable event or outcome occurring in a group of patients receiving experimental treatment compared with a comparison (**control**) group. The term **relative risk** is sometimes used as a synonym of risk ratio.
Sample	A part of the study's **target population** from which the subjects of the study will be recruited. If subjects are drawn in an unbiased way from a particular population, the results can be generalised from the sample to the population as a whole.
Sampling	The way participants are selected for inclusion in a study.
Scottish Intercollegiate Guidelines Network (SIGN)	SIGN was established in 1993 to sponsor and support the development of evidence-based clinical guidelines for the NHS in Scotland.
Selection bias	Selection bias has occurred if: • the characteristics of the **sample** differ from those of the wider population from which the sample has been drawn, or • there are systematic differences between comparison groups of patients in a study in terms of prognosis or responsiveness to treatment.
Selection criteria	Explicit standards used by guideline development groups to decide which studies should be included and excluded from consideration as potential sources of evidence.
Semi-structured interview	Structured interviews involve asking people pre-set questions. A semi-structured interview allows more flexibility than a structured interview. The interviewer asks a number of open-ended questions, following up areas of interest in response to the information given by the respondent.
Sensitivity	In diagnostic testing, sensitivity is the proportion of true positive results that are correctly identified as positive by the test. 100% sensitivity means that all those with a negative test result do not have the disease. **Specificity** should be considered alongside sensitivity to fully judge the accuracy of a test.
Severe hypoglycaemia	Hypoglycaemia requiring help from another person.
Shoulder dystocia	Any documented evidence of difficulty with delivering the shoulders after delivery of the baby's head.
Single-blind study	A study in which *either* the subject (patient/participant) *or* the observer (clinician/investigator) is not aware of which treatment or intervention the subject is receiving.
Singleton	One fetus or baby.

Sliding scale	Intravenous insulin and dextrose infusions with a set of instructions for adjusting the dose of insulin on the basis of blood glucose test results.
Specificity	In diagnostic testing, specificity is the proportion of true negative results that are correctly identified as negative by the test. 100% specificity means that all those with a positive test result have the disease. **Sensitivity** should be considered alongside specificity to fully judge the accuracy of a test.
Standard deviation	A measure of the spread, scatter or variability of a set of measurements. Usually used with the mean (average) to describe numerical data.
Statistical power	The ability of a study to demonstrate an association or **causal relationship** between two **variables**, given that an association exists. For example, 80% power in a clinical trial means that the study has a 80% chance of ending up with a **P value** of less than 5% in a statistical test (i.e. a statistically significant treatment effect) if there really was an important difference (e.g. 10% versus 5% mortality) between treatments. If the statistical power of a study is low, the study results will be questionable (the study might have been too small to detect any differences). By convention, 80% is an acceptable level of power. See also **P value**.
Stillbirth	Legal definition: a child that has issued forth from its mother after the 24th week of pregnancy and which did not at any time after being completely expelled from its mother breathe or show any other signs of life (Section 41 of the Births and Deaths Registration Act 1953 as amended by the Stillbirth Definition Act 1992).
Study checklist	A list of questions addressing the key aspects of the research methodology that must be in place if a study is to be accepted as valid. A different checklist is required for each study type. These checklists are used to ensure a degree of consistency in the way that studies are evaluated.
Study population	People who have been identified as the subjects of a study.
Study quality	See **methodological quality**.
Study type	The kind of design used for a study. **Randomised controlled trials**, **case–control studies**, and **cohort studies** are all examples of study types.
Subject	A person who takes part in an experiment or research study.
Survey	A study in which information is systematically collected from people (usually from a sample within a defined population).
Systematic	Methodical, according to plan; not random.
Systematic error	Refers to the various errors or biases inherent in a study. See also **bias**.
Systematic review	A review in which evidence from scientific studies has been identified, appraised and synthesised in a methodical way according to predetermined criteria. May or may not include a **meta-analysis**.
Target population	The people to whom guideline recommendations are intended to apply. Recommendations may be less valid if applied to a population with different characteristics from the participants in the research study, for example in terms of age, disease state, social background.
Technology appraisal (TA)	A technology appraisal, as undertaken by NICE, is the process of determining the clinical and cost-effectiveness of a **health technology**. NICE technology appraisals are designed to provide patients, health professionals and managers with an authoritative source of advice on new and existing health technologies.
Thrombosis	The formation or presence of a clot of coagulated blood in a blood vessel.
Transitional care unit	A unit providing care of term or near-term babies not needing high-dependency or intensive care, which can be safely delivered without babies being separated from their mothers.
Trimester	One of the 3 month periods into which pregnancy is divided. The first trimester is 0–13 weeks of gestation, the second trimester is 14–26 weeks of gestation, and the third trimester is 27 weeks of gestation until birth.
Triple-blind study	A study in which the statistical analysis is carried out without knowing which treatment patients received, in addition to the patients and investigators/**clinicians** being unaware which treatment patients were getting.
Type 1 diabetes	There is an absolute deficiency of insulin production, due to autoimmune destruction of the insulin-producing beta cells in the islets of Langerhans in the pancreas. It accounts for 5–15% of all people with diabetes.

Type 2 diabetes   There is a relative deficiency of insulin production, and/or the insulin produced is not effective (insulin resistance). It accounts for 85–95% of all people with diabetes.

Variable   A measurement that can vary within a study, e.g. the age of participants. Variability is present when differences can be seen between different people or within the same person over time with respect to any characteristic or feature that can be assessed or measured.

1 Introduction

1.1 Diabetes in pregnancy

Diabetes is a disorder of carbohydrate metabolism that requires immediate changes in lifestyle. In its chronic forms, diabetes is associated with long-term vascular complications, including retinopathy, nephropathy, neuropathy and vascular disease. Approximately 650000 women give birth in England and Wales each year,[1] and 2–5% of pregnancies involve women with diabetes.[2,3,20] Pre-existing type 1 diabetes and pre-existing type 2 diabetes account for 0.27% and 0.10% of births, respectively.[2] The prevalence of type 1 and type 2 diabetes is increasing. In particular, type 2 diabetes is increasing in certain minority ethnic groups (including people of African, black Caribbean, South Asian, Middle Eastern and Chinese family origin).[2] There is a lack of data about the prevalence of gestational diabetes, which may or may not resolve after pregnancy. The clinical experience of the guideline development group (GDG) suggests that the average prevalence in England and Wales is approximately 3.5% (the precise figure varies from region to region, depending on factors such as ethnic origin, with certain minority ethnic groups being at increased risk; see Section 4.1). Approximately 87.5% of pregnancies complicated by diabetes are, therefore, estimated to be due to gestational diabetes, with 7.5% being due to type 1 diabetes and the remaining 5% being due to type 2 diabetes.

Diabetes in pregnancy is associated with risks to the woman and to the developing fetus.[4,5] Miscarriage, pre-eclampsia and preterm labour are more common in women with pre-existing diabetes. In addition, diabetic retinopathy can worsen rapidly during pregnancy. Stillbirth, congenital malformations, macrosomia, birth injury, perinatal mortality and postnatal adaptation problems (such as hypoglycaemia) are more common in babies born to women with pre-existing diabetes.

This clinical guideline contains recommendations for the management of diabetes and its complications in women who wish to conceive and those who are already pregnant. The guideline builds on existing clinical guidelines for routine care during the antenatal, intrapartum and postnatal periods. It focuses on areas where additional or different care should be offered to women with diabetes and their newborn babies.

1.2 Aim of the guideline

Clinical guidelines have been defined as 'systematically developed statements which assist clinicians and patients in making decisions about appropriate treatment for specific conditions'.[6] This clinical guideline concerns the management of diabetes and its complications from preconception to the postnatal period. It has been developed with the aim of providing guidance on:

- preconception information
- diagnosis and management of gestational diabetes
- glycaemic control in the preconception, antenatal and intrapartum periods
- changes to medications for diabetes and its complications before or during pregnancy
- management of diabetic emergencies (for example, hypoglycaemia and ketoacidosis) and diabetic complications (such as retinopathy) during pregnancy
- the timetable of antenatal appointments to be offered to women with diabetes
- timing and mode of birth (including induction of labour, caesarean section, analgesia and anaesthesia, and the use of steroids for fetal lung maturation)
- initial care of the newborn baby
- management of diabetes and its complications during the postnatal period.

1.3 Areas outside the remit of the guideline

This guideline does not address:

- aspects of routine antenatal, intrapartum and postnatal care that apply equally to women with or without diabetes
- aspects of routine care for women with diabetes that do not change during the preconception, antenatal, intrapartum or postnatal periods
- advice about contraceptive methods for women with diabetes
- management of morbidity in newborn babies of women with diabetes beyond initial assessment and diagnosis.

1.4 For whom is the guideline intended?

This guideline is of relevance to those who work in or use the National Health Service (NHS) in England, Wales and Northern Ireland, in particular:

- healthcare professionals involved in the care of women with diabetes and their newborn babies (including general practitioners (GPs), nurses and midwives, obstetricians, diabetes physicians and neonatal paediatricians)
- those responsible for commissioning and planning healthcare services, including primary care trust commissioners, Health Commission Wales commissioners, and public health, trust and care-home managers
- women with diabetes and their families.

A version of this guideline for women with diabetes and the public is available from the NICE website (www.nice.org.uk/CG063publicinfo) or from NICE publications on 0845 003 7783 (quote reference number N1485).

1.5 Who has developed the guideline?

The National Collaborating Centre for Women's and Children's Health (NCC-WCH) was commissioned by the National Institute for Health and Clinical Excellence (NICE) to establish a multi-professional and lay working group (the GDG) to develop the guideline. The membership of the GDG was determined by the NCC-WCH and NICE, and included the following:

- two obstetricians
- two diabetes physicians
- two diabetes specialist midwives
- a diabetes specialist nurse
- a GP
- a neonatal paediatrician
- two patient/carer representatives.

Staff from the NCC-WCH provided methodological support for the guideline development process by undertaking systematic searches, retrieving and appraising the evidence, health economic modelling and writing successive drafts of the guideline. The neonatal paediatrician appointed to the GDG at the beginning of the development process resigned in October 2007 due to ill health and was replaced by another neonatal paediatrician.

During the development of the guideline, the GDG identified a need for expert advice in relation to obstetric analgesia and anaesthesia, diabetic retinopathy and data relating to pregnancy in women with pre-existing diabetes held by the Confidential Enquiry into Maternal and Child Health (CEMACH), which covers England, Wales and Northern Ireland. Expert advisers were appointed by the GDG to advise on each of these issues, although they were not involved in the final decisions regarding formulation of recommendations.

All GDG members' and external advisers' potential and actual conflicts of interest were recorded on declaration forms provided by NICE and are presented in Appendix A. The forms covered personal pecuniary interests (including consultancies, fee-paid work, shareholdings, fellowships and support from the healthcare industry), personal non-pecuniary interests (including research interests), personal family interests (including shareholdings) and non-personal pecuniary interests (including funding from the healthcare industry for research projects and meetings). The GDG chair and NCC-WCH project director considered all the declarations and concluded that none of the declared interests constituted a material conflict of interest that would influence the recommendations developed by the GDG.

Organisations with interests in the management of diabetes and its complications from preconception to the postnatal period were encouraged to register as stakeholders for the guideline. Registered stakeholders were consulted throughout the guideline development process. The process of stakeholder registration was managed by NICE. The different types of organisations that were eligible to register as stakeholders included:

- national patient and carer organisations that directly or indirectly represent the interests of women with diabetes and their families before and during pregnancy
- national organisations that represent the healthcare professionals who provide services for women with diabetes before and during pregnancy
- companies that manufacture the preparations or products used in the management of diabetes in pregnancy
- providers and commissioners of health services in England, Wales and Northern Ireland
- statutory organisations such as the Department of Health and the Welsh Assembly Government
- research organisations that have done nationally recognised research in relation to the topics covered in the guideline.

1.6   Other relevant documents

This guideline is intended to complement other existing and proposed works of relevance, including the following NICE guidance.

- Clinical guidelines
  - Type 1 diabetes: diagnosis and management of type 1 diabetes in children, young people and adults[7]
  - Type 2 diabetes: the management of type 2 diabetes (to replace separate guidelines on blood glucose, blood pressure and blood lipids, renal disease and retinopathy)[8]
  - Antenatal care: routine care for the healthy pregnant woman (the section of the antenatal care guideline that addresses screening for gestational diabetes has been developed in parallel with the development of this guideline; see Chapter 4).[9]
  - Intrapartum care: management and delivery of care to women in labour[10]
  - Postnatal care: routine postnatal care of women and their babies[11]
  - Induction of labour (this diabetes in pregnancy guideline replaces the part of the induction of labour guideline that relates to women with diabetes)[12]
  - Caesarean section.[13]
- Technology appraisals (TAs)
  - Guidance on the use of continuous subcutaneous insulin infusion for diabetes[14]
  - Guidance on the use of glitazones for the treatment of type 2 diabetes[15]
  - Guidance on the use of long-acting insulin analogues for the treatment of diabetes – insulin glargine[17]
  - Guidance on the use of patient-education models for diabetes.[18]
- Public health guidance
  - Improving the nutrition of pregnant and breastfeeding mothers and children in low-income households.[19]

The guideline also complements and updates the National Service Framework (NSF) for diabetes.[20]

1.7   Guideline methodology

This guideline was developed in accordance with the NICE guideline development process outlined in the 2005 technical manual[21] and the 2006 and 2007 editions of the NICE guidelines manual.[22,23] Table 1.1 summarises the key stages of the guideline development process and which version of the process was followed at each stage.

Literature search strategy

Initial scoping searches were executed to identify relevant guidelines (local, national and international) produced by other development groups. The reference lists in these guidelines were checked against subsequent searches to identify missing evidence.

Relevant published evidence to inform the guideline development process and answer the clinical questions was identified by systematic search strategies. The clinical questions are presented in Appendix B. Additionally, stakeholder organisations were invited to submit evidence for consideration by the GDG provided it was relevant to the topics included in the scope and of equivalent or better quality than evidence identified by the search strategies.

Systematic searches to answer the clinical questions formulated and agreed by the GDG were executed using the following databases via the 'Ovid' platform: Medline (1966 onwards), Embase (1980 onwards), Cumulative Index to Nursing and Allied Health Literature (CINAHL; 1982 onwards), and PsycINFO (1967 onwards). The most recent search conducted for the three Cochrane databases (Cochrane Central Register of Controlled Trials, Cochrane Database of Systematic Reviews and the Database of Abstracts of Reviews of Effects) was undertaken in Quarter 1, 2007. Searches to identify economic studies were undertaken using the above databases and the NHS Economic Evaluation Database (NHS EED).

Search strategies combined relevant controlled vocabulary and natural language in an effort to balance sensitivity and specificity. Unless advised by the GDG, searches were not date specific. Language restrictions were not applied to searches, although publications in languages other than English were not appraised. Both generic and specially developed methodological search filters were used appropriately.

There was no systematic attempt to search grey literature (conferences, abstracts, theses and unpublished trials). Hand searching of journals not indexed on the databases was not undertaken.

Towards the end of the guideline development process, searches were updated and re-executed, thereby including evidence published and included in the databases up to 21 March 2007.

Table 1.1   Stages in the NICE guideline development process and the versions followed at each stage

Stage	2005 version[21]	2006 version[22]	2007 version[23]
Scoping the guideline (determining what the guideline would and would not cover)	✓		
Preparing the work plan (agreeing timelines, milestones, guideline development group constitution, etc.)	✓		
Forming and running the guideline development group	✓		
Developing clinical questions	✓		
Identifying the evidence		✓	
Reviewing and grading the evidence		✓	
Incorporating health economics		✓	
Making group decisions and reaching consensus			✓
Linking guidance to other NICE guidance			✓
Creating guideline recommendations			✓
Developing clinical audit criteria			✓
Writing the guideline			✓
Validation (stakeholder consultation on the draft guideline)			✓
Declaration of interests[a]	✓	✓	✓

[a] The process for declaring interests was extended in November 2006 to cover NCC-WCH staff and to include personal family interests.

Evidence published after this date has not been included in the guideline. This date should be considered the starting point for searching for new evidence for future updates to this guideline.

Further details of the search strategies, including the methodological filters employed, are provided on the accompanying CD-ROM.

Appraisal and synthesis of clinical effectiveness evidence

Evidence relating to clinical effectiveness was reviewed using established guides[24–30] and classified using the established hierarchical system presented in Table 1.2.[22] This system reflects the susceptibility to bias that is inherent in particular study designs.

The type of clinical question dictates the highest level of evidence that may be sought. In assessing the quality of the evidence, each study was assigned a quality rating coded as '++', '+' or '−'. For issues of therapy or treatment, the highest possible evidence level (EL) is a well-conducted systematic review or meta-analysis of randomised controlled trials (RCTs; EL = 1++) or an individual RCT (EL = 1+). Studies of poor quality were rated as '−'. Usually, studies rated as '−' should not be used as a basis for making a recommendation, but they can be used to inform recommendations. For issues of prognosis, the highest possible level of evidence is a cohort study (EL = 2). A level of evidence was assigned to each study appraised during the development of the guideline.

For each clinical question, the highest available level of evidence was selected. Where appropriate, for example, if a systematic review, meta-analysis or RCT existed in relation to a question, studies of a weaker design were not considered. Where systematic reviews, meta-analyses and RCTs did not exist, other appropriate experimental or observational studies were sought. For diagnostic tests, test evaluation studies examining the performance of the test were used if the effectiveness (accuracy) of the test was required, but where an evaluation of the effectiveness of the test in the clinical management of patients and the outcome of disease was required, evidence from RCTs or cohort studies was optimal. For studies evaluating the accuracy of a diagnostic test, sensitivity, specificity, positive predictive values (PPVs) and negative predictive values (NPVs) were calculated or quoted where possible (see Table 1.3).

Table 1.2 Levels of evidence for intervention studies

Level	Source of evidence
1++	High-quality meta-analyses, systematic reviews of randomised controlled trials (RCTs), or RCTs with a very low risk of bias
1+	Well-conducted meta-analyses, systematic reviews of RCTs, or RCTs with a low risk of bias
1−	Meta-analyses, systematic reviews of RCTs, or RCTs with a high risk of bias
2++	High-quality systematic reviews of case–control or cohort studies; high-quality case–control or cohort studies with a very low risk of confounding, bias or chance and a high probability that the relationship is causal
2+	Well-conducted case–control or cohort studies with a low risk of confounding, bias or chance and a moderate probability that the relationship is causal
2−	Case–control or cohort studies with a high risk of confounding, bias or chance and a significant risk that the relationship is not causal
3	Non-analytical studies (for example, case reports, case series)
4	Expert opinion, formal consensus

Table 1.3 '2 × 2' table for calculation of diagnostic accuracy parameters

	Reference standard positive	Reference standard negative	Total
Test positive	a (true positive)	b (false positive)	a+b
Test negative	c (false negative)	d (true negative)	c+d
Total	a+c	b+d	a+b+c+d = N (total number of tests in study)

Sensitivity = a/(a+c), specificity = d/(b+d), PPV = a/(a+b), NPV = d/(c+d)

The system described above covers studies of treatment effectiveness. However, it is less appropriate for studies reporting accuracy of diagnostic tests. In the absence of a validated ranking system for this type of test, NICE has developed a hierarchy of evidence that takes into account the various factors likely to affect the validity of these studies (see Table 1.4).[22]

Clinical evidence for individual studies was extracted into evidence tables (provided on the accompanying CD-ROM) and a brief description of each study was included in the guideline text. The body of evidence identified for each clinical question was synthesised qualitatively in clinical evidence statements that accurately reflected the evidence. Quantitative synthesis (meta-analysis) was not performed for this guideline because there were no clinical questions for which sufficient numbers of similar studies were identified to merit such analysis.

Specific considerations for this guideline

Where the evidence supports it, the guideline makes separate recommendations for women with pre-existing diabetes (type 1 diabetes, type 2 diabetes and other forms of diabetes, such as maturity-onset diabetes of the young)[31] and gestational diabetes.

The term 'women' is used in the guideline to refer to all females of childbearing age, including young women who have not yet transferred from paediatric to adult services.

For this guideline, the effectiveness of interventions has been assessed against the following outcome domains.

- Neonatal outcomes
    - miscarriage, stillbirth, neonatal or infant death
    - congenital malformation
    - macrosomia, small for gestational age (SGA), low birthweight
    - shoulder dystocia, birth trauma (bone fracture, nerve palsy)
    - admission to intensive care unit, high-dependency unit, special care unit or transitional care unit
    - hypoglycaemia, respiratory distress, sepsis, transient heart failure, resuscitation, jaundice, hypocalcaemia, polycythaemia, hypoxic ischaemic encephalopathy, impairment of neurodevelopment.
- Maternal outcomes
    - preterm birth
    - mode of birth (spontaneous vaginal, instrumental, caesarean section)
    - mode of infant feeding
    - maternal health-related quality of life (validated questionnaire)
    - maternal satisfaction with experience of pregnancy and birth
    - perineal trauma, wound healing
    - maternal death
    - maternal obstetric complications (haemorrhage, infection, thrombosis, admission to intensive care unit, incontinence)
    - maternal diabetic complications (glycaemic control (glycosylated haemoglobin; HbA_{1c}), hypoglycaemic episodes, diabetic ketoacidosis (DKA), retinopathy, nephropathy, macrovascular disease)
    - development of type 2 diabetes.

CEMACH has conducted a three-part enquiry programme relating to diabetes in pregnancy. The programme, which started in 2002, focused on pre-existing diabetes (type 1 and type 2 diabetes; i.e. gestational diabetes was excluded). The three parts of the programme were:

- a survey of diabetes maternity services, which assessed the quality of maternity service provision against standards set out in the NSF for diabetes[20,32]
- a descriptive study of 3808 pregnancies followed until 28 days after birth in women with pre-existing diabetes who booked or gave birth between 1 March 2002 and 28 February 2003[2]
- a national confidential enquiry of demographic, social and lifestyle factors and clinical care in 442 pregnancies complicated by pre-existing diabetes.[33]

Results from the CEMACH diabetes in pregnancy programme were considered systematically by the GDG alongside other evidence and particularly as an indicator of current clinical practice.

Table 1.4 Levels of evidence for studies of the accuracy of diagnostic tests

Level	Type of evidence
Ia	Systematic review (with homogeneity)[a] of level-1 studies[b]
Ib	Level-1 studies[b]
II	Level-2 studies[c]; systematic reviews of level-2 studies
III	Level-3 studies[d]; systematic reviews of level-3 studies
IV	Consensus, expert committee reports or opinions and/or clinical experience without explicit critical appraisal; or based on physiology, bench research or 'first principles'

[a] Homogeneity means there are no or minor variations in the directions and degrees of results between individual studies that are included in the systematic review.

[b] Level-1 studies are studies that use a blind comparison of the test with a validated reference standard (gold standard) in a sample of patients that reflects the population to whom the test would apply.

[c] Level-2 studies are studies that have only one of the following:
  - narrow population (the sample does not reflect the population to whom the test would apply)
  - use a poor reference standard (defined as that where the 'test' is included in the 'reference', or where the 'testing' affects the 'reference')
  - the comparison between the test and reference standard is not blind
  - case–control studies.

[d] Level-3 studies are studies that have at least two or three of the features listed above.

Health economics considerations

The aims of the economic input to the guideline were to inform the GDG of potential economic issues relating to the management of diabetes and its complications from preconception to the postnatal period, and to ensure that recommendations represented cost-effective use of healthcare resources.

The GDG prioritised a number of clinical questions where it was thought that economic considerations would be particularly important in formulating recommendations. A systematic search for published economic evidence was undertaken for these questions. For economic evaluations, no standard system of grading the quality of evidence exists and included papers were assessed using a quality assessment checklist based on good practice in economic evaluation.[34] Reviews of the very limited relevant published economic literature are presented alongside the clinical reviews or as part of appendices detailing original economic analyses (see below).

Health economic considerations were aided by original economic analysis undertaken as part of the development of the guideline where robust clinical effectiveness data were available and UK cost data could be obtained. For this guideline the areas prioritised for economic analysis were:

- self-management programmes for women with diabetes who are planning a pregnancy (see Section 3.9)
- treatment for gestational diabetes (see Section 4.3) – this was addressed through a unified analysis of screening, diagnosis and treatment for gestational diabetes involving joint work with the NICE antenatal care GDG
- screening for congenital malformations (see Section 5.6)
- monitoring fetal growth and wellbeing (see Section 5.7)
- criteria for admission to a neonatal intensive care unit (NICU) or special care unit (see Section 7.1).

The results of each economic analysis are summarised briefly in the guideline text. Detailed descriptions of the methods used for assessing the cost-effectiveness of self-management programmes are presented in Appendix C. The methods used for assessing the cost-effectiveness of screening, diagnosis and treatment for gestational diabetes are presented in Appendix D and those for assessing the cost-effectiveness of screening for congenital cardiac malformations are described in Appendix E.

GDG interpretation of the evidence and formulation of recommendations

For each clinical question, recommendations for clinical care were derived using, and linked explicitly to, the evidence that supported them. In the first instance, informal consensus methods were used by the GDG to agree clinical and cost-effectiveness evidence statements. Statements summarising the GDG's interpretation of the evidence and any extrapolation from the evidence used to form recommendations were also prepared. In areas where no substantial clinical research evidence was identified, the GDG considered other evidence-based guidelines and consensus statements or used their collective experience to identify good practice. The health economics justification in areas of the guideline where the use of NHS resources (interventions) was considered was based on GDG consensus in relation to the likely cost-effectiveness implications of the recommendations. The GDG also identified areas where evidence to answer their clinical questions was lacking and used this information to formulate recommendations for future research.

Towards the end of the guideline development process, formal consensus methods were used to consider all the clinical care recommendations and research recommendations that had been drafted previously. The GDG identified nine key priorities for implementation (key recommendations), which (in accordance with the criteria specified in the NICE guidelines manual[23]) were those recommendations expected to have the biggest impact on care and outcomes for pregnant women with diabetes and their babies in the NHS as a whole. The key priorities were selected using a variant of the nominal group technique. Each GDG member submitted an electronic form indicating their top five recommendations in order of priority. The GDG members' votes were collated and a shortlist of priority recommendations was obtained by including all recommendations that had been voted for by at least one GDG member. The shortlisted recommendations were discussed at subsequent GDG meetings, and the final selection was made by retaining the recommendations that had received most votes and distilling the important issues contained in some long recommendations into more succinct recommendations.

The GDG also identified five key priorities for research (again using criteria set out in the NICE guidelines manual), which were the most important research recommendations, again using a variant of the nominal group technique. Each GDG member submitted an electronic form indicating their top five research recommendations in order of priority. The GDG members' votes were collated and a shortlist of priority recommendations was obtained using the same criteria that were used to shortlist recommendations for clinical care. The shortlisted recommendations were discussed at subsequent GDG meetings, and the final selection was made by retaining the recommendations that had received most votes.

1.8 Stakeholder involvement in the guideline development process

Registered stakeholder organisations were invited to comment on the scope of the guideline during the scoping stage of development and on the evidence and recommendations in the validation stage (see Table 1.1).

The GDG carefully considered and responded to all of the comments received from stakeholders during the consultation periods. The comments and responses, which were reviewed independently by a guideline review panel convened by NICE, are published on the NICE website.

1.9 Schedule for updating the guideline

Clinical guidelines commissioned by NICE are published with a review date 4 years from the date of publication. Reviewing may begin earlier than 4 years if significant evidence that affects guideline recommendations is identified sooner. The updated guideline will be available within 2 years of the start of the review process.

2 Summary of recommendations and algorithm

2.1 Key priorities for implementation (key recommendations)

Chapter 3   Preconception care

Outcomes and risks for the woman and baby
Women with diabetes who are planning to become pregnant should be informed that establishing good glycaemic control before conception and continuing this throughout pregnancy will reduce the risk of miscarriage, congenital malformation, stillbirth and neonatal death. It is important to explain that risks can be reduced but not eliminated.

Importance of planning pregnancy and the role of contraception
The importance of avoiding unplanned pregnancy should be an essential component of diabetes education from adolescence for women with diabetes.

Self-management programmes
Women with diabetes who are planning to become pregnant should be offered preconception care and advice before discontinuing contraception.

Chapter 5   Antenatal care

Target ranges for blood glucose during pregnancy
If it is safely achievable, women with diabetes should aim to keep fasting blood glucose between 3.5 and 5.9 mmol/litre and 1 hour postprandial blood glucose below 7.8 mmol/litre during pregnancy.

Management of diabetes during pregnancy
Women with insulin-treated diabetes should be advised of the risks of hypoglycaemia and hypoglycaemia unawareness in pregnancy, particularly in the first trimester.

During pregnancy, women who are suspected of having diabetic ketoacidosis should be admitted immediately for level 2 critical care*, where they can receive both medical and obstetric care.

Screening for congenital malformations
Women with diabetes should be offered antenatal examination of the four chamber view of the fetal heart and outflow tracts at 18–20 weeks.

Chapter 7   Neonatal care

Initial assessment and criteria for admission to intensive/special care
Babies of women with diabetes should be kept with their mothers unless there is a clinical complication or there are abnormal clinical signs that warrant admission for intensive or special care.

Chapter 8   Postnatal care

Information and follow-up after birth
Women who were diagnosed with gestational diabetes should be offered lifestyle advice (including weight control, diet and exercise) and offered a fasting plasma glucose measurement (but not an oral glucose tolerance test) at the 6 week postnatal check and annually thereafter.

---

* Level 2 critical care is defined as care for patients requiring detailed observation or intervention, including support for a single failing organ system or postoperative care and those 'stepping down' from higher levels of care.

2.2 Summary of recommendations

Chapter 3 Preconception care

Outcomes and risks for the woman and baby
Healthcare professionals should seek to empower women with diabetes to make the experience of pregnancy and childbirth a positive one by providing information, advice and support that will help to reduce the risks of adverse pregnancy outcomes for mother and baby.

Women with diabetes who are planning to become pregnant should be informed that establishing good glycaemic control before conception and continuing this throughout pregnancy will reduce the risk of miscarriage, congenital malformation, stillbirth and neonatal death. It is important to explain that risks can be reduced but not eliminated.

Women with diabetes who are planning to become pregnant and their families should be offered information about how diabetes affects pregnancy and how pregnancy affects diabetes. The information should cover:

- the role of diet, body weight and exercise
- the risks of hypoglycaemia and hypoglycaemia unawareness during pregnancy
- how nausea and vomiting in pregnancy can affect glycaemic control
- the increased risk of having a baby who is large for gestational age, which increases the likelihood of birth trauma, induction of labour and caesarean section
- the need for assessment of diabetic retinopathy before and during pregnancy
- the need for assessment of diabetic nephropathy before pregnancy
- the importance of maternal glycaemic control during labour and birth and early feeding of the baby in order to reduce the risk of neonatal hypoglycaemia
- the possibility of transient morbidity in the baby during the neonatal period, which may require admission to the neonatal unit
- the risk of the baby developing obesity and/or diabetes in later life.

The importance of planning pregnancy and the role of contraception
The importance of avoiding unplanned pregnancy should be an essential component of diabetes education from adolescence for women with diabetes.

Women with diabetes who are planning to become pregnant should be advised:

- that the risks associated with pregnancies complicated by diabetes increase with the duration of diabetes
- to use contraception until good glycaemic control (assessed by HbA_{1c}*) has been established
- that glycaemic targets, glucose monitoring, medications for diabetes (including insulin regimens for insulin-treated diabetes) and medications for complications of diabetes will need to be reviewed before and during pregnancy
- that additional time and effort is required to manage diabetes during pregnancy and that there will be frequent contact with healthcare professionals. Women should be given information about the local arrangements for support, including emergency contact numbers.

Diet, dietary supplements, body weight and exercise
Women with diabetes who are planning to become pregnant should be offered individualised dietary advice.

Women with diabetes who are planning to become pregnant and who have a body mass index above 27 kg/m² should be offered advice on how to lose weight in line with 'Obesity: guidance on the prevention, identification, assessment and management of overweight and obesity in adults and children' (NICE clinical guideline 43), available from www.nice.org.uk/CG043.

Women with diabetes who are planning to become pregnant should be advised to take folic acid (5 mg/day) until 12 weeks of gestation to reduce the risk of having a baby with a neural tube defect.

---

* Diabetes Control and Complications Trial (DCCT)-aligned haemoglobin A_{1c} (HbA_{1c}) test.

Target ranges for blood glucose in the preconception period
Individualised targets for self-monitoring of blood glucose should be agreed with women who have diabetes and are planning to become pregnant, taking into account the risk of hypoglycaemia.

If it is safely achievable, women with diabetes who are planning to become pregnant should aim to maintain their HbA_{1c} below 6.1%. Women should be reassured that any reduction in HbA_{1c} towards the target of 6.1% is likely to reduce the risk of congenital malformations.

Women with diabetes whose HbA_{1c} is above 10% should be strongly advised to avoid pregnancy.

Monitoring blood glucose and ketones in the preconception period
Women with diabetes who are planning to become pregnant should be offered monthly measurement of HbA_{1c}.

Women with diabetes who are planning to become pregnant should be offered a meter for self-monitoring of blood glucose.

Women with diabetes who are planning to become pregnant and who require intensification of hypoglycaemic therapy should be advised to increase the frequency of self-monitoring of blood glucose to include fasting and a mixture of pre- and postprandial levels.

Women with type 1 diabetes who are planning to become pregnant should be offered ketone testing strips and advised to test for ketonuria or ketonaemia if they become hyperglycaemic or unwell.

The safety of medications for diabetes before and during pregnancy
Women with diabetes may be advised to use metformin* as an adjunct or alternative to insulin in the preconception period and during pregnancy, when the likely benefits from improved glycaemic control outweigh the potential for harm. All other oral hypoglycaemic agents should be discontinued before pregnancy and insulin substituted.

Healthcare professionals should be aware that the rapid-acting insulin analogues (aspart and lispro*) are safe to use during pregnancy.

Women with insulin-treated diabetes who are planning to become pregnant should be informed that there is insufficient evidence about the use of long-acting insulin analogues during pregnancy. Therefore isophane insulin* (also known as NPH insulin) remains the first choice for long-acting insulin during pregnancy.

The safety of medications for diabetic complications before and during pregnancy
Angiotensin-converting enzyme inhibitors and angiotensin-II receptor antagonists should be discontinued before conception or as soon as pregnancy is confirmed. Alternative antihypertensive agents suitable for use during pregnancy should be substituted.

Statins should be discontinued before pregnancy or as soon as pregnancy is confirmed.

Removing barriers to the uptake of preconception care and when to offer information
Women with diabetes should be informed about the benefits of preconception glycaemic control at each contact with healthcare professionals, including their diabetes care team, from adolescence.

The intentions of women with diabetes regarding pregnancy and contraceptive use should be documented at each contact with their diabetes care team from adolescence.

Preconception care for women with diabetes should be given in a supportive environment and the woman's partner or other family member should be encouraged to attend.

Self-management programmes
Women with diabetes who are planning to become pregnant should be offered a structured education programme as soon as possible if they have not already attended one (see 'Guidance on the use of patient-education models for diabetes' [NICE technology appraisal guidance 60], available from www.nice.org.uk/TA060†.

---

* This drug does not have UK marketing authorisation specifically for pregnant and breastfeeding women at the time of publication (March 2008). Informed consent should be obtained and documented.

† The clinical guideline 'Type 2 diabetes: the management of type 2 diabetes' will update the information on type 2 diabetes in this technology appraisal. It is currently in development and is expected to be published in April 2008.

Women with diabetes who are planning to become pregnant should be offered preconception care and advice before discontinuing contraception.

Retinal assessment in the preconception period
Women with diabetes seeking preconception care should be offered retinal assessment at their first appointment (unless an annual retinal assessment has occurred within the previous 6 months) and annually thereafter if no diabetic retinopathy is found.

Retinal assessment should be carried out by digital imaging with mydriasis using tropicamide*, in line with the UK National Screening Committee's recommendations for annual mydriatic two-field digital photographic screening as part of a systematic screening programme.

Women with diabetes who are planning to become pregnant should be advised to defer rapid optimisation of glycaemic control until after retinal assessment and treatment have been completed.

Renal assessment in the preconception period
Women with diabetes should be offered a renal assessment, including a measure of microalbuminuria, before discontinuing contraception. If serum creatinine is abnormal (120 micromol/litre or more), or the estimated glomerular filtration rate (eGFR) is less than 45 ml/minute/1.73 m², referral to a nephrologist should be considered before discontinuing contraception.

Chapter 4   Gestational diabetes

Risk factors for gestational diabetes
Healthcare professionals should be aware that the following have been shown to be independent risk factors for gestational diabetes:

- body mass index above 30 kg/m²
- previous macrosomic baby weighing 4.5 kg or above
- previous gestational diabetes
- family history of diabetes (first-degree relative with diabetes)
- family origin with a high prevalence of diabetes:
    - South Asian (specifically women whose country of family origin is India, Pakistan or Bangladesh)
    - black Caribbean
    - Middle Eastern (specifically women whose country of family origin is Saudi Arabia, United Arab Emirates, Iraq, Jordan, Syria, Oman, Qatar, Kuwait, Lebanon or Egypt).

Screening, diagnosis, and treatment for gestational diabetes
Screening for gestational diabetes using risk factors is recommended in a healthy population. At the booking appointment, the following risk factors for gestational diabetes should be determined:†

- body mass index above 30 kg/m²
- previous macrosomic baby weighing 4.5 kg or above
- previous gestational diabetes
- family history of diabetes (first-degree relative with diabetes)
- family origin with a high prevalence of diabetes:
    - South Asian (specifically women whose country of family origin is India, Pakistan or Bangladesh)
    - black Caribbean
    - Middle Eastern (specifically women whose country of family origin is Saudi Arabia, United Arab Emirates, Iraq, Jordan, Syria, Oman, Qatar, Kuwait, Lebanon or Egypt).
Women with any one of these risk factors should be offered testing for gestational diabetes.

---

*   This drug does not have UK marketing authorisation specifically for pregnant and breastfeeding women at the time of publication (March 2008). Informed consent should be obtained and documented.

†   This recommendation is taken from 'Antenatal care: routine care for the healthy pregnant woman' (NICE clinical guideline 62), available from www.nice.org.uk/CG062.

In order to make an informed decision about screening and testing for gestational diabetes, women should be informed that:*

- in most women, gestational diabetes will respond to changes in diet and exercise
- some women (between 10% and 20%) will need oral hypoglycaemic agents or insulin therapy if diet and exercise are not effective in controlling gestational diabetes
- if gestational diabetes is not detected and controlled there is a small risk of birth complications such as shoulder dystocia
- a diagnosis of gestational diabetes may lead to increased monitoring and interventions during both pregnancy and labour.

Screening for gestational diabetes using fasting plasma glucose, random blood glucose, glucose challenge test and urinalysis for glucose should not be undertaken.*

The 2 hour 75 g oral glucose tolerance test (OGTT) should be used to test for gestational diabetes and diagnosis made using the criteria defined by the World Health Organization†. Women who have had gestational diabetes in a previous pregnancy should be offered early self-monitoring of blood glucose or OGTT at 16–18 weeks, and a further OGTT at 28 weeks if the results are normal. Women with any of the other risk factors for gestational diabetes should be offered an OGTT at 24–28 weeks.

Women with gestational diabetes should be instructed in self-monitoring of blood glucose. Targets for blood glucose control should be determined in the same way as for women with pre-existing diabetes.

Women with gestational diabetes should be informed that good glycaemic control throughout pregnancy will reduce the risk of fetal macrosomia, trauma during birth (to themselves and the baby), induction of labour or caesarean section, neonatal hypoglycaemia and perinatal death.

Women with gestational diabetes should be offered information covering:

- the role of diet, body weight and exercise
- the increased risk of having a baby who is large for gestational age, which increases the likelihood of birth trauma, induction of labour and caesarean section
- the importance of maternal glycaemic control during labour and birth and early feeding of the baby in order to reduce the risk of neonatal hypoglycaemia
- the possibility of transient morbidity in the baby during the neonatal period, which may require admission to the neonatal unit
- the risk of the baby developing obesity and/or diabetes in later life.

Women with gestational diabetes should be advised to choose, where possible, carbohydrates from low glycaemic index sources, lean proteins including oily fish and a balance of polyunsaturated fats and monounsaturated fats.

Women with gestational diabetes whose pre-pregnancy body mass index was above 27 kg/m² should be advised to restrict calorie intake (to 25 kcal/kg/day or less) and to take moderate exercise (of at least 30 minutes daily).

Hypoglycaemic therapy should be considered for women with gestational diabetes if diet and exercise fail to maintain blood glucose targets during a period of 1–2 weeks.

Hypoglycaemic therapy should be considered for women with gestational diabetes if ultrasound investigation suggests incipient fetal macrosomia (abdominal circumference above the 70th percentile) at diagnosis.

Hypoglycaemic therapy for women with gestational diabetes (which may include regular insulin‡, rapid-acting insulin analogues [aspart and lispro‡] and/or hypoglycaemic agents [metformin‡ and gliben-clamide‡]) should be tailored to the glycaemic profile of, and acceptability to, the individual woman.

---

* This recommendation is taken from 'Antenatal care: routine care for the healthy pregnant woman' (NICE clinical guideline 62), available from www.nice.org.uk/CG062.

† Fasting plasma venous glucose concentration greater than or equal to 7.0 mmol/lite or 2 hour plasma venous glucose concentration greater than or equal to 7.8 mmol/litre. World Health Organization Department of Noncommunicable Disease Surveillance (1999) *Definition, diagnosis and classification of diabetes mellitus and its complications. Report of a WHO consultation. Part 1: diagnosis and classification of diabetes mellitus.* Geneva: World Health Organization.

‡ This drug does not have UK marketing authorisation specifically for pregnant and breastfeeding women at the time of publication (March 2008). Informed consent should be obtained and documented.

Chapter 5   Antenatal care

Target ranges for blood glucose during pregnancy
Individualised targets for self-monitoring of blood glucose should be agreed with women with diabetes in pregnancy, taking into account the risk of hypoglycaemia.

If it is safely achievable, women with diabetes should aim to keep fasting blood glucose between 3.5 and 5.9 mmol/litre and 1 hour postprandial blood glucose below 7.8 mmol/litre during pregnancy.

HbA_{1c} should not be used routinely for assessing glycaemic control in the second and third trimesters of pregnancy.

Monitoring blood glucose and ketones during pregnancy
Women with diabetes should be advised to test fasting blood glucose levels and blood glucose levels 1 hour after every meal during pregnancy.

Women with insulin-treated diabetes should be advised to test blood glucose levels before going to bed at night during pregnancy.

Women with type 1 diabetes who are pregnant should be offered ketone testing strips and advised to test for ketonuria or ketonaemia if they become hyperglycaemic or unwell.

Management of diabetes during pregnancy
Healthcare professionals should be aware that the rapid-acting insulin analogues (aspart and lispro[*]) have advantages over soluble human insulin[*] during pregnancy and should consider their use.

Women with insulin-treated diabetes should be advised of the risks of hypoglycaemia and hypoglycaemia unawareness in pregnancy, particularly in the first trimester.

During pregnancy, women with insulin-treated diabetes should be provided with a concentrated glucose solution and women with type 1 diabetes should also be given glucagon; women and their partners or other family members should be instructed in their use.

During pregnancy, women with insulin-treated diabetes should be offered continuous subcutaneous insulin infusion (CSII or insulin pump therapy) if adequate glycaemic control is not obtained by multiple daily injections of insulin without significant disabling hypoglycaemia.[†]

During pregnancy, women with type 1 diabetes who become unwell should have diabetic ketoacidosis excluded as a matter of urgency.

During pregnancy, women who are suspected of having diabetic ketoacidosis should be admitted immediately for level 2 critical care[‡], where they can receive both medical and obstetric care.

Retinal assessment during pregnancy
Pregnant women with pre-existing diabetes should be offered retinal assessment by digital imaging with mydriasis using tropicamide[*] following their first antenatal clinic appointment and again at 28 weeks if the first assessment is normal. If any diabetic retinopathy is present, an additional retinal assessment should be performed at 16–20 weeks.

If retinal assessment has not been performed in the preceding 12 months, it should be offered as soon as possible after the first contact in pregnancy in women with pre-existing diabetes.

Diabetic retinopathy should not be considered a contraindication to rapid optimisation of glycaemic control in women who present with a high HbA_{1c} in early pregnancy.

Women who have preproliferative diabetic retinopathy diagnosed during pregnancy should have ophthalmological follow-up for at least 6 months following the birth of the baby.

Diabetic retinopathy should not be considered a contraindication to vaginal birth.

---

[*] This drug does not have UK marketing authorisation specifically for pregnant and breastfeeding women at the time of publication (March 2008). Informed consent should be obtained and documented.

[†] For the purpose of this guidance, 'disabling hypoglycaemia' means the repeated and unpredicted occurrence of hypoglycaemia requiring third-party assistance that results in continuing anxiety about recurrence and is associated with significant adverse effect on quality of life

[‡] Level 2 critical care is defined as care for patients requiring detailed observation or intervention, including support for a single failing organ system or postoperative care and those 'stepping down' from higher levels of care.

Renal assessment during pregnancy
If renal assessment has not been undertaken in the preceding 12 months in women with pre-existing diabetes, it should be arranged at the first contact in pregnancy. If serum creatinine is abnormal (120 micromol/litre or more) or if total protein excretion exceeds 2 g/day, referral to a nephrologist should be considered (eGFR should not be used during pregnancy). Thromboprophylaxis should be considered for women with proteinuria above 5 g/day (macroalbuminuria).

Screening for congenital malformations
Women with diabetes should be offered antenatal examination of the four chamber view of the fetal heart and outflow tracts at 18–20 weeks.

Monitoring fetal growth and wellbeing
Pregnant women with diabetes should be offered ultrasound monitoring of fetal growth and amniotic fluid volume every 4 weeks from 28 to 36 weeks.

Routine monitoring of fetal wellbeing before 38 weeks is not recommended in pregnant women with diabetes, unless there is a risk of intrauterine growth restriction.

Women with diabetes and a risk of intrauterine growth restriction (macrovascular disease and/or nephropathy) will require an individualised approach to monitoring fetal growth and wellbeing.

Timetable of antenatal appointments
Women with diabetes who are pregnant should be offered immediate contact with a joint diabetes and antenatal clinic.

Women with diabetes should have contact with the diabetes care team for assessment of glycaemic control every 1–2 weeks throughout pregnancy.

Antenatal appointments for women with diabetes should provide care specifically for women with diabetes, in addition to the care provided routinely for healthy pregnant women (see 'Antenatal care: routine care for the healthy pregnant woman' [NICE clinical guideline 62], available from www.nice.org.uk/CG062). Table 5.7 describes where care for women with diabetes differs from routine antenatal care. At each appointment women should be offered ongoing opportunities for information and education.

Preterm labour in women with diabetes
Diabetes should not be considered a contraindication to antenatal steroids for fetal lung maturation or to tocolysis.

Women with insulin-treated diabetes who are receiving steroids for fetal lung maturation should have additional insulin according to an agreed protocol and should be closely monitored.

Betamimetic drugs should not be used for tocolysis in women with diabetes.

Chapter 6   Intrapartum care

Timing and mode of birth
Pregnant women with diabetes who have a normally grown fetus should be offered elective birth through induction of labour, or by elective caesarean section if indicated, after 38 completed weeks.

Diabetes should not in itself be considered a contraindication to attempting vaginal birth after a previous caesarean section.

Pregnant women with diabetes who have an ultrasound-diagnosed macrosomic fetus should be informed of the risks and benefits of vaginal birth, induction of labour and caesarean section.

Analgesia and anaesthesia
Women with diabetes and comorbidities such as obesity or autonomic neuropathy should be offered an anaesthetic assessment in the third trimester of pregnancy.

If general anaesthesia is used for the birth in women with diabetes, blood glucose should be monitored regularly (every 30 minutes) from induction of general anaesthesia until after the baby is born and the woman is fully conscious.

Table 5.7   Specific antenatal care for women with diabetes

Appointment	Care for women with diabetes during pregnancy[a]
First appointment (joint diabetes and antenatal clinic)	Offer information, advice and support in relation to optimising glycaemic control. Take a clinical history to establish the extent of diabetes-related complications. Review medications for diabetes and its complications. Offer retinal and/or renal assessment if these have not been undertaken in the previous 12 months.
7–9 weeks	Confirm viability of pregnancy and gestational age.
Booking appointment (ideally by 10 weeks)	Discuss information, education and advice about how diabetes will affect the pregnancy, birth and early parenting (such as breastfeeding and initial care of the baby).
16 weeks	Offer retinal assessment at 16–20 weeks to women with pre-existing diabetes who showed signs of diabetic retinopathy at the first antenatal appointment.
20 weeks	Offer four chamber view of the fetal heart and outflow tracts plus scans that would be offered at 18–20 weeks as part of routine antenatal care.
28 weeks	Offer ultrasound monitoring of fetal growth and amniotic fluid volume. Offer retinal assessment to women with pre-existing diabetes who showed no diabetic retinopathy at their first antenatal clinic visit.
32 weeks	Offer ultrasound monitoring of fetal growth and amniotic fluid volume. Offer to nulliparous women all investigations that would be offered at 31 weeks as part of routine antenatal care.
36 weeks	Offer ultrasound monitoring of fetal growth and amniotic fluid volume. Offer information and advice about: • timing, mode and management of birth • analgesia and anaesthesia • changes to hypoglycaemic therapy during and after birth • management of the baby after birth • initiation of breastfeeding and the effect of breastfeeding on glycaemic control • contraception and follow-up.
38 weeks	Offer induction of labour, or caesarean section if indicated, and start regular tests of fetal wellbeing for women with diabetes who are awaiting spontaneous labour.
39 weeks	Offer tests of fetal wellbeing.
40 weeks	Offer tests of fetal wellbeing.
41 weeks	Offer tests of fetal wellbeing.

[a] Women with diabetes should also receive routine care according to the schedule of appointments in 'Antenatal care: routine care for the healthy pregnant woman' (NICE clinical guideline 62), including appointments at 25 weeks (for nulliparous women) and 34 weeks, but with the exception of the appointment for nulliparous women at 31 weeks.

Glycaemic control during labour and birth

During labour and birth, capillary blood glucose should be monitored on an hourly basis in women with diabetes and maintained at between 4 and 7 mmol/litre.

Women with type 1 diabetes should be considered for intravenous dextrose and insulin infusion from the onset of established labour.

Intravenous dextrose and insulin infusion is recommended during labour and birth for women with diabetes whose blood glucose is not maintained at between 4 and 7 mmol/litre.

Chapter 7   Neonatal care

Initial assessment and criteria for admission to intensive or special care

Women with diabetes should be advised to give birth in hospitals where advanced neonatal resuscitation skills are available 24 hours a day.

Babies of women with diabetes should be kept with their mothers unless there is a clinical complication or there are abnormal clinical signs that warrant admission for intensive or special care.

Blood glucose testing should be carried out routinely in babies of women with diabetes at 2–4 hours after birth. Blood tests for polycythaemia, hyperbilirubinaemia, hypocalcaemia and hypomagnesaemia should be carried out for babies with clinical signs.

Babies of women with diabetes should have an echocardiogram performed if they show clinical signs associated with congenital heart disease or cardiomyopathy, including heart murmur. The timing of the examination will depend on the clinical circumstances.

Babies of women with diabetes should be admitted to the neonatal unit if they have:

- hypoglycaemia associated with abnormal clinical signs
- respiratory distress
- signs of cardiac decompensation due to congenital heart disease or cardiomyopathy
- signs of neonatal encephalopathy
- signs of polycythaemia and are likely to need partial exchange transfusion
- need for intravenous fluids
- need for tube feeding (unless adequate support is available on the postnatal ward)
- jaundice requiring intense phototherapy and frequent monitoring of bilirubinaemia
- been born before 34 weeks (or between 34 and 36 weeks if dictated clinically by the initial assessment of the baby and feeding on the labour ward).

Babies of women with diabetes should not be transferred to community care until they are at least 24 hours old, and not before healthcare professionals are satisfied that the babies are maintaining blood glucose levels and are feeding well.

Prevention and assessment of neonatal hypoglycaemia

All maternity units should have a written policy for the prevention, detection and management of hypoglycaemia in babies of women with diabetes.

Babies of women with diabetes should have their blood glucose tested using a quality-assured method validated for neonatal use (ward-based glucose electrode or laboratory analysis).

Babies of women with diabetes should feed as soon as possible after birth (within 30 minutes) and then at frequent intervals (every 2–3 hours) until feeding maintains pre-feed blood glucose levels at a minimum of 2.0 mmol/litre.

If blood glucose values are below 2.0 mmol/litre on two consecutive readings despite maximal support for feeding, if there are abnormal clinical signs or if the baby will not feed orally effectively, additional measures such as tube feeding or intravenous dextrose should be given. Additional measures should only be implemented if one or more of these criteria are met.

Babies of women with diabetes who present with clinical signs of hypoglycaemia should have their blood glucose tested and be treated with intravenous dextrose as soon as possible.

Chapter 8   Postnatal care

Breastfeeding and effects on glycaemic control

Women with insulin-treated pre-existing diabetes should reduce their insulin immediately after birth and monitor their blood glucose levels carefully to establish the appropriate dose.

Women with insulin-treated pre-existing diabetes should be informed that they are at increased risk of hypoglycaemia in the postnatal period, especially when breastfeeding, and they should be advised to have a meal or snack available before or during feeds.

Women who have been diagnosed with gestational diabetes should discontinue hypoglycaemic treatment immediately after birth.

Women with pre-existing type 2 diabetes who are breastfeeding can resume or continue to take metformin* and glibenclamide* immediately following birth but other oral hypoglycaemic agents should be avoided while breastfeeding.

Women with diabetes who are breastfeeding should continue to avoid any drugs for the treatment of diabetes complications that were discontinued for safety reasons in the preconception period.

---

* This drug does not have UK marketing authorisation specifically for pregnant and breastfeeding women at the time of publication (March 2008). Informed consent should be obtained and documented.

Information and follow-up after birth
Women with pre-existing diabetes should be referred back to their routine diabetes care arrangements.

Women who were diagnosed with gestational diabetes should have their blood glucose tested to exclude persisting hyperglycaemia before they are transferred to community care.

Women who were diagnosed with gestational diabetes should be reminded of the symptoms of hyperglycaemia.

Women who were diagnosed with gestational diabetes should be offered lifestyle advice (including weight control, diet and exercise) and offered a fasting plasma glucose measurement (but not an OGTT) at the 6 week postnatal check and annually thereafter.

Women who were diagnosed with gestational diabetes (including those with ongoing impaired glucose regulation) should be informed about the risks of gestational diabetes in future pregnancies and they should be offered screening (OGTT or fasting plasma glucose) for diabetes when planning future pregnancies.

Women who were diagnosed with gestational diabetes (including those with ongoing impaired glucose regulation) should be offered early self-monitoring of blood glucose or an OGTT in future pregnancies. A subsequent OGTT should be offered if the test results in early pregnancy are normal.

Women with diabetes should be reminded of the importance of contraception and the need for preconception care when planning future pregnancies.

2.3 Key priorities for research

Chapter 4   Gestational diabetes

Screening, diagnosis and treatment for gestational diabetes

What is the clinical and cost-effectiveness of the three main available screening techniques for gestational diabetes: risk factors, two-stage screening by the glucose challenge test and OGTT, and universal OGTT (with or without fasting)?

Why this is important
Following the Australian carbohydrate intolerance study in pregnant women (ACHOIS) it seems that systematic screening for gestational diabetes may be beneficial to the UK population. A multicentre randomised controlled trial is required to test the existing screening techniques, which have not been systematically evaluated for clinical and cost-effectiveness (including acceptability) within the UK.

Chapter 5   Antenatal care

Monitoring blood glucose and ketones during pregnancy

How effective is ambulatory continuous blood glucose monitoring in pregnancies complicated by diabetes?

Why this is important
The technology for performing ambulatory continuous blood glucose monitoring is only just becoming available, so there is currently no evidence to assess its effectiveness outside the laboratory situation. Research is needed to determine whether the technology is likely to have a place in the clinical management of diabetes in pregnancy. The new technology may identify women in whom short-term postprandial peaks of glycaemia are not detected by intermittent blood glucose testing. The aim of monitoring is to adjust insulin regimens to reduce the incidence of adverse outcomes of pregnancy (for example, fetal macrosomia, caesarean section and neonatal hypoglycaemia), so these outcomes should be assessed as part of the research.

Management of diabetes during pregnancy

Do new-generation continuous subcutaneous insulin infusion (CSII) pumps offer an advantage over traditional intermittent insulin injections in terms of pregnancy outcomes in women with type 1 diabetes?

Why this is important
Randomised controlled trials have shown no advantage or disadvantage of using CSII pumps over intermittent insulin injections in pregnancy. A new generation of CSII pumps may offer technological advantages that would make a randomised controlled trial appropriate, particularly with the availability of insulin analogues (which may have improved the effectiveness of intermittent insulin injections).

Monitoring fetal growth and wellbeing

How can the fetus at risk of intrauterine death be identified in women with diabetes?

Why this is important
Unheralded intrauterine death remains a significant contributor to perinatal mortality in pregnancies complicated by diabetes. Conventional tests of fetal wellbeing (umbilical artery Doppler ultrasound, cardiotocography and other biophysical tests) have been shown to have poor sensitivity for predicting such events. Alternative approaches that include measurements of liquor erythropoietin and magnetic resonance imaging spectroscopy may be effective, but there is currently insufficient clinical evidence to evaluate them. Well-designed randomised controlled trials that are sufficiently powered are needed to determine whether these approaches are clinically and cost-effective.

Chapter 6   Intrapartum care

Glycaemic control during labour and birth

What is the optimal method for controlling glycaemia during labour and birth?

Why this is important
Epidemiological studies have shown that poor glycaemic control during labour and birth is associated with adverse neonatal outcomes (in particular, neonatal hypoglycaemia and respiratory distress). However, no randomised controlled trials have compared the effectiveness of intermittent subcutaneous insulin injections and/or CSII with that of intravenous dextrose plus insulin during labour and birth. The potential benefits of intermittent insulin injections and/or CSII over intravenous dextrose plus insulin during the intrapartum period include patient preference due to the psychological effect of the woman feeling in control of her diabetes and having increased mobility. Randomised controlled trials are therefore needed to evaluate the safety of intermittent insulin injections and/or CSII during labour and birth compared with that of intravenous dextrose plus insulin.

2.4   Summary of research recommendations

Chapter 3   Preconception care

Self-management programmes

What is the most clinically and cost-effective form of preconception care and advice for women with diabetes?

Why this is important
Preconception care and advice for women with pre-existing diabetes is recommended because a health economic analysis has demonstrated cost-effectiveness of attendance at a preconception clinic. Due to limitations in the clinical evidence available to inform the health economic modelling it was not possible to establish the optimal form of preconception care and advice for this group of women. Future research should seek to establish the clinical and cost-effectiveness of different models of preconception care and advice for women with pre-existing diabetes. Specifically it should evaluate different forms of content (i.e. what topics are covered), frequency and timing of contact with healthcare professionals (for example, whether

one long session is more clinically and cost-effective than a series of shorter sessions), which healthcare professionals should be involved (for example, whether preconception care and advice provided by a multidisciplinary team is more clinically and cost-effective than contact with one healthcare professional), and format (for example, whether group sessions are more clinically and cost-effective than providing care and advice for each woman separately). The research should also seek to establish whether women with type 1 and type 2 diabetes have different needs in terms of preconception care and advice, and how different models of care and advice compare to structured education programmes already offered to women with type 1 and type 2 diabetes.

Chapter 4   Gestational diabetes

Screening, diagnosis and treatment for gestational diabetes

What is the clinical and cost-effectiveness of the three main available screening techniques for gestational diabetes: risk factors, two-stage screening by the glucose challenge test and OGTT, and universal OGTT (with or without fasting)?

Why this is important
Following the Australian carbohydrate intolerance study in pregnant women (ACHOIS) it seems that systematic screening for gestational diabetes may be beneficial to the UK population. A multicentre randomised controlled trial is required to test the existing screening techniques, which have not been systematically evaluated for clinical and cost-effectiveness (including acceptability) within the UK.

Chapter 5   Antenatal care

Monitoring blood glucose and ketones during pregnancy

How effective is ambulatory continuous blood glucose monitoring in pregnancies complicated by diabetes?

Why this is important
The technology for performing ambulatory continuous blood glucose monitoring is only just becoming available, so there is currently no evidence to assess its effectiveness outside the laboratory situation. Research is needed to determine whether the technology is likely to have a place in the clinical management of diabetes in pregnancy. The new technology may identify women in whom short-term postprandial peaks of glycaemia are not detected by intermittent blood glucose testing. The aim of monitoring is to adjust insulin regimens to reduce the incidence of adverse outcomes of pregnancy (for example, fetal macrosomia, caesarean section and neonatal hypoglycaemia), so these outcomes should be assessed as part of the research.

Management of diabetes during pregnancy

Do new-generation continuous subcutaneous insulin infusion (CSII) pumps offer an advantage over traditional intermittent insulin injections in terms of pregnancy outcomes in women with type 1 diabetes?

Why this is important
Randomised controlled trials have shown no advantage or disadvantage of using CSII pumps over intermittent insulin injections in pregnancy. A new generation of CSII pumps may offer technological advantages that would make a randomised controlled trial appropriate, particularly with the availability of insulin analogues (which may have improved the effectiveness of intermittent insulin injections).

Retinal assessment during pregnancy

Should retinal assessment during pregnancy be offered to women diagnosed with gestational diabetes who are suspected of having pre-existing diabetes?

Why this is important
Women with gestational diabetes may have previously unrecognised type 2 diabetes with retinopathy. At present this is not screened for because of the difficulty in identifying these

women amongst the larger group who have reversible gestational diabetes. The benefit of recognising such women is that treatment for diabetic retinopathy is available and could prevent short- or long-term deterioration of visual acuity. The research needed would be an observational study of retinal assessment in women newly diagnosed with gestational diabetes to determine whether there is a significant amount of retinal disease present. The severity of any abnormality detected might identify women most at risk for appropriate retinal assessment.

Renal assessment during pregnancy

Does identification of microalbuminuria during pregnancy offer the opportunity for appropriate pharmacological treatment to prevent progression to pre-eclampsia in women with pre-existing diabetes?

Why this is important
Microalbuminuria testing is available, but it is not performed routinely in antenatal clinics for women with pre-existing diabetes because a place for prophylactic treatment of pre-eclampsia in microalbuminuria-positive women has not been investigated. The benefit of clinically and cost-effective prophylactic treatment would be to significantly improve pregnancy outcomes in this group of women.

Screening for congenital malformations

How reliable is first-trimester screening for Down's syndrome incorporating levels of pregnancy-associated plasma protein (PAPP-A) in women with pre-existing diabetes?

Why this is important
Several screening tests for Down's syndrome incorporate measurements of PAPP-A. However, two clinical studies have reported conflicting results in terms of whether levels of PAPP-A in women with type 1 diabetes are lower than those in other women. Current practice is to adjust PAPP-A measurements in women with diabetes on the assumption that their PAPP-A levels are indeed lower than those of other women. Further research is, therefore, needed to evaluate the diagnostic accuracy and effect on pregnancy outcomes of screening tests for Down's syndrome incorporating measurements of PAPP-A in women with pre-existing diabetes.

How effective is transvaginal ultrasound for the detection of congenital malformations in women with diabetes and coexisting obesity?

Why this is important
Obstetric ultrasound signals are attenuated by the woman's abdominal wall fat. Many women with diabetes (and particularly women with type 2 diabetes) are obese, and this may limit the sensitivity of abdominal ultrasound screening for congenital malformations. Vaginal ultrasound does not have this difficulty, but there is currently no evidence that it is more effective than abdominal ultrasound. Research studies are, therefore, needed to evaluate the diagnostic accuracy and affect on pregnancy outcomes of vaginal ultrasound in women with diabetes and coexisting obesity. This is important because women with diabetes are at increased risk of having a baby with a congenital malformation.

Monitoring fetal growth and wellbeing

How can the fetus at risk of intrauterine death be identified in women with diabetes?

Why this is important
Unheralded intrauterine death remains a significant contributor to perinatal mortality in pregnancies complicated by diabetes. Conventional tests of fetal wellbeing (umbilical artery Doppler ultrasound, cardiotocography and other biophysical tests) have been shown to have poor sensitivity for predicting such events. Alternative approaches that include measurements of liquor erythropoietin and magnetic resonance imaging spectroscopy may be effective, but there is currently insufficient clinical evidence to evaluate them. Well-designed randomised controlled trials that are sufficiently powered are needed to determine whether these approaches are clinically and cost-effective.

Chapter 6   Intrapartum care

Analgesia and anaesthesia

What are the risks and benefits associated with analgesia and anaesthesia in women with diabetes?

Why this is important
The increasing number of women with diabetes and the high rate of intervention during birth emphasise the need for clinical studies to determine the most effective methods for analgesia and anaesthesia in this group of women. The research studies should investigate the effect of analgesia during labour, and the cardiovascular effects of spinal anaesthesia and vasopressors on diabetic control.

Glycaemic control during labour and birth

What is the optimal method for controlling glycaemia during labour and birth?

Why this is important
Epidemiological studies have shown that poor glycaemic control during labour and birth is associated with adverse neonatal outcomes (in particular, neonatal hypoglycaemia and respiratory distress). However, no randomised controlled trials have compared the effectiveness of intermittent subcutaneous insulin injections and/or CSII with that of intravenous dextrose plus insulin during labour and birth. The potential benefits of intermittent insulin injections and/or CSII over intravenous dextrose plus insulin during the intrapartum period include patient preference due to the psychological effect of the woman feeling in control of her diabetes and having increased mobility. Randomised controlled trials are therefore needed to evaluate the safety of intermittent insulin injections and/or CSII during labour and birth compared with that of intravenous dextrose plus insulin.

Chapter 7   Neonatal care

Prevention and assessment of neonatal hypoglycaemia

Is systematic banking of colostrum antenatally of any benefit in pregnancies complicated by diabetes?

Why this is important
Babies of women with diabetes are at increased risk of neonatal hypoglycaemia and may need frequent early feeding to establish and maintain normoglycaemia. Additionally, the opportunity for early skin-to-skin contact and initiation of breastfeeding is not always achieved in pregnancies complicated by diabetes because of the increased risk of neonatal complications requiring admission to intensive/special care. Antenatal expression and storage of colostrum may, therefore, be of benefit to babies of women with diabetes. There have been no clinical studies to evaluate the effectiveness of antenatal banking of colostrum in women with diabetes. Randomised controlled trials are needed to determine whether this practice is clinically and cost-effective. Encouraging women with diabetes to express and store colostrum before birth might be viewed as an additional barrier to breastfeeding in this group of women who already have lower breastfeeding rates than the general maternity population. There is also a putative risk of precipitating uterine contractions through antenatal expression of colostrum and an accompanying release of oxytocin. These factors should be explored in the randomised controlled trials.

Chapter 8   Postnatal care

Information and follow-up after birth

Are there suitable long-term pharmacological interventions to be recommended postnatally for women who have been diagnosed with gestational diabetes to prevent the onset of type 2 diabetes?

Why this is important
Oral hypoglycaemic agents such rosiglitazone and metformin offer the possibility of pharmacological treatment for prevention of progression to type 2 diabetes in women who have been diagnosed with gestational diabetes. As yet there have been no clinical studies to

investigate the effectiveness of oral hypoglycaemic agents in this context. Randomised controlled trials are needed to determine the clinical and cost-effectiveness of such treatments compared with diet and exercise.

2.5 Algorithm

The algorithm for specific antenatal care for women with diabetes on the following four pages is reproduced from the Quick Reference Guide version of this guideline.

Diabetes in pregnancy

Antenatal care

Key:

● Appointment including specific diabetes care

● Appointment including routine care only

● No routine care appointment

Antenatal care

See also the NICE clinical guideline on antenatal care (www.nice.org.uk/CG062).

Offer:

● immediate referral to a joint diabetes and antenatal clinic

● contact with the diabetes care team every 1–2 weeks to assess glycaemic control

● advice on where to have the birth, which should be in a hospital with advanced neonatal resuscitation skills available 24 hours a day

● information and education at each appointment

● care specifically for women with diabetes, in addition to routine antenatal care, as described below.

Specific antenatal care for women with diabetes

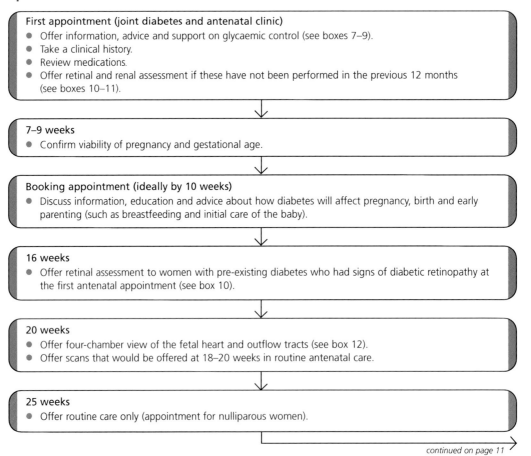

First appointment (joint diabetes and antenatal clinic)
● Offer information, advice and support on glycaemic control (see boxes 7–9).
● Take a clinical history.
● Review medications.
● Offer retinal and renal assessment if these have not been performed in the previous 12 months (see boxes 10–11).

7–9 weeks
● Confirm viability of pregnancy and gestational age.

Booking appointment (ideally by 10 weeks)
● Discuss information, education and advice about how diabetes will affect pregnancy, birth and early parenting (such as breastfeeding and initial care of the baby).

16 weeks
● Offer retinal assessment to women with pre-existing diabetes who had signs of diabetic retinopathy at the first antenatal appointment (see box 10).

20 weeks
● Offer four-chamber view of the fetal heart and outflow tracts (see box 12).
● Offer scans that would be offered at 18–20 weeks in routine antenatal care.

25 weeks
● Offer routine care only (appointment for nulliparous women).

continued on page 11

Diabetes in pregnancy | Antenatal care

28 weeks
- Offer ultrasound monitoring of fetal growth and amniotic fluid volume (see box 12).
- Offer retinal assessment to women with pre-existing diabetes who did not have diabetic retinopathy at their first antenatal clinic visit.

31 weeks
- No appointment (routine care offered to nulliparous women at 32 weeks).

32 weeks
- Offer ultrasound monitoring of fetal growth and amniotic fluid volume.
- Offer investigations that would be offered to nulliparous women at 31 weeks in routine antenatal care.

34 weeks
- Offer routine care only.

36 weeks
- Offer ultrasound monitoring of fetal growth and amniotic fluid volume.
- Offer information and advice about:
  - timing, mode and management of birth
  - analgesia and anaesthesia (including anaesthetic assessment for women with comorbidities, such as obesity or autonomic neuropathy)
  - changes to hypoglycaemic therapy during and after birth
  - initial care of the baby
  - initiation of breastfeeding and the effect of breastfeeding on glycaemic control
  - contraception and follow-up.

38 weeks
- Offer induction of labour, or caesarean section if indicated.
- Offer tests of fetal well-being for women waiting for spontaneous labour.

39 weeks
- Offer tests of fetal well-being for women waiting for spontaneous labour.

40 weeks
- Offer tests of fetal well-being for women waiting for spontaneous labour.

41 weeks
- Offer tests of fetal well-being for women waiting for spontaneous labour.

Diabetes in pregnancy   Antenatal care

Box 7 Blood glucose targets and monitoring

- Advise women to test fasting and 1-hour postprandial blood glucose levels after every meal during pregnancy.
- Agree individualised targets for self-monitoring.
- Advise women to aim for a fasting blood glucose of between 3.5 and 5.9 mmol/litre and 1-hour postprandial blood glucose below 7.8 mmol/litre.
- The presence of diabetic retinopathy should not prevent rapid optimisation of glycaemic control in women with a high HbA_{1c} in early pregnancy.
- Do not use HbA_{1c} routinely in the second and third trimesters.

Box 8 Additional care for women taking insulin

Offer:

- concentrated oral glucose solution to all women taking insulin
- glucagon to women with type 1 diabetes
- insulin pump therapy if glycaemic control using multiple injections is not adequate and the woman experiences significant disabling hypoglycaemia.

Advise:

- women to test their blood glucose before going to bed at night
- on the risks of hypoglycaemia and hypoglycaemia unawareness, especially in the first trimester
- women and their partners or family members on the use of oral glucose solutions and glucagon for hypoglycaemia.

Box 9 Detecting and managing diabetic ketoacidosis

If diabetic ketoacidosis is suspected during pregnancy, admit women immediately for level 2 critical care[1], where both medical and obstetric care are available.

For women with type 1 diabetes:

- offer ketone testing strips and advise women to test their ketone levels if they are hyperglycaemic or unwell
- exclude diabetic ketoacidosis as a matter of urgency in women who become unwell.

---

[1] Level 2 critical care is defined as care for patients requiring detailed observation or intervention, including support for a single failing organ system or postoperative care and those 'stepping down' from higher levels of care.

Diabetes in pregnancy

Antenatal care

Box 10 Retinal assessment for women with pre-existing diabetes

Offer retinal assessment:

- as soon as possible after the first contact in pregnancy if it has not been performed in the past 12 months
- following the first antenatal clinic appointment
- at 28 weeks if the first assessment is normal
- at 16–20 weeks if any diabetic retinopathy is present.

Retinal assessment should be carried out by digital imaging with mydriasis using tropicamide*.

Box 11 Renal assessment for women with pre-existing diabetes

Offer:

- renal assessment at the first contact in pregnancy if it has not been performed in the past 12 months.

Consider:

- referral to a nephrologist if serum creatinine is abnormal (120 micromol/litre or more) or total protein excretion exceeds 2 g/day
- thromboprophylaxis if proteinuria is above 5 g/day.

Do not offer:

- eGFR during pregnancy.

Box 12 Monitoring and screening fetal development

Offer:

- antenatal examination of the four-chamber view of the fetal heart and outflow tracts at 18–20 weeks
- ultrasound monitoring of fetal growth and amniotic fluid volume every 4 weeks from 28 to 36 weeks
- individualised monitoring of fetal well-being to women at risk of intrauterine growth restriction (those with macrovascular disease or nephropathy).

Do not offer:

- tests of fetal well-being before 38 weeks, unless there is a risk of intrauterine growth restriction.

---

* Drug names are marked with an asterisk if they do not have UK marketing authorisation specifically for pregnant and breastfeeding women at the time of publication (March 2008). Informed consent should be obtained and documented.

3 Preconception care

3.1 Outcomes and risks for the woman and baby

Description of the evidence

No specific searches were undertaken for this section of the guideline. The evidence is drawn from publications identified in searches for other sections.

How diabetes affects pregnancy

Women with type 1 and type 2 diabetes have an increased risk of adverse pregnancy outcomes, including miscarriage, fetal congenital anomaly and perinatal death.[2] [EL = 3]

Factors associated with poor pregnancy outcome (defined as a singleton baby with a major congenital anomaly born at any gestational age and/or a baby who died between 20 weeks of gestation and 28 days after birth) in women with type 1 and type 2 diabetes have been documented in the final report of the CEMACH diabetes in pregnancy programme.[33] [EL = 3–4]

Maternal social deprivation is associated with poor pregnancy outcome for women with type 1 or type 2 diabetes (odds ratio (OR) 1.2, 95% confidence interval (CI) 1.1 to 1.4), but ethnicity (Black, Asian or Other Ethnic Minority group) is not (OR 0.9, 95% CI 0.5 to 1.5).[33] [EL = 3–4] This differs from the general maternity population in which both factors are associated with poor pregnancy outcomes.[32] [EL = 2+]

Women with pre-existing complications of diabetes are more likely to have a poor pregnancy outcome (OR 2.6, 95% CI 1.3 to 4.9) than women without.[33] [EL = 3–4] However, nephropathy (OR 2.0, 95% CI 1.0 to 4.2), recurrent hypoglycaemia (OR 1.1, 95% CI 0.7 to 1.7) and severe hypoglycaemia (OR 1.3, 95% CI 0.7 to 2.3) during pregnancy were not associated with poor pregnancy outcome. Antenatal evidence of fetal growth restriction was associated with poor pregnancy outcome (OR 2.9, 95% CI 1.4 to 6.3), but antenatal evidence of fetal macrosomia was not (OR 0.8, 95% CI 0.5 to 1.3).

Certain social and lifestyle factors have also been shown to be associated with poor pregnancy outcome:[33] unplanned pregnancy (OR 1.8, 95% CI 1.0 to 2.9), no contraceptive use in the 12 months prior to pregnancy (OR 2.3, 95% CI 1.3 to 4.0), no preconception folic acid (OR 2.2, 95% CI 1.3 to 3.9), smoking (OR 1.9 95% CI 1.2 to 3.2), sub-optimal approach of the woman to her diabetes prior to pregnancy (OR 4.9, 95% CI 2.7 to 8.8) and sub-optimal approach of the woman to her diabetes during pregnancy (OR 3.9, 95% CI 2.5 to 6.1). However, a body mass index (BMI) of at least 30 kg/m^2 was not associated with poor pregnancy outcomes (OR 1.1, 95% CI 0.6 to 1.9). [EL = 3–4] The importance of planning pregnancy and the role of contraception is considered further in Section 3.2. Diet and dietary supplements are considered further in Section 3.3.

A lack of local glycaemic control targets (OR 2.0, 95% CI 1.0 to 3.8) and sub-optimal glycaemic control before and during pregnancy were also associated with poor pregnancy outcome (preconception OR 3.9, 95% CI 2.2 to 7.0; first trimester OR 3.4, 95% CI 2.1 to 5.7; after first trimester OR 5.2, 95% CI 3.3 to 8.2).[33] [EL = 3–4]

Specific diabetes care risk factors, maternity care risk factors and postnatal care risk factors were also identified in the CEMACH final report.[33] [EL = 3–4] These issues are discussed in Chapters 5 (diabetes care during pregnancy and antenatal care for women with diabetes), 6 (intrapartum care) and 8 (postnatal care for women with diabetes).

How pregnancy affects diabetes

Pregnancy can affect the control and complications of diabetes. There is increased frequency of hypoglycaemia and decreased hypoglycaemia awareness during pregnancy. Nausea and vomiting in pregnancy can disrupt blood glucose control and severe nausea and vomiting (hyperemesis gravidarum) in women with diabetes can lead to ketoacidosis (see Section 5.3).

Pregnancy is associated with progression of diabetic retinopathy. Progression of retinopathy is more likely in women with more severe retinopathy, poor glycaemic control and hypertension (see Section 5.4).

Pregnancy may accelerate progression to end-stage renal disease in women with moderate to advanced diabetic nephropathy (see Section 5.5).

General anaesthesia in women with diabetes leads to a high risk of hypoglycaemia and a higher rate of Mendelson syndrome due to the higher resting gastric volume compared to women without diabetes (see Section 6.2).

Ethnicity

The CEMACH descriptive study found that maternal ethnic origin of pregnant women with type 1 and type 2 diabetes (considered together) was not significantly different to the general maternity population of England, which reports 80.3% White, 5.8% Black (Black Caribbean, Black African and Black Other), 10.5% Asian (Indian, Pakistani and Bangladeshi) and 3.4% Chinese and other ethnic background. However, a much higher proportion of women with type 2 diabetes were of Black, Asian or Other Ethnic Minority origin compared to women with type 1 diabetes (48.5% versus 8.5%).[2] [EL = 3]

The CEMACH data suggested that ethnicity is not associated with poorer pregnancy outcome for women with type 1 or type 2 diabetes (Black, Asian or Other Ethnic Minority group, OR 0.9, 95% CI 0.5 to 1.5). However, women from ethnic minority groups are more likely to develop gestational diabetes (see Section 4.1). They are also more likely to have unplanned pregnancies and less likely to have a measure of long-term glycaemic control in the 6 months before pregnancy (see Section 3.8).[33] [EL = 3–4]

The CEMACH data for England showed that in women of white ethnic origin there was a clear increase in the number of women with type 2 diabetes with increasing quintile of social deprivation (6.8% in least and 45.1% in most-deprived quintile). This trend was not statistically significant in women of white ethnic origin with type 1 diabetes (18.3% in least-deprived quintile and 21.9% in most-deprived quintile). For women of Black or Other Ethnic Minority origin, this association was stronger and seen in women with type 1 diabetes (4.7% in least-deprived quintile and 35.6% in most-deprived quintile) and type 2 diabetes (3.4% in least-deprived quintile and 59.4% in most-deprived quintile).[2] [EL = 3]

Evidence statement

Women with pre-existing type 1 and type 2 diabetes have an increased risk of adverse pregnancy outcomes, including miscarriage, fetal congenital anomaly and perinatal death. The following factors are associated with adverse pregnancy outcome: maternal social deprivation, unplanned pregnancy and lack of contraceptive use in the 12 months prior to pregnancy, lack of preconception folic acid, smoking, sub-optimal approach of the woman to her diabetes before or during pregnancy and sub-optimal glycaemic control before or during pregnancy, antenatal evidence of fetal growth restriction, pre-existing diabetes complications, lack of local glycaemic control targets, lack of discussion of diabetes-specific issues related to alcohol intake, lack of discussion of fetal risks in diabetic pregnancy, lack of a baseline retinal examination in the 12 months before pregnancy and sub-optimal preconception care (excluding glycaemic control). [EL = 3–4]

Pregnancy can affect glycaemic control in women with diabetes, increasing the frequency of hypoglycaemia and hypoglycaemia unawareness, and the risk of ketoacidosis. General anaesthesia in women with diabetes can also increase the risk of hypoglycaemia. The progression of certain complications of diabetes, specifically diabetic retinopathy and diabetic nephropathy, can be accelerated by pregnancy.

Existing guidance

The standard set by the NSF for diabetes[20] in relation to diabetes in pregnancy was for the NHS to develop, implement and monitor policies to empower and support women with pre-existing diabetes and women with gestational diabetes to optimise pregnancy outcomes. The NSF stated that maternity care should ensure that all pregnant women have a positive experience of pregnancy and childbirth, and that they should receive care that promotes their physical and psychological wellbeing and optimises the health of their babies. The NSF highlighted that maternity care for women with diabetes may be perceived as highly 'medicalised' with a tendency towards intervention in labour and birth and that this could make the experience negative or frightening. It was suggested that keeping women with diabetes and their partners fully informed and involved in decision making would help to ensure that their experience of pregnancy and childbirth would be a positive one.

From evidence to recommendations

As no systematic searches were conducted for this section of the guideline, the GDG's recommendations are based on its consensus view of what information should be offered to women with pre-existing diabetes before pregnancy to support and explain its substantive recommendations regarding management options before, during and after pregnancy, both in terms of maternity care and management of diabetes during these periods and to reinforce the recommendations of the NSF for diabetes.[20]

Recommendations for outcomes and risks for the woman and baby

Healthcare professionals should seek to empower women with diabetes to make the experience of pregnancy and childbirth a positive one by providing information, advice and support that will help to reduce the risks of adverse pregnancy outcomes for mother and baby.

Women with diabetes who are planning to become pregnant should be informed that establishing good glycaemic control before conception and continuing this throughout pregnancy will reduce the risk of miscarriage, congenital malformation, stillbirth and neonatal death. It is important to explain that risks can be reduced but not eliminated.

Women with diabetes who are planning to become pregnant and their families should be offered information about how diabetes affects pregnancy and how pregnancy affects diabetes. The information should cover:

- the role of diet, body weight and exercise
- the risks of hypoglycaemia and hypoglycaemia unawareness during pregnancy
- how nausea and vomiting in pregnancy can affect glycaemic control
- the increased risk of having a baby who is large for gestational age, which increases the likelihood of birth trauma, induction of labour and caesarean section
- the need for assessment of diabetic retinopathy before and during pregnancy
- the need for assessment of diabetic nephropathy before pregnancy
- the importance of maternal glycaemic control during labour and birth and early feeding of the baby in order to reduce the risk of neonatal hypoglycaemia
- the possibility of transient morbidity in the baby during the neonatal period, which may require admission to the neonatal unit
- the risk of the baby developing obesity and/or diabetes in later life.

There were no research recommendations relating to the information that should be offered about outcomes and risks for the woman and the baby.

3.2 The importance of planning pregnancy and the role of contraception

Description of the evidence

No specific searches were undertaken for this section of the guideline. The evidence is drawn from publications identified in searches for other sections.

The CEMACH diabetes in pregnancy programme provides data on current practice in England, Wales and Northern Ireland in relation to planning pregnancy, use of contraception and preconception counselling in women with type 1 and type 2 diabetes.[33] [EL = 3–4]

The CEMACH descriptive study found 38.2% of women with type 1 diabetes and 24.8% of women with type 2 diabetes had pre-pregnancy counselling documented.[2] A pre-pregnancy glycaemic test in the 6 months before pregnancy was recorded for 40% of the women with type 1 diabetes and 29.4% of the women with type 2 diabetes. [EL = 3]

The CEMACH enquiry reported that pre-pregnancy counselling included a discussion about:

- glycaemic control in 51% of women with poor pregnancy outcome and 56% with good pregnancy outcome
- diet in 42% of women with poor pregnancy outcome and 48% with good pregnancy outcome
- contraception in 19% of women with poor pregnancy outcome and 36% with good pregnancy outcome
- retinopathy in 30% of women with poor pregnancy outcome and 39% with good pregnancy outcome
- nephropathy in 23% of women with poor pregnancy outcome and 25% with good pregnancy outcome
- hypertension in 22% of women with poor pregnancy outcome and 28% with good pregnancy outcome
- alcohol intake in 20% of women with poor pregnancy outcome and 25% with good pregnancy outcome
- need for increased pregnancy surveillance in 54% of women with poor pregnancy outcome and 62% with good pregnancy outcome
- fetal risks in 42% of women with poor pregnancy outcome and 58% with good pregnancy outcome
- the increased chance of induction of labour for 32% of women with poor pregnancy outcome and 51% with good pregnancy outcome
- the increased possibility of caesarean section for 39% of women with poor pregnancy outcome and 53% with good pregnancy outcome.

Note that poor pregnancy outcome was defined as a singleton baby with a major congenital anomaly who gave birth at any gestation and/or a baby who died from 20 weeks of gestation up to 28 days after birth. Good pregnancy outcome was defined as a singleton baby without a congenital anomaly who survived to day 28 after birth.

The CEMACH enquiry found an association between poor pregnancy outcome and a lack of discussion of diabetes-specific issues related to alcohol intake (OR 2.5, 95% CI 1.1 to 5.4), lack of discussion of fetal risks in diabetic pregnancy (OR 2.9, 95% CI 1.1 to 8.2), lack of a baseline retinal examination in the 12 months before pregnancy (OR 2.3, 95% CI 1.2 to 4.5) and assessment of sub-optimal preconception care (excluding glycaemic control; OR 5.2, 95% CI 2.7 to 10.1).[33] [EL = 3–4]

However, the CEMACH enquiry found no association between poor pregnancy outcome and a lack of contraceptive advice before pregnancy (OR 1.7, 95% CI 0.8 to 3.5), lack of discussion about diet (OR 1.8, 95% CI 0.8 to 4.1), poor glycaemic control (OR 1.2, 95% CI 0.5 to 2.5), retinopathy (OR 1.1, 95% CI 0.6 to 2.3), nephropathy (OR 0.8, 95% CI 0.4 to 1.7), hypertension (OR 1.1, 95% CI 0.5 to 2.3), lack of discussion of increased diabetes surveillance (OR 1.7, 95% CI 0.6 to 4.5), increased pregnancy surveillance (OR 1.5, 95% CI 0.6 to 4.0), increased risk of induction of labour (OR 2.2, 95% CI 1.0 to 4.9) or possible caesarean section (OR 2.4, 95% CI 1.0 to 5.8), lack of dietetic review before pregnancy (OR 1.2, 95% CI 0.7 to 2.1), lack of a baseline test of renal function (OR 2.0, 95% CI 0.9 to 4.3) or assessment of albuminuria (OR 1.5, 95% CI 0.8 to 2.8).[33] [EL = 3–4]

As noted in Section 3.1, social and lifestyle factors, such as unplanned pregnancy and lack of contraceptive use in the last 12 months, are associated with poor pregnancy outcome. In the general maternity population, 42% of women did not plan their last pregnancy. The CEMACH enquiry found 51% (72/141) of the women with poor pregnancy outcome and 38% (55/144) of the women with good pregnancy outcome were documented as having not planned their last pregnancy (OR 1.8, 95% CI 1.0 to 2.9).[33] [EL = 3–4] Sixty-six percent (71/108) of the women with poor pregnancy outcome and 45% (54/121) of the women with good pregnancy outcome were not documented as using any type of contraception in the 12 months before conception (OR 2.3, 95% CI 1.3 to 4.0).

The CEMACH enquiry (comparison of women with type 1 and type 2 diabetes) reported that 38% (32/84) of women with type 2 diabetes and 40% (50/121) of women with type 1 diabetes were documented as having not planned their last pregnancy compared with 42% in the general maternity population. Contraceptive use in the 12 months prior to pregnancy was lower in women with type 2 diabetes (32%) compared with women with type 1 diabetes (59%, $P = 0.001$).[33] [EL = 3–4]

The CEMACH enquiry (comparison of women with type 1 and type 2 diabetes) reported that there was no difference between women with type 1 or type 2 diabetes with regard to whether they had a test for glycaemic control in the 12 months prior to pregnancy (83% versus 81%, $P = 0.66$).[33] Women with type 1 diabetes were more likely to have sub-optimal preconception glycaemic control (75%) than women with type 2 diabetes (60%) ($P = 0.013$). [EL = 3–4]

There are advantages to the woman and baby in planning pregnancy. Optimising glycaemic control before conception and in the first few weeks of pregnancy is of prime importance. Poor glycaemic control before pregnancy and in early pregnancy is associated with congenital malformations and miscarriage (see Section 3.4).

The CEMACH enquiry found that a greater number of women with poor pregnancy outcomes (69%) compared with women with good pregnancy outcome (50%) were not documented as having commenced folic acid supplementation before pregnancy (adjusted OR 2.2, 95% CI 1.3 to 3.9).[33] Only 32% (33/103) of women taking folic acid were on the high dose (5 mg/day). [EL = 3–4]

The CEMACH enquiry (comparison of women with type 1 and type 2 diabetes) reported there was no difference between the number of women with type 1 diabetes and those with type 2 diabetes who were documented as having commenced folic acid supplementation in the 12 months before pregnancy (45% [32/71] of women with type 2 diabetes and 49% [54/110] of women with type 1 diabetes, $P = 0.6$).[33] [EL = 3–4]

Women with diabetes are at an increased risk of having a baby with a neural tube defect. Women with diabetes who are planning to get pregnant are recommended to supplement their diet with folic acid until 12 weeks of gestation (see Section 3.3).

Some medications used to treat complications of diabetes can increase the risk of congenital malformation if used in the early stages of pregnancy. These medications include angiotensin-converting enzyme (ACE) inhibitors used to treat hypertension and nephropathy, angiotensin-II receptor blockers (ARBs) (also known as angiotensin-II receptor antagonists) used to treat hypertension and statins used to treat elevated cholesterol. These medications should be discontinued before pregnancy to reduce the risk of congenital malformations and safe alternative medications should be prescribed if appropriate (see Section 3.7).

Because of the importance of planning future pregnancies in women with diabetes, it is recommended that information and advice about contraception and the importance of planned pregnancy is offered to the women with diabetes in the postnatal period (see Section 8.2).

Since development of the fetal organs occurs during the first 3 months of pregnancy and good glycaemic control in the preconception period and the first trimester of pregnancy decreases the risk of congenital anomaly and miscarriage (see Section 3.4),[35,36] planning pregnancy is particularly important for women with diabetes. However, women with diabetes are less likely to plan pregnancy than women without diabetes and young women with diabetes lack awareness of the importance of planning pregnancy and the role of preconception care (see Section 3.8).

Evidence statement

Women with pre-existing diabetes who have preconception care and advice involving a discussion of glycaemic control, diet, contraception, retinopathy, nephropathy, hypertension, alcohol intake, the need for increased pregnancy surveillance, fetal risks, the chance of induction of labour and caesarean section have better pregnancy outcomes than women who do not have preconception care and advice.

Development of the fetal organs occurs in the first 3 months of pregnancy, and so good glycaemic control and avoidance of medications that could harm the developing fetus should be established before discontinuing contraception.

From evidence to recommendations

As no systematic searches were conducted for this section of the guideline, the GDG's recommendations are based on its consensus view of what information should be offered to women with diabetes in relation to planning pregnancy and the role of contraception to support and explain its substantive recommendations regarding management options before, during and after pregnancy.

> **Recommendations for the importance of planning pregnancy and the role of contraception**
>
> The importance of avoiding unplanned pregnancy should be an essential component of diabetes education from adolescence for women with diabetes.
>
> Women with diabetes who are planning to become pregnant should be advised:
>
> - that the risks associated with pregnancies complicated by diabetes increase with the duration of diabetes
> - to use contraception until good glycaemic control (assessed by HbA$_{1c}$*) has been established
> - that glycaemic targets, glucose monitoring, medications for diabetes (including insulin regimens for insulin-treated diabetes) and medications for complications of diabetes will need to be reviewed before and during pregnancy
> - that additional time and effort is required to manage diabetes during pregnancy and that there will be frequent contact with healthcare professionals. Women should be given information about the local arrangements for support, including emergency contact numbers.

There were no research recommendations relating to the information that should be offered about the importance of planning pregnancy and the role of contraception.

3.3 Diet, dietary supplements, body weight and exercise

Description of the evidence

Diet
The aims of dietary advice for women with diabetes who are planning a pregnancy are:

- optimisation of glycaemic control, avoiding large fluctuations of blood glucose, especially postprandial blood glucose, while avoiding ketosis and hypoglycaemia in women taking insulin
- provision of sufficient energy and nutrients to allow normal fetal growth while avoiding accelerated fetal growth patterns.[37]

Hyperglycaemia in early pregnancy is associated with congenital malformations and miscarriage (see Section 3.4). In later pregnancy it is implicated in accelerated fetal growth, stillbirth, and neonatal hypoglycaemia and hypocalcaemia (see Sections 3.4 and 5.1).

Targeting postprandial hyperglycaemia is particularly important during pregnancy. Adjusting treatment to postprandial blood glucose levels is associated with better outcomes in women with type 1 diabetes or gestational diabetes than responding to fasting blood glucose (FBG) levels (see Sections 3.4, 4.3 and 5.1).

Dose Adjustment for Normal Eating (DAFNE) is an example of a structured education programme for people with type 1 diabetes in the UK (see Section 3.4).

Low glycaemic index (GI) diets appear to reduce postprandial hyperglycaemia and women on low GI diets have been reported to have babies with lower birthweights compared with women on high GI diets (see Sections 3.4 and 5.1).

---

* Diabetes Control and Complications Trial (DCCT)-aligned haemoglobin A$_{1c}$ (HbA$_{1c}$) test.

A meta-analysis was identified that compared the effect on HbA_{1c} of low GI diets with that of high GI diets.[38,39] The meta-analysis included 14 studies and 356 nonpregnant people (203 with type 1 diabetes and 153 with type 2 diabetes). The meta-analysis found that low GI diets reduced HbA_{1c} by 0.43 percentage points (95% CI 0.72 to 0.13) over and above that produced by high GI diets. Taking HbA_{1c} and fructosamine data together and adjusting for baseline differences, glycated proteins were reduced 7.4% more on the low GI diet than on the high GI diet (95% CI 8.8 to 6.0). [EL = 1++]

A prospective randomised study[40] was performed in 15 women with glucose intolerance diagnosed early in the third trimester of pregnancy. The results showed that the mean plasma glucose concentrations of the diet-treated women were significantly greater than those of the controls (pregnant women with a normal glucose tolerance who ate according to appetite) at 10 a.m., 2 p.m. and 8 p.m. as compared with significantly lower in the insulin-treated group than the controls at 6 p.m., 2 a.m., 4 a.m. and 6 a.m. The mean 2 hour neonatal plasma glucose concentration of the diet-treated group was significantly higher than that of other groups. [EL = 1−]

Nausea and vomiting in pregnancy can disrupt blood glucose control (see Section 5.3).

Dietary supplements
Women with diabetes have an increased risk of having a baby with a neural tube defect (see Section 5.6).

The CEMACH enquiry found 69% (83/120) of the women with poor pregnancy outcome and 50% (66/131) of the women with good pregnancy outcome were documented as not having commenced folic acid supplementation before pregnancy (this is similar to the general maternity population), but only 33 women were on the 'high dose' (5 mg) of folic acid. Not commencing folic acid supplements prior to pregnancy led to an increased risk of poor pregnancy outcome (OR 2.2, 95% CI 1.3 to 3.9).[33] [EL = 3–4]

The CEMACH enquiry (comparison of women with type 1 and type 2 diabetes) reported that 45% (32/71) of women with type 2 diabetes and 49% (54/110) of women with type 1 diabetes were documented as having commenced folic acid supplementation before pregnancy.[33] [EL = 3–4]

A case–control study compared folate metabolism in 31 pregnant women with diabetes to that in 54 pregnant women without diabetes.[39] The study found no significant differences for any measures of folate metabolism. [EL = 2+]

Body weight
Obesity is an independent risk factor for a number of adverse pregnancy outcomes including:[37]

• impaired glucose tolerance (IGT)
• hypertensive disorders
• caesarean section
• perinatal mortality
• macrosomia
• preterm birth
• congenital malformations. [EL = 2+]

A cohort study included 196 women with pre-existing diabetes and 428 women with gestational diabetes.[41] After controlling for type of diabetes, maternal age, parity and obstetric history, the study found that, when compared with pre-pregnancy BMI less than 20 kg/m², pre-pregnancy BMI 30 kg/m² or more was independently associated with caesarean section (OR 3.5, 95% CI 1.4 to 8.6) and preterm birth at less than 37 weeks of gestation (OR 5.1, 95% CI 1.4 to 18.6). Weight gain during pregnancy was independently associated with hypertensive disorders of pregnancy (OR 1.4, 95% CI 1.2 to 1.7) and large-for-gestational-age (LGA) babies (OR 1.3, 95% CI 1.1 to 1.6). [EL = 2++]

A prospective cohort study collected data on pre-pregnancy exposures and pregnancy outcome in 22 951 women (574 with diabetes, 1974 with a BMI 28 kg/m² or more).[42] There was no increased risk of major defects in the offspring of women without diabetes who were obese (relative risk (RR) 0.95, 95% CI 0.62 to 1.5) and no increased risk among women with diabetes who were not obese (RR 0.98, 95% CI 0.43 to 2.2). The offspring of women with diabetes and coexisting obesity were three times as likely to have a major defect (RR 3.1, 95% CI 1.2 to 7.6) than those of women without diabetes, suggesting that obesity and diabetes may act synergistically in the pathogenesis of congenital malformations. [EL = 2++]

A prospective population-based cohort study[43] of 1041 Latino mother–baby pairs assessed the combined influence of maternal weight and other anthropometric and metabolic characteristics on the birthweights of babies. The results showed that there was an increased risk of adverse maternal and infant outcomes associated with excessive maternal weight, weight gain and glucose intolerance. [EL = 2+]

A retrospective cohort study[44] examined the relationship between gestational weight gain and adverse neonatal outcomes among term babies (37 weeks of gestation or more). The results showed that the gestational weight gain above Institute of Medicine guidelines was common and associated with multiple adverse neonatal outcomes, whereas gestational weight gain below guidelines was only associated with SGA babies. [EL = 2–]

A prospective cohort study[45] evaluated the independent influence of pre-pregnancy BMI and glucose tolerance status on the presentation of diabetes-related adverse pregnancy outcomes in Spanish women. The results showed that pre-pregnancy maternal BMI exhibited a much stronger influence than abnormal blood glucose tolerance on macrosomia, caesarean section, pregnancy-induced hypertension and LGA newborns. [EL = 2++]

Exercise

Moderate exercise has been found to improve blood glucose control in women with gestational diabetes (see Section 4.3). No studies were identified in the population of pregnant women with pre-existing type 1 or type 2 diabetes.

A meta-analysis included six studies involving a total of 322 women with type 2 diabetes.[46] All studies compared dietary advice with dietary advice plus exercise. On average there was more weight loss in the dietary advice plus exercise groups. HbA_{1c} decreased more in the women in the dietary advice plus exercise group than in those in the dietary advice group alone. Dietary advice plus exercise was associated with a statistically significant mean decrease in HbA_{1c} of 0.9% at 6 months (95% CI 0.4 to 1.3) and 1% at 12 months (95% CI 0.4 to 1.5). [EL = 1++]

A Cochrane systematic review[47] aimed to evaluate the effect of exercise programmes alone or in conjunction with other therapies such as diet, compared with no specific programme or with other therapies, in pregnant women with diabetes on perinatal and maternal morbidity and mortality. The review found no significant difference between exercise and the other regimens in any of the outcomes evaluated. [EL = 1+]

Existing guidance

The NICE antenatal care guideline[9] recommends that healthy pregnant women (and those intending to become pregnant) should be informed that dietary supplementation with folic acid, before conception and up to 12 weeks of gestation, reduces the risk of having a baby with neural tube defects. The recommended dose is 400 micrograms per day for the general maternity population. An Expert Advisory Group report issued by the Department of Health[48] recommended that women with no history of neural tube defects should take 400 micrograms per day, whereas women with a history of neural tube defects should take a higher dose (5 mg per day).

NICE has developed public health guidance on maternal and child nutrition,[19] which aims to improve the nutrition of pregnant and breastfeeding mothers and children in low-income households. The guidance recommends that women with diabetes who may become pregnant and those who are in the early stages of pregnancy should be prescribed 5 mg of folic acid per day.

Evidence statement

Low GI diets reduce postprandial glycaemia.

Obesity is a risk factor for a number of adverse perinatal outcomes. In cohort studies of women with gestational diabetes who are obese undergoing moderate calorie restriction, good outcomes were achieved without ketoacidosis.

Exercise can help women with diabetes to lose weight and improve glycaemic control.

Folic acid supplementation reduces the prevalence of neural tube defects. Women with diabetes have an increased risk of neural tube defects, and there is no evidence that folic acid metabolism differs from that of women who do not have diabetes.

From evidence to recommendations

A number of factors interact during pregnancy to influence glycaemic control including physiological changes during pregnancy, comorbidities, changes in lifestyle, insulin treatment and dietary factors.[37] It follows that dietary advice should be given on an individual basis from someone with appropriate training and expertise.

Given the evidence that obesity is linked to a number of adverse perinatal outcomes, women with diabetes who are obese and intending to become pregnant should be advised of the risks to their own health and that of their babies and encouraged to start a supervised weight reduction diet.

Folic acid is particularly important for women with diabetes planning a pregnancy because of the increased risk of congenital malformations, which include neural tube defects. At present there is no evidence to suggest that these women would benefit from a larger dose than is recommended for women who do not have diabetes. However, the GDG's view was that women with diabetes should take the higher dose of 5 mg per day, as for other women with increased risk of neural tube defects, when intending to become pregnant.

Recommendations for diet, dietary supplements, body weight and exercise

Women with diabetes who are planning to become pregnant should be offered individualised dietary advice.

Women with diabetes who are planning to become pregnant and who have a body mass index above 27 kg/m² should be offered advice on how to lose weight in line with 'Obesity: guidance on the prevention, identification, assessment and management of overweight and obesity in adults and children' (NICE clinical guideline 43), available from www.nice.org.uk/CG043.

Women with diabetes who are planning to become pregnant should be advised to take folic acid (5 mg/day) until 12 weeks of gestation to reduce the risk of having a baby with a neural tube defect.

There were no research recommendations relating to the information that should be offered about diet, dietary supplements, body weight and exercise.

3.4   Target ranges for blood glucose in the preconception period

Description of the evidence

Congenital malformations
Fourteen studies were identified that examined the effect of preconception glycaemic control on congenital malformations. All studies found a positive relationship between poor preconception glycaemic control and congenital malformations.

A non-randomised controlled trial and five cohort studies compared rates of congenital malformations in women attending for preconception care with those in non-attenders. Here, preconception care means intensive treatment aimed at optimising blood glucose control prior to conception.

The non-randomised controlled trial[49] compared 94 women originally assigned to intensive treatment (intensive treatment group) with 86 women originally assigned to conventional treatment (conventional treatment group). All women originally assigned to conventional treatment were changed to intensive treatment during pregnancy; 26 changed before conception and 60 changed after conception. The goals for all pregnant women were fasting glucose level 3.9–5.5 mmol/litre and 1 hour postprandial glucose level 7.7 mmol/litre or less. The mean HbA$_{1c}$ at conception in the intensive treatment group was 7.4% ± 1.3% compared with 8.1% ± 1.7% in the conventional treatment group ($P = 0.0001$). Nine congenital malformations were identified, eight in the conventional treatment group ($P = 0.06$). [EL = 2++]

The five cohort studies compared women with type 1 diabetes attending a preconception clinic with non-attenders.[36,50–53] All five studies found significantly more congenital malformations in the non-attending group ($P < 0.05$). Four of these studies reported first-trimester HbA$_{1c}$ levels. In all cases the first-trimester HbA$_{1c}$ was significantly higher in the non-attending group ($P < 0.05$). [EL = 2++]

Nine studies examined the relationship between first-trimester HbA$_{1c}$ and the incidence of congenital malformations.

A cohort study of 691 pregnancies and 709 babies of 488 women with type 1 diabetes[35] found first-trimester HbA$_{1c}$ to be associated with occurrence of malformations ($P = 0.02$ after adjusting for White's classification of diabetes, age at onset of diabetes, duration of diabetes, parity, smoking and participation in preconception 'counselling', no description of preconception counselling reported). The RR, when compared with women without diabetes, for different gradients of first-trimester HbA$_{1c}$ are presented in Table 3.1. [EL = 2++]

Table 3.1 Relative risk of congenital malformations for different gradients of first-trimester HbA$_{1c}$ for women with type 1 diabetes compared with women without diabetes[35]

HbA$_{1c}$ at less than 14 weeks of gestation (%)	Congenital malformations	RR (95% CI)
< 5.6	1/47	1.6 (0.3–9.5)
5.6–6.8	7/170	3.0 (1.2–7.5)
6.9–8.0	8/252	2.3 (1.0–5.7)
8.1–9.3	6/133	3.3 (1.3–8.6)
≥ 9.4	4/61	4.8 (1.6–13.9)

A study of 435 pregnant women[54] (289 with type 1 diabetes and 146 with type 2 diabetes) compared women with first-trimester HbA$_{1c}$ more than 8% with women with first-trimester HbA$_{1c}$ less than 8%. Women with first-trimester HbA$_{1c}$ more than 8% had higher rates of congenital malformations (8.3% versus 2.5%, OR 3.5, 95% CI 1.3 to 8.9, $P < 0.01$). [EL = 2++]

A cohort study of 303 pregnant women with type 1 diabetes[55] found the rate of major malformations increased significantly in women whose first-trimester HbA$_1$ values exceeded 12.7% (normal mean 5.9%, standard deviation (SD) 0.57) or 12 SD above the mean (see Table 3.2). [EL = 2++]

Table 3.2 Relative risk of congenital malformations in women with raised HbA$_1$ compared with women with HbA$_1$ of 9.3% or less[55]

First-trimester HbA$_1$ (%)	Congenital malformations	RR (95% CI)
≤ 9.3	3/99 (3%)	1.0
9.4–11.0	4/77 (5.2%)	1.7 (0.4–1.7)
11.1–12.7	2/46 (4.3%)	1.4 (0.3–8.3)
12.8–14.4	7/18 (38.9%)	12.8 (4.7–35.0)
> 14.4	4/10 (40%)	13.2 (4.3–40.4)

In a cohort study of 142 women with type 1 diabetes[56] 17/142 pregnancies were complicated by malformation (six minor and 11 major). The mean initial HbA$_{1c}$ was significantly higher in the group with minor malformations (9.3%, SD 1.9, $P < 0.05$) and in the group with major malformations (9.6%, SD 1.8, $P < 0.001$) than in the group without malformations (8.0%, SD 1.4). There were 4.8% (3/63) of congenital malformations in women with initial HbA$_{1c}$ less than 8.0%, 12.9% (8/62) in women with initial HbA$_{1c}$ in the range 8.0–9.9% and 35.3% (6/17) in women with HbA$_{1c}$ 10.0% or more. [EL = 2++]

A cohort study of 116 women with type 1 diabetes[57] found HbA_{1c} was significantly higher in the group with major congenital malformations (13) than in the group without (9.5 ± 1.0 versus 8.5 ± 1.6, $P < 0.01$). There were no malformations (0/19) in women with HbA_{1c} 6.9% or less compared with malformations in 5.1% (2/39) of women with HbA_{1c} in the range 7.0–8.5%, 22.9% (8/35) of women with HbA_{1c} in the range 8.6–9.9% and 21.7% (5/23) of women with HbA_{1c} 10.0% or more. [EL = 2++]

A cohort study of 105 women with type 1 diabetes[58] found a significant increase in the incidence of malformation above a first-trimester HbA_{1a+b+c} of 9.2% (normal non-diabetic mean 6%, range 5.0–6.9%, $P = 0.05$). Ten of the 14 malformations occurred in 42 women whose levels exceeded this value, compared with four malformations in the 45 women with lower values. [EL = 2++]

A cohort study of 83 pregnant women[59] (63 with type 1 diabetes and 20 with type 2 diabetes) examined the effect of first-trimester HbA_{1c} on congenital malformations. There were nine congenital malformations, all occurring in women with first-trimester HbA_{1c} more than 9.5%. Seven of the nine malformations were in women whose HbA_{1c} was more than 11.5% and six were in women whose HbA_{1c} was more than 13.5%. The normal non-diabetic mean (SD) HbA_{1c} was 5.1% (1.1%). [EL = 2++]

In a cohort study of 229 women with type 1 diabetes,[60] 6.1% (14) of women had babies with congenital malformations. The threshold for increased risk of malformation was a preprandial glucose concentration of 6.6 mmol/litre or an initial HbA_1 of 13% (6.2 SD above the normal mean; $P < 0.05$). The normal non-diabetic mean (SD) HbA_1 in the laboratory used in the study was 7.0% (0.8%). [EL = 2++]

Miscarriage
Eight studies were identified that examined the effect of preconception glycaemic control on miscarriage. One non-randomised trial and two cohort studies compared rates of miscarriage in women who received preconception care with rates in women with no preconception care.

The non-randomised controlled trial[49] compared 94 women originally assigned to intensive treatment (intensive treatment group) with 86 women originally assigned to conventional treatment (conventional treatment group). All women originally assigned to conventional treatment were changed to intensive treatment during pregnancy; 26 changed before conception and 60 changed after conception. The goals for all pregnant women were fasting glucose level 3.85–5.5 mmol/litre and 1 hour postprandial glucose level 7.7 mmol/litre or less. The mean HbA_{1c} at conception in the intensive treatment group was 7.4% ± 1.3% compared with 8.1% ± 1.7% in the conventional treatment group ($P = 0.0001$). There was no significant difference between the rates of miscarriage in the intensive and conventional treatment groups (13.3% [18] versus 10.4% [14]). [EL = 2++]

A cohort study compared pregnancy outcomes in relation to glycaemic control in 386 women with type 1 diabetes and 432 women without diabetes.[61] The percentage of women who enrolled before conception was 75.9%; the remaining 24.1% enrolled less than 21 days after conception. Sixteen percent (62/386) of women with diabetes had miscarriages as did 16% (70/432) of women without diabetes. Within the normal range, there was no relationship between the level of HbA_{1c} and the rate of pregnancy loss in women with diabetes or without diabetes. Above the normal range, loss rates in women with diabetes increased in an approximately linear fashion with increasing levels of HbA_{1c} ($y = 0.7x - 19.1$, $P = 0.015$). Fasting ($P = 0.01$) and postprandial ($P = 0.004$) blood glucose levels were significantly higher in women who miscarried and were significant predictors of loss when analysed by logistic regression. [EL = 2++]

A cohort study of 99 pregnant women with type 1 diabetes[62] compared outcomes in 28 women who had attended a preconception clinic with those in 71 women who had enrolled after conception. HbA_{1c} levels were significantly lower in the preconception care group at the first antenatal visit ($P = 0.0008$) and at 9 weeks of gestation ($P = 0.002$) and 14 weeks of gestation ($P = 0.02$). The rate of miscarriage was significantly lower in the preconception care group (7% versus 24%, $P = 0.04$). HbA_{1c} at the first antenatal visit and at 9 weeks of and 14 weeks of gestation were significantly higher in women who had miscarriages ($P = 0.005$, $P = 0.02$, $P = 0.02$). [EL = 2++]

A cohort study of 94 women with type 1 diabetes[63] compared 59 women who attended a preconception clinic with 35 non-attenders. Miscarriage occurred in 5/59 women who attended the preconception clinic and in 10/35 non-attenders ($P < 0.001$). The initial glucose and HbA_{1c} values of women who had no preconception care and who had a miscarriage were significantly higher compared with women who received preconception care and whose pregnancies progressed beyond 22 weeks of gestation ($P < 0.001$). [EL = 2++]

The remaining five studies examined the effect of first-trimester HbA_{1c} on miscarriage. A cohort study of 105 women with type 1 diabetes[58] reported miscarriage in 18 women. The mean first-trimester HbA_{1c} was 9.4% ± 2.3%, which was not significantly different from the mean HbA_{1c} values of those pregnancies resulting in a malformation (10.3 ± 1.9%) or no adverse outcome (8.9% ± 2.3%). The normal non-diabetic range of HbA_{1c} was 5.5–8.5%. The rate of miscarriage may be underestimated in this study. The range of gestational age at entry was 6–16 completed weeks. Some women may experience miscarriage before enrolling for antenatal care. [EL = 2++]

A cohort study of 303 women with type 1 diabetes[55] found miscarriage rates were significantly increased when first-trimester HbA_1 was greater than 11.0% (normal non-diabetic mean (SD) 5.9% (0.57%)). [EL = 2++]

A cohort study of 83 women[59] included 63 women with type 1 diabetes and 20 with type 2 diabetes. Miscarriages occurred in 22 pregnancies (26.5%). No miscarriages occurred in women with first-trimester HbA_{1c} less than 7.5%, 1/22 occurred in women whose HbA_{1c} was 7.5–9.4%, 21/22 occurred in women whose HbA_{1c} was more than 11.5% and 19/22 occurred in women whose HbA_{1c} was more than 13.5%. The normal non-diabetic mean (SD) HbA_{1c} was 5.1% (1.1%). [EL = 2++]

A cohort study of 84 pregnancies in 68 women with type 1 diabetes[64] measured HbA_1 (normal non-diabetic range 5.5–8.5%), glycosylated proteins and glycosylated albumin at 9 weeks of gestation. Women who had a miscarriage had significantly higher HbA_1 (12.0 ± 0.6) than women whose pregnancies progressed beyond 20 weeks (10.7 ± 0.3, $P < 0.05$). There was no association with glycosylated proteins or glycosylated albumin. The findings suggest that poor metabolic control around conception, rather than in the weeks immediately preceding the miscarriage, is the important factor. [EL = 2++]

In a cohort study of 215 women with type 1 diabetes,[60] 52 women (24%) had miscarriages. The threshold for increased risk of miscarriage rate was a preprandial glucose concentration of 7.15 mmol/litre or an initial HbA_1 of 12% (6.2 SD above the normal mean, $P < 0.05$). The normal non-diabetic mean (SD) HbA_1 was 7.0% (0.8%). [EL = 2++]

A cohort study of 116 pregnancies in 75 women with type 1 diabetes[65] found that miscarriages were significantly more likely to occur when HbA_1 was 12% or more ($P < 0.05$). [EL = 2++]

Other neonatal outcomes

A cohort study of 1218 pregnancies in 990 women[66] considered the effect of glycaemic control at different times before and during pregnancy on adverse outcomes (perinatal death and/or congenital malformation). The median HbA_{1c} 0–3 months before conception was 8.0 (interquartile range 7.3–9.1) in the adverse outcome group compared with 7.6 (6.8–8.5) in the other group ($P = 0.005$). Women in the adverse outcome group were also less likely to have preconception guidance (42% versus 59%, $P = 0.002$) and to measure glucose daily at conception (23% versus 35%, $P = 0.019$). [EL = 2++]

A cohort study of 83 women[59] included 63 women with type 1 diabetes and 20 with type 2 diabetes. This study considered miscarriages and congenital malformation together and calculated predictive values for adverse outcome as follows: HbA_{1c} more than 7.5%, sensitivity 100%, specificity 14%, PPV 0.41, NPV 1; HbA_{1c} more than 9.5%, sensitivity 97%, specificity 82%, PPV 0.74, NPV 0.89; HbA_{1c} more than 13.5%, sensitivity 55%, specificity 94%, PPV 0.85, NPV 0.77; HbA_{1c} more than 15.5%, PPV 1. The normal non-diabetic HbA_{1c} level was 5.1% (1.1%). [EL = 2++]

A study of 57 births in women with type 1 diabetes examined effect of glycaemic control at different times before and during pregnancy on birthweight.[67] Multiple regression found a correlation with HbA_{1c} at 0–12 weeks of gestation (multiple $r = 0.48$, $F = 0.00005$). [EL = 2+]

Maternal hypoglycaemia
Three studies were identified that reported maternal hypoglycaemia as an outcome.

A cohort study of 239 women with type 1 diabetes[51] compared 143 women who attended a pre-pregnancy clinic with 96 women managed over the same period who had not received pre-pregnancy care. The first-trimester mean HbA_{1c} was significantly lower in the preconception care group (8.4% versus 10.5%, $P < 0.0001$). Hypoglycaemia was significantly more common in women in the preconception care group (26.5% versus 8.3%, $\chi^2=11.1$, $P < 0.001$). One of the 12 women who had a baby with a malformation had experienced hypoglycaemia in the first 9 weeks of pregnancy. The other 45 women who had severe hypoglycaemia had no abnormal outcomes. [EL = 2++]

A cohort study of 84 pregnant women with type1 diabetes[68] recruited before 9 weeks of gestation found hypoglycaemia requiring third-party assistance occurred in 71% of women, with a peak incidence at 10–15 weeks. Consequences of maternal hypoglycaemia included several grand mal seizures, five episodes of cerebral oedema, two road traffic accidents and comminuted fracture of the tibia and fibula. Although all women in the study were undergoing intensive insulin therapy there was no association between hypoglycaemia and glycaemic control as measured by preprandial glucose, postprandial glucose or glycohaemoglobin concentrations. There was no association between hypoglycaemia and early pregnancy loss or major malformations in babies. [EL = 2++]

A cohort study of 84 women recruited prior to conception and 110 women referred at 6–8 weeks of gestation[36] found that at 2–8 weeks of gestation in the preconception group 42% recorded no hypoglycaemic episodes, 35% recorded one or two episodes per week and 23% experienced several episodes per week. One woman experienced loss of consciousness requiring a glucagon injection and intravenous glucose therapy in an emergency department. One other woman required second-party assistance by administration of juice in the home. [EL = 2++]

A UK RCT[69] evaluated a course teaching flexible intensive insulin treatment. The course provided skills to enable adults with type 1 diabetes to replace insulin by matching it to a desired carbohydrate intake on a meal-by-meal basis. The HbA_{1c} at 6 months in adults who attended a 5 day training course (immediate DAFNE group) was 8.4% as compared with 9.4% in those who received usual care for 6 months and then attended a training course (delayed DAFNE group). The impact of diabetes on 'freedom to eat as I wish' significantly improved in the immediate DAFNE group as compared with the delayed group. There was a significant improvement in general wellbeing and treatment satisfaction in the immediate DAFNE group but no difference in severe hypoglycaemia, weight or lipids. [EL = 1+]

Current practice
Fifty-eight percent (218/379) of women in the CEMACH diabetes in pregnancy enquiry were reported to have had a test of glycaemic control in the 12 months before pregnancy.[33] [EL 3–4] This compares with 37% of 3808 women with diabetes in the full cohort having had a test of glycaemic control in the 6 months before pregnancy. It is important to note that the data for these two groups of women were collected in different ways, namely, from review of the medical records and from questionnaires sent to health professionals involved in their care. Sixteen percent of the 379 women did not have a glycaemic control test in the year before pregnancy and for more than a quarter (27%, 101/379) of women there was no documentation available. There was evidence that targets for glycaemic control had been set before pregnancy for only 28% of 369 women. For 52% of women there was no documentation in the medical records about glycaemic control targets. It was assessed that 79% of 354 women with available documentation had sub-optimal glycaemic control before pregnancy. Women who had sub-optimal preconception glycaemic control were more likely to go on to have a poor pregnancy outcome (OR 3.89, 95% CI 2.15 to 7.02, adjusted for maternal age and deprivation). The main concerns of the enquiry panels were a lack of timely clinical input by heath professionals to improve glycaemic control and that insulin regimens advised were inadequate to achieve control.

The 2002 CEMACH enquiry found that of units expected to provide maternity care for women with diabetes in England, Wales and Northern Ireland, 91% (194/213) used HbA_{1c} to monitor glycaemic control, either alone or in combination with other tests, 6% (13/213) used HbA_1, and 1% (3/213) used fructosamine as the only test. Only 74% (158/213) of the units used an HbA_{1c} assay aligned with the Diabetes Control and Complications Trial (DCCT).[32] Of the women in the CEMACH descriptive study of 3808 diabetic pregnancies who had a HbA_{1c} measurement before conception, 28% had a value below 7%. [EL = 3]

Existing guidance

The NSF for diabetes[20] recommends 'Women should be encouraged and supported to monitor their blood glucose regularly, and to adjust their insulin dosage in order to maintain their blood glucose levels within the normal (non-diabetic) range. The aim should be for the woman to maintain her HbA_{1c} below 7.0%.'

Evidence statement

A large number of high-quality cohort studies have established an association between blood glucose control before conception and the incidence of miscarriage and congenital malformations. Threshold values for increased risk of miscarriage and congenital malformations are difficult to identify because of differences between studies in measures of glycosylated haemoglobin and the normal non-diabetic range. In general, the risk of miscarriage and congenital malformations increases as first-trimester HbA_{1c} increases above the normal range. There is a substantial increase in the incidence of miscarriages and congenital malformations in women whose first-trimester DCCT-aligned HbA_{1c} exceeds 10%.

From evidence to recommendations

Evidence shows that the risk of congenital malformations increases with increasing values of HbA_{1c} above the normal (non-diabetic) range. Therefore women are advised to aim to keep their HbA_{1c} within the normal non-diabetic range; where HbA_{1c} is aligned with the DCCT this is below 6.1%. Women should be reassured that any reduction in HbA_{1c} towards the target of 6.1% is likely to reduce the risk of congenital malformations.

Very high levels of HbA_{1c} (more than 10%) susbtantially increase the risk of adverse outcomes and it is the GDG's view that pregnancy should be avoided when DCCT-aligned HBA_{1c} exceeds 10%.

Good glycaemic control before conception puts the woman at an increased risk of hypoglycaemia, and women may be attempting to achieve optimal glycaemic control for several months until conception occurs. Targets for blood glucose monitoring should, therefore, be agreed with the individual taking into account the risk of hypoglycaemia.

Recommendations for target ranges for blood glucose in the preconception period

Individualised targets for self-monitoring of blood glucose should be agreed with women who have diabetes and are planning to become pregnant, taking into account the risk of hypoglycaemia.

If it is safely achievable, women with diabetes who are planning to become pregnant should aim to maintain their HbA_{1c} below 6.1%. Women should be reassured that any reduction in HbA_{1c} towards the target of 6.1% is likely to reduce the risk of congenital malformations.

Women with diabetes whose HbA_{1c} is above 10% should be strongly advised to avoid pregnancy.

There were no research recommendations relating to target ranges for blood glucose in the preconception period.

3.5 Monitoring blood glucose and ketones in the preconception period

Description of the evidence

No studies were identified that assessed how blood glucose or ketones should be monitored in the preconception period.

The DCCT compared intensive treatment with conventional treatment where intensive treatment was a package of care that included self-monitoring of blood glucose at least four times a day and a monthly measurement of HbA_{1c}.[70] The DCCT involved 1441 people with type 1 diabetes. The goal of intensive therapy was blood glucose concentrations as close to the non-diabetic range as possible. HbA$_{1c}$ was maintained at a significantly lower level in the intensive treatment group compared with the conventional treatment group ($P < 0.0001$). The mean ± SD value for all glucose profiles in the intensive therapy group was 8.6 ± 1.7 mmol/litre compared with 12.8 ± 3.1 mmol/litre in the conventional therapy group ($P < 0.001$). The study found intensive therapy delayed the onset of complications of diabetes and slowed their progression. [EL = 1++]

The DCCT protocol required that women in the conventional treatment group change to intensive therapy while attempting to become pregnant and during pregnancy. An ancillary study compared pregnancy outcomes in 94 women originally assigned to intensive treatment with 86 women originally assigned to conventional treatment.[49] All women originally assigned to conventional treatment were changed to intensive treatment during pregnancy; 26 changed before conception and 60 changed after conception. The mean HbA$_{1c}$ at conception in the intensive treatment group was 7.4% ± 1.3% compared with 8.1% ± 1.7% in the conventional treatment group ($P = 0.0001$). Nine congenital malformations were identified, eight of which were in the conventional treatment group ($P = 0.06$). [EL = 2++]

Evidence statement

No studies were identified on how to monitor blood glucose and ketones in the preconception period. An RCT found that a package of care that included self-monitoring of blood glucose at least four times a day and a monthly measurement of HbA$_{1c}$ improved blood glucose control in people with type 1 diabetes and reduced the progression of complications of diabetes. An ancillary study found that the incidence of congenital malformations in the babies of women with type 1 diabetes was also reduced.

No studies were identified on monitoring for ketones in the preconception period.

From evidence to recommendations

In the absence of direct evidence for the effectiveness of self-monitoring of blood glucose in the preconception period, an approach to blood glucose monitoring based on that included in the intensive treatment package from the DCCT is recommended (self-monitoring of blood glucose at least four times a day and a monthly measurement of HbA$_{1c}$).

Evidence of the effectiveness of self-management of blood glucose using meters supports the provision of meters (see Section 5.2). Therefore, women with insulin-treated diabetes should be offered meters to facilitate frequent monitoring alongside intensified insulin regimens, the aim being to avoid hypoglycaemia.

A mixture of pre- and postprandial testing will give a more accurate picture of the blood glucose profile than preprandial testing alone (see Sections 3.4, 5.1 and 5.2). The GDG's view is that the same monitoring regimen should be used in the preconception period and during pregnancy.

In pregnancy there is accelerated ketosis (see Section 5.3). In the absence of any evidence for the effectiveness of self-monitoring of ketones in the preconception period, the GDG's view is that recommendations should be based on best current practice. Therefore the GDG recommends that women should be advised in the use of ketone strips as part of preconception care.

Recommendations for monitoring blood glucose and ketones in the preconception period

Women with diabetes who are planning to become pregnant should be offered monthly measurement of HbA$_{1c}$.

Women with diabetes who are planning to become pregnant should be offered a meter for self-monitoring of blood glucose.

Women with diabetes who are planning to become pregnant and who require intensification of hypoglycaemic therapy should be advised to increase the frequency of self-monitoring of blood glucose to include fasting and a mixture of pre- and postprandial levels.

Women with type 1 diabetes who are planning to become pregnant should be offered ketone testing strips and advised to test for ketonuria or ketonaemia if they become hyperglycaemic or unwell.

There were no research recommendations relating to monitoring blood glucose and ketones in the preconception period.

3.6 The safety of medications for diabetes before and during pregnancy

The safety of diabetes medications (including oral hypoglycaemic agents and insulin preparations) for use during pregnancy is considered in this section. The effectiveness of insulin preparations and regimens (including continuous subcutaneous insulin infusion (CSII) pumps) is considered in Section 5.3).

Description of the evidence

Oral hypoglycaemic agents

Oral hypoglycaemic agents are used to maintain blood glucose control in people with type 2 diabetes. There are four main categories of oral hypoglycaemic agents: sulphonylureas (chlorpropamide, glibenclamide (also known as glyburide), gliclazide, glimepiride, glipizide, gliquidone and tolbutamide), biguanides (metformin), α-glucosidase inhibitors (acarbose) and thiazolidinediones (pioglitazone and rosiglitazone). Two other medications are used to stimulate insulin release (nateglinide and repaglinide). Each works in a different way and is suitable for different clinical situations.

A systematic review and meta-analysis examined the relationship between first-trimester exposure to oral hypoglycaemic agents and subsequent congenital abnormalities and neonatal mortality.[71] The review sought to account for the potential confounding effect of maternal glycaemic control. The meta-analysis included ten studies which reported on 471 women exposed to oral hypoglycaemic agents in the first trimester and 1344 women not exposed. There were three prospective cohort studies, three retrospective cohort studies, three case series and one case–control study. The oral hypoglycaemic agents used in the studies included chlorpropamide (eight studies), tolbutamide (six studies), glibenclamide (four studies), metformin (five studies) and phenformin (three studies). Six studies were rated as of 'poor' quality, two were 'fair' and two were 'good'. Most women in the studies had type 2 diabetes. Women with type 1 diabetes and gestational diabetes were also present in some studies. There was no significant difference in the rate of major malformations between those exposed to oral hypoglycaemic agents and those not exposed (10 studies, OR 1.05, 95% CI 0.65 to 1.70). [EL = 2++]

A further systematic review included seven additional studies that looked at the use of metformin in the first trimester of pregnancy.[72] All the studies were small observational studies, six in women with polycystic ovary syndrome and one in women with type 2 diabetes. There were no reports of birth defects, increased incidence of pre-eclampsia or other adverse maternal or neonatal outcomes. The use of metformin during pregnancy in women with polycystic ovary syndrome is associated with a reduction in miscarriage in early pregnancy, weight loss, a reduction in fasting serum insulin levels and in the incidence of gestational diabetes. [EL = 2+]

Another systematic review evaluated the safety of metformin in pregnancy for women with diabetes and polycystic ovary syndrome.[73] The review reported that metformin use during the first trimester of pregnancy was not associated with an increased risk of major malformations. [EL = 2+]

An RCT compared glibenclamide with insulin for the treatment of gestational diabetes.[74] The study involved 404 women with gestational diabetes. Approximately 83% were Hispanic, 12% were white and 5% were black. Women were randomly assigned between 11 and 33 weeks of gestation to receive either glibenclamide (*n* = 201) or insulin (*n* = 203). The mean blood glucose concentrations during treatment were 5.9 ± 0.9 mmol/litre in the glibenclamide group and 5.9 ± 1.0 mmol/litre in the insulin group (*P* = 0.99). Eight women (4%) in the glibenclamide group required insulin treatment. There were no significant differences between the glibenclamide and insulin groups in the percentage of babies who were LGA (12% versus 13%), macrosomic (7% versus 4%), had lung complications (8% versus 6%) or neonatal hypoglycaemia (9% versus 6%), were admitted to a NICU (6% versus 7%), or had fetal anomalies (2% and 2%). Cord-serum insulin concentrations were similar in the two groups and glibenclamide was not detected in the cord serum of any baby in the glibenclamide group. [EL = 1++]

An RCT of metformin for the treatment of gestational diabetes (the Metformin in Gestational Diabetes (MIG) trial) is due to report soon. A pilot study randomised 14 women to insulin and 16 to metformin. There were no differences in perinatal outcomes.[75] [EL = 1−]

A retrospective cohort study examined the effects of oral hypoglycaemic agents in 379 singleton pregnancies of women with type 2 diabetes.[76] The women were subdivided into: oral hypoglycaemic agents alone ($n = 93$ pregnancies); converted from oral hypoglycaemic agents to insulin ($n = 249$); and insulin alone or converted from diet alone to insulin ($n = 37$). The oral hypoglycaemic agents assessed were metformin and glibenclamide. Fetal anomaly rates were similar across the three groups, whereas perinatal mortality rates (per 1000 births) were higher in the group that used oral hypoglycaemic agents alone (125, $P = 0.003$). Conversion from oral hypoglycaemic agents to insulin was protective for perinatal mortality compared with oral hypoglycaemic agents alone (OR 0.220, 95% CI 0.061 to 0.756, $P = 0.024$). The data suggest that metformin and glibenclamide are not teratogenic. [EL = 2+]

A reference guide to drugs in pregnancy and lactation reported that there were limited data on the use of metformin, acarbose, nateglinide, glimepiride, glipizide and glibenclamide in pregnant women and suggested they present a low risk to the fetus. No data were found on the use of repaglinide or pioglitazone in pregnant women, but it was suggested that they present a moderate risk to the fetus. No comparative studies were found on the use of rosiglitazone in pregnant women, but it was suggested that it presents a risk to the fetus. Evidence suggested that chlorpropamide and tolbutamide present a risk to the fetus if taken by women in the third trimester of pregnancy. Gliclazide and gliquidone were not reviewed.[77] [EL = 3]

The reference guide reported that 14 small observational studies had investigated the use of metformin in pregnant women with diabetes. Metformin has been shown to cross the placenta. The observational studies identified congenital malformations in some babies of women taking metformin, but the rate was not compared with the expected rate of congenital malformations in babies born to women with diabetes who were not taking metformin. The reference guide suggested that use of metformin may decrease fetal and infant morbidity and mortality in developing countries where the proper use of insulin is problematic, but that insulin is still the treatment of choice.[77] [EL = 3]

The reference guide reported that three observational studies had investigated the use of acarbose in pregnant women with diabetes. The observational studies identified congenital malformations in some babies of women taking acarbose, and the rate was not compared with the expected rate of congenital malformations in babies born to women with diabetes who were not taking acarbose. The reference guide noted that high maternal blood glucose is associated with maternal and fetal effects, including congenital abnormalities, and that insulin is the treatment of choice to prevent hyperglycaemia.[77] [EL = 3]

The reference guide stated that one case report had investigated the use of nateglinide in a pregnant woman with diabetes. It is not known whether nateglinide can cross the placenta, and the reference guide suggested that it presents a low risk of developmental toxicity.[77] [EL = 3]

The reference guide reported that no studies had investigated the use of glimepiride in pregnant women. It is not known whether glimepiride can cross the placenta, but the reference guide suggested that it may present a risk of skeletal deformities, growth retardation and intrauterine death.[77] [EL = 3]

The reference guide reported that case reports had investigated the use of glipizide in pregnant women. Glipizide has been shown to cross the placenta. An observational study that looked at the incidence of congenital malformation in women with type 2 diabetes found no association between oral hypoglycaemic agents and organogenesis or congenital malformations.[77] [EL = 3]

The reference guide reported that several observational studies had investigated the use of glibenclamide in pregnant women. Small amounts of glibenclamide may cross the placenta. The observational studies suggested that use of glibenclamide may decrease fetal and infant morbidity and mortality in developing countries where the proper use of insulin is problematic, and the reference guide suggested that it may be an acceptable alternative to insulin for women with gestational diabetes.[77] [EL = 3]

The reference guide reported that no studies had investigated the use of repaglinide in pregnant women. It is not known whether repaglinide can cross the placenta, and the reference guide suggested that it may affect fetal growth.[77] [EL = 3]

The reference guide reported that no studies had investigated the use of pioglitazone in pregnant women. It is not known whether pioglitazone can cross the placenta, but the reference guide suggested that it may result in post-implantation losses, delayed development and reduced fetal weight.[77] [EL = 3]

The reference guide stated that one case report had investigated the use of rosiglitazone in a pregnant woman with diabetes. It is not known whether rosiglitazone can cross the placenta, but the reference guide suggested that it may present a risk of placental toxicity, fetal death and growth retardation.[77] [EL = 3]

The reference guide stated that case reports had investigated the use of chlorpropamide and tolbutamide in pregnant women with diabetes. Chlorpropamide and tolbutamide have been shown to cross the placenta. Out of 74 case reports identified, four babies of women who had taken chlorpropamide experienced prolonged, symptomatic neonatal hypoglycaemia and one baby experienced prolonged neonatal hypoglycaemia and seizures. Several case series looked at the incidence of congenital malformations and found that chlorpropamide did not appear to be related to congenital abnormalities in pregnant women. However, the reference guide suggested that insulin is still the treatment of choice. Ten case reports relating to tolbutamide use identified no increase in the rate of congenital abnormalities over and above that expected in women with diabetes, although another four case reports attributed congenital malformations to tolbutamide. One case of prolonged hypoglycaemia in a baby following maternal treatment with tolbutamide was identified.[77] [EL = 3]

The British National Formulary recommends that metformin, acarbose and repaglinide should be avoided during pregnancy and are normally substituted with insulin.[78] The manufacturers of nateglinide, pioglitazone and rosiglitazone advise pregnant women to avoid them, and insulin is normally substituted in women with diabetes. Sulphonylureas can lead to neonatal hypoglycaemia, and insulin is normally substituted in women with diabetes. If oral hypoglycaemic drugs are used then therapy should be stopped at least 2 days before birth.

There is information on the use of oral hypoglycaemic agents during breastfeeding in Section 8.1.

Insulin

Insulin has been shown to be compatible with pregnancy and is recommended as the drug of choice for pregnant women with diabetes.[77] [EL = 3]

Insulin analogues

Insulin analogues are synthetic insulins created by modifying the chemical structure of insulin to produce either faster acting preprandial insulin or longer acting basal insulin. The insulin analogues currently licensed for use in the UK are the rapid-acting analogues lispro, aspart and glulisine and the long-acting analogues detemir and glargine. No studies were identified in relation to the effectiveness and safety of insulin glulisine or insulin detemir in pregnancy, although some research is in progress.

Insulin aspart:
Insulin aspart is licensed for use in pregnancy.

An RCT compared 157 pregnant women with type 1 diabetes treated using insulin aspart with 165 pregnant women with type 1 diabetes treated using human insulin.[79] There were fewer episodes of nocturnal hypoglycaemia (RR 0.48, 95% CI 0.20 to 1.14, $P = 0.10$) and severe hypoglycaemia (RR 0.72, 95% CI 0.36 to 1.46, $P = 0.36$) in the aspart group. Prandial increments (mean: breakfast, lunch and dinner) were significantly lower with insulin aspart in the first and third trimester. No differences were observed in 24 hour mean plasma glucose profiles or HbA_{1c} values. Progression of retinopathy and perinatal complications were similar in both groups. [EL = 1++]

A small RCT randomised 27 women with gestational diabetes to either insulin aspart or human insulin.[80] The trial period extended from the diagnosis of gestational diabetes (18–28 weeks) to 6 weeks postpartum. There was no significant difference in mean reduction in HbA_{1c} over the trial period ($0.3 \pm 0.5\%$ for the insulin aspart group versus $0.1 \pm 0.4\%$ for human insulin). The safety profile for both groups was similar. [EL = 1+]

An observational study compared ten pregnant women with type 1 diabetes treated using insulin aspart with ten pregnant women treated using human insulin.[81] Groups did not differ in terms of age, weight, duration of diabetes or gestational age at the time of booking. HbA_{1c} was lower in the insulin aspart group at booking ($7.0 \pm 1.0\%$ versus $8.6 \pm 1.0\%$, $P < 0.05$), throughout pregnancy and at birth ($5.8 \pm 0.8\%$ versus $6.7 \pm 0.7\%$, $P < 0.05$). FBG values (4.3 ± 1.4 versus 5.4 ± 2.0 mmol/litre, $P < 0.01$) and pre-lunch blood glucose values (4.5 ± 1.7 versus 5.1 ± 2.3 mmol/litre, $P < 0.01$) were lower with insulin aspart. There was no significant difference in birthweight between the insulin aspart and human insulin groups (3.4 ± 0.5 kg versus 3.89 ± 0.7 kg, $P = 0.13$). [EL = 2+]

A pilot study randomised five women with gestational diabetes to receive insulin aspart and five women to receive human insulin.[82] There was no difference between the two groups in mean plasma glucose level, insulin dose or mean birthweight. There were no adverse maternal or fetal outcomes in either group. [EL = 1+]

Insulin lispro:
An *in vitro* perfusion study of the transfer of insulin lispro across the placenta found no transfer at or below a maternal concentration of 200 microU/ml (corresponding to 26 units of insulin).[83] A small placental transfer was observed at maternal concentration of 580 microU/ml (75 units) and 1000 microU/ml (130 units) when maintained for 60 minutes (this duration does not occur in the clinical setting due to the short elimination half-life of insulin lispro). [EL = 3]

A systematic review summarised 42 RCTs that compared rapid-acting insulin analogues (lispro and aspart) with regular insulin in 7933 people (including pregnant women) with type 1 diabetes, type 2 diabetes and gestational diabetes.[84] The review showed no differences between treatments in pregnant women with type 1 diabetes, women with gestational diabetes, or people with type 2 diabetes. One study included in the review assessed pregnant women with type 1 diabetes and found the reduction in HbA_{1c} levels to be similar with rapid-acting insulin analogues and regular insulin. However, biochemical hypoglycaemia was significantly more frequent in women who used insulin analogue compared with those who used regular insulin ($P < 0.05$). One study that assessed women with gestational diabetes found the total number of hypoglycaemic events did not differ between the groups. Twenty studies involving women with type 1 diabetes assessed post-treatment HbA_{1c} levels and found weighted mean difference of HbA_{1c} values to be -0.12% (95% CI -0.17% to -0.07%) in favour of rapid-acting insulin analogues compared with regular insulin. One study involving young women with type 1 diabetes did not show any significant reduction in HbA_{1c} levels between rapid-acting insulin analogues compared with regular insulin. [EL = 1++]

An RCT that was included in the systematic review provided additional data not reported by the systematic review.[85] In this study 24 women with gestational diabetes treated using insulin lispro were compared with 24 women treated using regular human insulin and 50 women with normal glucose challenge test (GCT). The 1 hour postprandial blood glucose values were significantly higher in the regular group than in the lispro or control groups. The rate of babies with a cranial : thoracic circumference ratio between the 10th and the 25th percentile was significantly higher in the group treated using regular insulin compared with the lispro and control groups. There were no other differences between the three groups in neonatal outcomes. [EL = 1+]

An open RCT involving 33 women with type 1 diabetes assessed the effectiveness and safety of preprandial administration of insulin lispro and regular rapid-acting insulin.[86] Blood glucose was determined six times daily and HbA_{1c} every 4 weeks. Blood glucose was significantly lower ($P < 0.01$) after breakfast in the insulin lispro group, while there were no significant differences between the treatment groups in terms of glycaemic control during the rest of the day. Biochemical hypoglycaemia (blood glucose less than 3.0 mmol/litre) was more frequent in the insulin lispro than in the regular insulin group (5.5% versus 3.9%, respectively). HbA_{1c} values declined during the study period and were similar in both groups. Retinopathy progressed in both groups; one woman in the regular insulin group developed proliferative retinopathy. There was no perinatal mortality in either group. The study suggests that it is possible to achieve at least as adequate glycaemic control with lispro as with regular insulin therapy in pregnant women with type 1 diabetes. [EL = 1+]

An earlier systematic review[87] was found on the use of insulin lispro in pregnancy. The review included an RCT of 42 women with insulin-requiring gestational diabetes randomly allocated to either insulin lispro or regular insulin. The aim of the study was to investigate whether insulin lispro crosses the placenta. No insulin lispro was detected in umbilical cord blood and there was no difference between the two groups in insulin antibodies. The women receiving insulin lispro had significantly lower glucose excursions after a test meal and experienced fewer episodes of hypoglycaemia before breakfast. They also experienced fewer hyperglycaemic episodes. There was no difference in obstetric or fetal outcomes. [EL = 1+]

The review also included 12 observational studies involving 303 women (294 with type 1 diabetes, nine with type 2 diabetes). There were seven congenital malformations in 170 women (4.1%) with pre-existing type 1 or type 2 diabetes who had been exposed to insulin lispro during embryogenesis. In comparison there were 14 congenital malformations in 133 (10.5%) women treated using regular insulin. Three observational studies reported improved glycaemic control in pregnant women using insulin lispro compared with pregnant women using regular insulin. Two of these studies also reported fewer maternal hypoglycaemic episodes and one study reported greater maternal satisfaction with insulin lispro compared with regular insulin. One study reported the development of proliferative retinopathy in three women without background retinopathy at the beginning of pregnancy. However, other risk factors for progression of retinopathy were present. Nonetheless the development of proliferative retinopathy in people with no retinopathy is rare, although it has been observed in association with rapid and substantial improvement in glycaemic control. There is no theoretical basis for an increased risk of retinopathy with insulin lispro apart from facilitating rapid and/or substantial improvement in glycaemic control.[88] No other cases of progression of retinopathy in association with insulin lispro have been reported. [EL = 2++]

An open RCT involving 33 women with type 1 diabetes assessed the effectiveness and safety of preprandial administration of insulin lispro and regular rapid-acting insulin.[86] Blood glucose was determined six times daily and HbA_{1c} every 4 weeks. Blood glucose was significantly lower ($P < 0.01$) after breakfast in the lispro group, while there were no significant differences between the treatment groups in terms of glycaemic control during the rest of the day. Biochemical hypoglycaemia (blood glucose less than 3.0 mmol/litre) was more frequent in the insulin lispro group than in the regular insulin group (5.5% versus 3.9%, respectively). HbA_{1c} values declined during the study period and were similar in both groups. Retinopathy progressed in both groups; one woman in the regular insulin group developed proliferative retinopathy. There was no perinatal mortality in either group. The study suggests that it is possible to achieve at least as adequate glycaemic control with lispro as with regular insulin therapy in pregnant women with type 1 diabetes. [EL = 1+]

Four case series of women with type 1 diabetes exposed to insulin lispro in pregnancy ($n = 696$) were published since the systematic review.[89–92] These studies found that insulin lispro improved glycaemic control with no adverse maternal or fetal effects. [EL = 3]

Insulin glargine:
An observational study of the use of glargine in 22 centres in the UK reported outcomes from 122 babies in 127 pregnancies.[93] One hundred and fifteen women had type 1 diabetes, five had type 2 diabetes and seven had gestational diabetes. HbA_{1c} fell from 8.1 ± 0.2% at booking to 6.7 ± 0.1% during the third trimester. Background retinopathy developed in one woman, progressed in three women and laser photocoagulation was required in seven women. Hypoglycaemia requiring assistance occurred in nine (7%) and 16 (12%) had two or more episodes of hypoglycaemia. There were seven (6%) early miscarriages. All 122 babies were liveborn. There were three congenital malformations (positional talipes, ventricular septal defect and transposition of the great arteries (TGA)), two occurring in women taking glargine before pregnancy giving a congenital malformation rate of 2.5%. [EL = 3]

An observational study compared maternal and perinatal outcomes in 47 women with type 1 diabetes taking glargine before pregnancy to 50 women using long-acting insulin (protaphan).[94] Groups were matched for age, parity, duration of diabetes and diabetic complications. There was no difference in outcomes (gestational age at birth, pregnancy complications, neonatal birthweight, shoulder dystocia or respiratory distress). The decrease in HbA_{1c} between the first and third trimester was greater in the glargine group ($P = 0.04$) and there was a tendency towards fewer hypoglycaemic episodes (11/47 in glargine group versus 21/50 in protaphan group, $P = 0.07$). [EL = 2+]

A matched case–control study involving 64 pregnant women with diabetes investigated the association between insulin glargine use during pregnancy and incidence of fetal macrosomia or adverse neonatal outcomes.[95] There was no significant difference between the birthweight or centile birthweight of babies born to the women treated using insulin glargine and those born to the control group treated using intermediate-acting human insulin. Incidence of fetal macrosomia was 37.5% (12/32) in the insulin glargine group and 40.6% (13/32) in the control group. There was no significant difference in neonatal morbidity between the groups. The evidence suggests insulin glargine treatment during pregnancy does not appear to be associated with increased fetal macrosomia or neonatal morbidity. [EL = 2+]

Four case series (26 women with type 1 diabetes, four women with gestational diabetes) and two case reports (both in women with type 1 diabetes) found no adverse maternal or fetal outcomes associated with the use of glargine in pregnancy.[87,96–101] [EL = 3]

Existing guidance

The NSF for diabetes[20] recommends that women with type 2 diabetes who require treatment with oral hypoglycaemic agents to achieve good blood glucose control and who are planning to become pregnant or are already pregnant should be transferred to insulin therapy because of the theoretical risk associated with these drugs crossing the placenta.

Evidence statement

A laboratory study using validated methodology found glibenclamide did not cross the placenta. No high-quality studies have considered the use of oral hypoglycaemic agents in the first 7 weeks of pregnancy, i.e. during the period of organogenesis, although a meta-analysis of observational studies found no increased risk of congenital malformations.

Metformin crosses the placenta; however, a large number of observational studies of its use during pregnancy have found no teratogenic effect.

An RCT has found glibenclamide to be an effective alternative to insulin for the treatment of gestational diabetes.

Insulin aspart is licensed for use during pregnancy. A large number of studies have shown no indication that insulin lispro is teratogenic. There have been no clinical trials of glulisine, glargine or detemir in pregnancy.

From evidence to recommendations

Oral hypoglycaemic agents have a number of potential advantages over insulin for the treatment of type 2 diabetes during pregnancy and for the treatment of gestational diabetes. They are more convenient and less expensive than insulin and may improve the long-term prognosis of women with type 2 diabetes and gestational diabetes. The safety record of glibenclamide and metformin is sufficient for well-designed RCTs to be conducted on its use in early pregnancy. These studies are needed before they can be recommended for use in early pregnancy. Until this evidence is available the risks and benefits of metformin during pregnancy, including the risk of hypoglycaemia, should be weighed on an individual basis, promoting the principle of informed choice.

For some women insulin analogues may offer benefits over isophane insulin (also known as NPH insulin) in terms of flexibility and improved glycaemic control. Insulin aspart is licensed for use in pregnancy. Until sufficiently powered RCTs of insulin lispro in pregnancy have confirmed its safety and effectiveness, the risks and benefits of insulin lispro, including the risk of hypoglycaemia, should be weighed on an individual basis, promoting the principle of informed choice.

The use of other rapid- and long-acting insulin analogues (glulisine, detemir and glargine) during pregnancy should be avoided until more data are available on their safety.

Recommendations for the safety of medications for diabetes before and during pregnancy

Women with diabetes may be advised to use metformin* as an adjunct or alternative to insulin in the preconception period and during pregnancy, when the likely benefits from improved glycaemic control outweigh the potential for harm. All other oral hypoglycaemic agents should be discontinued before pregnancy and insulin substituted.

Healthcare professionals should be aware that the rapid-acting insulin analogues (aspart and lispro*) are safe to use during pregnancy.

Women with insulin-treated diabetes who are planning to become pregnant should be informed that there is insufficient evidence about the use of long-acting insulin analogues during pregnancy. Therefore isophane insulin* (also known as NPH insulin) remains the first choice for long-acting insulin during pregnancy.

There were no research recommendations relating to which medications for diabetes are safe for use during pregnancy and which should be discontinued.

3.7 The safety of medications for diabetic complications before and during pregnancy

Description of the evidence

Angiotensin-converting enzyme inhibitors
In people with diabetes, ACE inhibitors are used to treat hypertension and slow the progression of nephropathy.[102]

Two case series were identified that reported on the use of ACE inhibitors in women with diabetes and nephropathy who were planning a pregnancy and who discontinued treatment on confirmation of pregnancy.

Three cohort studies and two case series were identified that considered the maternal, fetal and neonatal effects of first-trimester exposure to ACE inhibitors.

Angiotensin-converting enzyme inhibitors before pregnancy:
In eight women with diabetic nephropathy[103] ACE inhibitors were used for a minimum of 6 months prior to conception. Women attempted conception when proteinuria was less than 500 mg/day and euglycaemia was achieved. At conception ACE inhibitors were discontinued. Before ACE inhibitor treatment proteinuria was 1633 ± 666 mg/day. At conception it was 273 ± 146 mg/day ($P < 0.0001$). Proteinuria increased gradually over each trimester to 593 ± 515, 783 ± 813 and 1000 ± 1185 mg/day, respectively ($P = 0.2$ between trimesters). Three months after birth proteinuria was 619 ± 411 mg/day. In two women (25%), proteinuria exceeded 1000 mg/day during pregnancy. There was no significant change in any other renal function test (creatinine clearance test, serum creatinine, uric acid, potassium). Women remained euglycaemic throughout pregnancy. There were three cases of pre-eclamptic toxaemia (PET) just prior to birth, which resolved immediately following birth. There were two LGA babies without complications. There were no other adverse maternal or neonatal outcomes. [EL = 3]

In a case series of 24 women with diabetic nephropathy and normal to mild renal impairment[104] all women received ACE inhibitors for at least 6 months prior to conception and maintained strict glycaemic control from at least 3 months prior to conception. Proteinuria was 1292 ± 656 mg/day before treatment, 202 ± 141 mg/day at conception ($P = 0.001$), 650 ± 502 mg/day in the first and second trimesters, 1012 ± 1206 mg/day in the third trimester and 590 ± 410 mg/day 6–8 weeks after birth. Mean serum creatinine and uric acid levels increased significantly in the first and third trimesters. Creatinine clearance and potassium remained stable. All women maintained blood glucose levels near to normal throughout pregnancy. There were 11/24 cases (46%) of superimposed

---

* This drug does not have UK marketing authorisation specifically for pregnant and breastfeeding women at the time of publication (March 2008). Informed consent should be obtained and documented.

pre-eclampsia, 4/24 cases (17%) of preterm birth and 5/24 cases (21%) of intrauterine growth restriction (IUGR). The rate of caesarean section was 62.5%. There was one intrauterine death at 24 weeks of gestation secondary to early severe IUGR. One baby was admitted to intensive care because of prematurity. No deterioration was observed in any of the women at 2 year follow-up. Two babies had cerebral palsy due to birth trauma secondary to LGA. [EL = 3]

ACE inhibitors in the first trimester:
A cohort study[105] included 29 507 babies, 209 of whom had been exposed to ACE inhibitors in the first trimester alone and 202 of whom had been exposed to other antihypertensive medication in the first trimester. Babies of women with diabetes, or who were exposed to ACE inhibitors after the first trimester, or who were exposed to any other potential teratogens, were excluded. Maternal use of prescribed medications was determined from pharmacy files, which included the date when the prescription was filled and the number of days for which the medicine was supplied. Major congenital malformations were identified from medical records. Babies with first-trimester-only exposure to ACE inhibitors had an increased risk of major congenital malformations (RR 2.71, 95% CI 1.72 to 4.27) as compared with babies who had no exposure to antihypertensive medications. In contrast, exposure to other antihypertensive medications during only the first trimester did not confer an increased risk (RR 0.66, 95% CI 0.25 to 1.75). [EL = 2+]

A second cohort study which assessed ACE inhibitor use before pregnancy and in early pregnancy assessed adverse pregnancy outcomes in 18 women and 19 pregnancies.[106] No congenital abnormalities or neonatal renal dysfunction were reported. Even in the six pregnancies in which ACE inhibitors were continued beyond 12 weeks of gestation (including one where therapy was continued until 25 weeks of gestation) there were no congenital abnormalities. [EL = 2++]

A third cohort study assessed the effect of prescription of ACE inhibitors at 5–15 weeks of gestation in 21 pregnant women in terms of adverse pregnancy outcomes.[107] There were no stillbirths or congenital malformations among the 21 babies. [EL = 2++]

A report of post-marketing surveillance for ACE inhibitors[108] reported outcomes of pregnancy in 66 women who self-enrolled to the registry after first-trimester-only exposure. There were 48 live births and 15 miscarriages (23%). Among the 48 live births there were three cases of IUGR. Another child had a patent ductus arteriosus that required surgical ligation at 18 months. Other known risk factors were present in the three cases of IUGR (i.e. multiple gestation or hypertension). [EL = 3]

A prospective case series[109] reported outcomes for eight women treated using ACE inhibitors in the first trimester. There were no major malformations. There were two cases of IUGR, one of which ended in an intrauterine death. This was attributed to severe disease in the mother rather than drug effect. [EL = 3]

A reference guide to drugs in pregnancy and lactation reported that data from studies involving pregnant women suggest a risk to the fetus if the ACE inhibitors enalapril, lisinopril, moexipril, perindopril, quinapril and trandolapril are used in the second or third trimesters of pregnancy. There was no information about captopril, cilazapril, fosinopril, imidapril or ramipril.[77] [EL = 3]

The British National Formulary recommends that ACE inhibitors should be avoided during pregnancy as they may adversely affect fetal and neonatal blood pressure control and renal function and they may cause skull defects and oligohydramnios.[78]

There is information on the use of ACE inhibitors during breastfeeding in Section 8.1.

Angiotensin-II receptor blockers
A reference guide to drugs in pregnancy and lactation reported that data from studies involving pregnant women suggest a risk to the fetus if ARBs are used in the second or third trimesters of pregnancy.[77] [EL = 3]

The British National Formulary recommends that ARBs should be avoided during pregnancy as they may adversely affect fetal and neonatal blood pressure control and renal function; they may also cause skull defects and oligohydramnios.[78]

There is information on the use of ARBs during breastfeeding in Section 8.1.

Statins

Statins (HMG CoA reductase inhibitors) are used to reduce elevated levels of cholesterol. Statins currently licensed for use in the UK include atorvastatin, fluvastatin, pravastatin, rosuvastatin and simvastatin.

A reference guide to drugs in pregnancy and lactation reported that atorvastatin, fluvastatin, pravastatin and simvastatin are contraindicated in pregnancy and lactation.[77] [EL = 3]

The reference guide reported that a small number of case reports and surveillance studies and a case series had investigated the use of atorvastatin, fluvastatin, pravastatin and simvastatin in pregnant women. The case series evaluated 20 cases of malformation in 54 cases of statin exposure reported to the US Food and Drug Administration between 1987 and 2001. The malformations included five major defects of the central nervous system (including two cases of holoprosencephaly) and five unilateral limb deficiencies. There was no review for rosuvastatin. [EL = 3]

The British National Formulary recommends that statins should be avoided during pregnancy as congenital malformations have been reported and decreased synthesis of cholesterol may affect fetal development.[78]

There is information on the use of statins during breastfeeding in Section 8.1.

Calcium-channel blockers

A cohort study examined the potential teratogenicity of calcium-channel blockers.[110] Six teratogen information services prospectively collected and followed up 78 women with first-trimester exposure to calcium-channel blockers. Pregnancy outcome was compared with that of a control group matched for maternal age and smoking habits. There was no increase in major malformation rates (calcium-channel blockers 3.0% (2/66); nonteratogenic controls 0%; $P = 0.27$). The defects reported were attributable to maternal diabetes or co-ingestion of teratogens. The increase in preterm birth (calcium-channel blockers 28%, nonteratogenic controls 9%, $P = 0.003$), attributed to maternal disease by stepwise regression, was the most important factor responsible for the observed decrease in birthweight (mean −334 g versus nonteratogenic controls, $P = 0.08$). This study suggests that calcium-channel blockers do not represent a major teratogenic risk. [EL = 2++]

Another cohort study investigated the effect of verapamil infused intravenously after plasma volume expansion with dextran-70 in nine women with severe gestational proteinuric hypertension.[111] The haemodynamic response in the women and adverse fetal effects were monitored. Verapamil produced a statistically significant reduction in mean arterial pressure and systemic vascular resistance without adversely affecting cardiac output. The decrease in blood pressure was smooth and controlled and was associated with an insignificant increase in heart rate. There were no adverse fetal effects, as evidenced by cardiotocographic monitoring. The apparent effectiveness of verapamil in this study justifies further investigation. [EL = 2+]

A reference guide to drugs in pregnancy and lactation reported that there were limited data for the use of diltiazem in pregnant women, and suggested that it presents a high risk to the fetus. There were no studies investigating the use of amlodipine or nisoldipine in pregnant women, and the reference guide suggested that these present a moderate risk to the fetus. There were limited data for the use of felodipine, nicardipine or nimodipine in pregnant women, and the reference guide suggested that they present a risk to the fetus. There were limited data for the use of isradipine in pregnant women and the reference guide suggested that it presents a low risk to the fetus. There were limited data for the use of nifedipine in pregnant women, and the reference guide suggested that it presents a low risk to the fetus. The reference guide suggested that verapamil is compatible with pregnancy. There was no review of lacidipine or lercanidipine.[77] [EL = 3]

The British National Formulary suggests that the calcium-channel blocker verapamil may reduce uterine blood flow leading to fetal hypoxia and that it may inhibit labour; the manufacturer advises women to avoid it in the first trimester of pregnancy unless absolutely necessary.[78] Amlodipine and nimodipine have no information available about possible harms; the manufacturers advise pregnant women to avoid them, but the risk to the fetus should be balanced against the risk of uncontrolled maternal hypertension. Isradipine, nifedipine and nicardipine may inhibit labour; the manufacturers advise pregnant women to avoid them, but the risk to the fetus should be balanced against the risk of uncontrolled maternal hypertension. Felodipine may inhibit labour and pregnant women are advised to avoid it. Nisoldipine should be avoided by pregnant women. Lacidipine may inhibit labour; the manufacturer advises pregnant women to avoid it. Lercanidipine and diltiazem have no information available; the manufacturer advises pregnant women to avoid them.

There is information on the use of calcium-channel blockers during breastfeeding in Section 8.1.

Obesity drugs
A reference guide to drugs in pregnancy and lactation reported that there were no data for the use of orlistat (a lipase inhibitor) or sibutramine (a centrally acting appetite suppressant) in pregnant women, and it suggested that they present a low risk to the fetus. There was no review for rimonabant, another centrally acting appetite suppressant.[77] [EL = 3]

The British National Formulary reports that the manufacturers of orlistat advise that it should be used with caution during pregnancy. The manufacturers of sibutramine and rimonabant recommend that they should be avoided in pregnancy.[78]

There is information on the use of obesity drugs during breastfeeding in Section 8.1.

Evidence statement

Two small case series reported on the use of ACE inhibitors until conception in women with diabetic nephropathy. Renal function did not appear to deteriorate during pregnancy. There was no evidence of teratogenic effect and evidence of moderate-to-good pregnancy outcomes associated with the use of ACE inhibitors.

Two small case series reporting on the use of ACE inhibitors in the first trimester of pregnancy did not detect a teratogenic effect. However a large, well-controlled cohort study that linked pregnancy outcomes to prescription records found that babies with first-trimester-only exposure to ACE inhibitors had an increased risk of major congenital malformations compared with babies who had no exposure to antihypertensive medications.

No clinical evidence was identified in relation to the safety of ARBs or statins in pregnancy. The British National Formulary recommends that ARBs and statins should be avoided during pregnancy.

Two small cohort studies suggest that calcium-channel blockers do not have a teratogenic effect, but no large-scale trials of their effectiveness and safety in pregnancy were identified. The British National Formulary recommends that they should be avoided in pregnancy.

No clinical evidence was identified in relation to the safety of obesity drugs in pregnancy. The British National Formulary recommends that orlistat should be used with caution in pregnancy and that other drugs for the treatment of obesity should be avoided.

From evidence to recommendations

ACE inhibitors and ARBs (angiotensin-II receptor antagonists) should be avoided throughout pregnancy because of the possible risk of congenital malformations. However, the benefits of continuing with ACE inhibitors until discontinuation of contraception for the purposes of protecting renal function should be considered. For women with microalbuminuria, the risk of progression to macroalbuminuria in the preconception period is thought to be small while the risk of pre-eclampsia is greatly increased.

Calcium-channel blockers should be avoided throughout pregnancy because of the risk of disruption to labour and fetal hypoxia. However, the risk to the fetus should be balanced against the risk of uncontrolled maternal hypertension in deciding whether to discontinue nifedipene.

As cholesterol and products synthesised during pregnancy are important to fetal development and as there is no apparent harm from interrupting cholesterol-lowering therapy during pregnancy,[77] statins should be avoided during pregnancy. [EL = 3]

Recommendations for the safety of medications for diabetic complications before and during pregnancy

Angiotensin-converting enzyme inhibitors and angiotensin-II receptor antagonists should be discontinued before conception or as soon as pregnancy is confirmed. Alternative antihypertensive agents suitable for use during pregnancy should be substituted.

Statins should be discontinued before pregnancy or as soon as pregnancy is confirmed.

There were no research recommendations relating to which medications for diabetic complications are safe for use during pregnancy and which should be discontinued.

3.8 Removing barriers to the uptake of preconception care and when to offer information

Preconception care is aimed at reducing congenital abnormalities by improving maternal glycaemic control before conception and during the first 7 weeks of pregnancy. 'Preconception care', 'preconception counselling' and 'preconception clinic' are often used interchangeably but most definitions include the following components:

- information and education for the woman and her partner
- support in improving glucose control before pregnancy through intensified insulin regimens, dietary advice and glucose monitoring
- preparation for pregnancy, including supplementation with folic acid; medication review; and assessment and treatment (if necessary) of diabetic complications.

Description of the evidence

A CEMACH audit from England, Wales and Northern Ireland and four studies undertaken in the USA were found that looked at the factors influencing uptake of preconception care in women with diabetes.

A CEMACH audit of pregnancy in women with pre-existing diabetes in England, Wales and Northern Ireland ($n = 3808$) found that only 35% of women received preconception counselling. Of these, 68% received counselling at the adult diabetes clinic, 13% at a preconception clinic and 4% from the GP (the service providing the counselling was not known for 15% of women). Folic acid was taken by 39% of women and 37% were reported as having a measure of long-term glycaemic control in the 6 months prior to pregnancy. Women with type 2 diabetes and women from a minority ethnic group were significantly less likely to have had a measure of long-term glycaemic control ($P < 0.001$).[2] [EL = 3]

A 2002 audit of units expected to provide maternity care for women with diabetes in England, Wales and Northern Ireland reported that there was no formal arrangement for preconception counselling in 16% of units; in 49% there was advice within the general diabetes clinic only; 17% of units had separate preconception clinics; the remaining units had other arrangements, advice within the general diabetes clinic and by an obstetrician within obstetric services, or advice by an obstetrician within the obstetric services only.[32] [EL = 3]

A population-based study recruited 85/122 (70%) women with diabetes who gave birth at 15 participating hospitals over 12 consecutive months.[112] Nonparticipants included women excluded from the study due to adverse pregnancy outcome. Study methods included: a review of medical records (for HbA_{1c} on entry to preconception care); a self-administered questionnaire (for information on demographics, access to health care, contraceptive behaviour and including the Marital Satisfaction Scale and the Health Locus of Control scale); and interviews (for responses on a range of topics potentially related to pregnancy planning behaviour). A planned pregnancy was defined as a pregnancy that was desired before conception, in which contraception was stopped or avoided for the purposes of becoming pregnant, and in which the woman stated that she attempted to achieve optimal blood glucose control before becoming pregnant. All other pregnancies were defined as unplanned. By this definition 41% (35/85) of pregnancies were planned. The results were as follows. [EL = 2+]

Background characteristics
The average SD above the laboratory mean for glycohaemoglobin at the first antenatal visit was significantly lower in planned than unplanned pregnancies (3.1 versus 5.8, $P = 0.004$). Women with planned pregnancies had significantly higher income ($P < 0.0001$), more education ($P = 0.05$), were more likely to be white ($P = 0.007$), to have private health insurance ($P < 0.001$), to have attended for diabetes care in the 6 months before conception ($P = 0.003$) and were less likely to smoke ($P < 0.001$).

Contraceptive behaviour and desire for motherhood
Among the 50 women with unplanned pregnancies, 70% (35) used contraception less than half the time. (There were five women who thought that diabetes made it more difficult to conceive). Seventy percent (35/50) of women with unplanned pregnancies said they were very happy when they found out they were pregnant.

Relationship with partner
Women with planned pregnancies were more satisfied with their relationship with their partner than were women with unplanned pregnancies. Logistic regression found a significant association between Marital Adjustment Scale score and pregnancy planning (OR 3.86, $P = 0.0002$). In the planned pregnancy group, 80% (28/35) of women believed that their partners were well informed about diabetes and pregnancy issues before the pregnancy. Many couples had attended appointments together and almost all women expressed a feeling of being supported. In contrast 16% (8/50) of women with unplanned pregnancies felt their partners were informed about diabetes and pregnancy before the pregnancy and most 'felt that their partners did not understand the enormity of effort required to achieve good diabetes control'.

Knowledge
Nearly all women with planned pregnancies (33/35, 94%) and 68% (34/50) of women with unplanned pregnancies knew they should be in good diabetes control before pregnancy. However, women with planned pregnancies were more likely to understand the specific association between high blood glucose levels and birth defects (83% versus 30%). Eight women with unplanned pregnancies could not recall hearing any information before pregnancy about diabetes and pregnancy. In women with unplanned pregnancies, 56% (28/50) had a previous pregnancy with diabetes. In the women with planned pregnancies, 49% (17/35) had a previous pregnancy with diabetes.

Personality
Women with unplanned pregnancies were significantly more likely to have an external locus of control (i.e. to attribute their health outcomes to the control of powerful others) than were women with planned pregnancies (OR 2.28, $P < 0.004$). There was no association between pregnancy planning and internal locus of control (the belief that health outcomes are largely under one's own control) or chance locus of control (the belief that health is due to luck or fate).

Advice from healthcare provider
Among women with planned pregnancies, 75% (26/35) felt they had received reassuring and encouraging advice from their providers before pregnancy. In contrast, 14% (7/50) of women with unplanned pregnancies received reassuring advice. Among women with unplanned pregnancies, 38% (19/50) recalled that pregnancy was discouraged.

Relationship with healthcare provider
A positive relationship with their healthcare provider was described by 75% (25/35) of women with planned pregnancies compared with 28% (14/50) of women with unplanned pregnancies. Women who described a positive relationship 'felt it was important that their doctor understood the difficulty of living with diabetes and did not judge them on their blood glucose control'. [EL = 2+]

A multicentre case–control study[113] compared women with pre-existing diabetes making their first preconception visit ($n = 57$, 53 type 1 diabetes, four type 2 diabetes) with those making their first antenatal visit without having received preconception care ($n = 97$, 79 type 1 diabetes, 18 type 2 diabetes). In the antenatal group only 24% of pregnancies were planned. After logistic regression the following variables were associated with seeking preconception care: education (OR 4.81,

$P < 0.01$), living with partner (OR 11.25, $P < 0.01$), visited a diabetes clinic in the last year (OR 8.25, $P < 0.01$), encouraged by provider to receive preconception care (OR 3.39, $P < 0.02$) and adherence to diabetes regimen (OR 3.03, $P < 0.03$). All women in the study completed a validated questionnaire on knowledge, attitudes, beliefs and behaviours regarding diabetes in pregnancy. Women in the preconception care group were significantly more likely to perceive that preconception care conferred benefits to the woman and child and to report instrumental social support (i.e. social support that involved practical, tangible aid offered by another individual). However these items were not significant when entered into a logistic regression model. [EL = 2+]

A 5 year longitudinal study involved 66 women with type 1 diabetes and 207 women without diabetes.[114] All women with diabetes were at least 1 year post diagnosis. Women were classified as being in one of four stages of the maternal diabetes lifecycle: (1) prevention of unplanned pregnancies; (2) reproductive decision making; (3) commencement of intensive metabolic control; or (4) treatment continuation with pregnancy. The study used annual questionnaires and interviews to assess knowledge, attitudes, personality and social support. In the prevention of unplanned pregnancy stage 82% of women with diabetes and 88% of women without diabetes used contraception. Women with diabetes were more likely to use condoms ($P = 0.05$). Themes that emerged during interviews included the belief that oral contraceptives were unsafe for women with diabetes and that diabetes made it difficult to conceive. In the 5 years of the study there were 23 pregnancies in women with diabetes, 78% (17) of which were unplanned. In women without diabetes there were 33 pregnancies, 48% (16) of which were unplanned. Consistent use of contraception was significantly associated with higher levels of social support for contraception ($P < 0.05$) and positive attitudes towards contraception ($P < 0.05$). There was no significant association with knowledge of contraception, knowledge of diabetes, locus of control or self-esteem. [EL = 2+]

A cross-sectional study surveyed 55 women with pre-existing diabetes attending a preconception clinic.[115] HbA_{1c} levels were determined either before conception or during the first trimester. Values in the normal range (4–6%) were considered 'optimal', values between 6% and 8% were considered 'adequate' and values greater than 8% were considered 'sub-optimal'. All women were given a questionnaire on preconception education and control of glycaemia. Sixty percent (33/55) of women had sub-optimal control while only 11% (6) had values in the normal range. Women with prior poor outcome of pregnancy were significantly more likely to enter pregnancy with poor glycaemic control ($P = 0.02$). Logistic regression revealed that not being advised to achieve target glucose or HbA_{1c} values (questionnaire response) was associated with entering pregnancy with poor glycaemic control ($P = 0.02$). Overall 29 women stated that they had planned their pregnancies but only 12 (22%) saw a physician before conception to modify insulin intake or glycaemic control. [EL = 2+]

No comparable studies were found for the UK, although two studies were found in women without diabetes. An interview study using a semi-structured questionnaire included 88 pregnant women and 40 non-pregnant women.[116] Among the pregnant women 45 had a planned pregnancy and 43 had an unplanned pregnancy. Life events, difficulties, quality of relationships, self-esteem and the 'secondary gain' inherent in becoming pregnant were examined. Secondary gain was used to refer to advantage or benefit that may arise from becoming pregnant, for example by alleviating previous problems. Examples of secondary gain included autonomy from parents, solidification of an unstable relationship, an excuse to leave a boring job and/or begin a new and important phase in their lives. Women with unplanned pregnancies were significantly more likely to be rated as having a 'high' chance of secondary gain than women with planned pregnancies ($\chi^2 = 29.41$, $P < 0.0001$). The study also found that women with planned pregnancies were significantly more likely to have a partnership rated 'high' in overall quality ($\chi^2 = 7.10$, $P < 0.05$). The authors concluded that women with unplanned pregnancy may in fact fall into a group of 'semi-planned' pregnancy 'who are indifferent or at worst ambivalent about the idea of pregnancy'. [EL = 2+]

An interview study with 47 women without diabetes[117] found that, when discussing the circumstances of their pregnancies, women did not use the terms 'planned' or 'unplanned' spontaneously. When asked to apply the terms, women applied the term 'planned' only when four criteria were met. Intending to become pregnant and stopping contraception were not sufficient. Agreeing to the pregnancy with their partner and reaching the right time in terms of lifestyle or life stage were also necessary. The term 'unplanned' covered a wide variety of circumstances. [EL = 2+]

Young women
A case–control study[118] examined knowledge, attitudes, intentions and behaviours regarding diabetes and reproductive issues, sexual activity and birth control in young women with diabetes as well in those without diabetes. The study results showed that having diabetes did not appear to significantly decrease the risk-taking behaviour of the young women. [EL = 2–]

A descriptive qualitative study[119] examined whether young women with type 1 diabetes were aware and concerned about pregnancy-related complications and how to prevent them. The study showed that young women with diabetes lacked awareness of pregnancy-related complications associated with diabetes, of the term 'preconception counselling' and its role in preventing such complications, and of the importance for women with diabetes to use a highly effective method of contraception for preventing unplanned pregnancy. [EL = 3]

Current practice
A CEMACH survey of maternity units in England, Wales and Northern Ireland assessed the quality of maternity service provision against standards set out in the NSF for diabetes.[32] It found that in 2002 only 17% of maternity units provided a preconception clinic; this proportion had remained largely unchanged from 1994 (16%). [EL = 2+]

Further information about current practice in terms of preconception care and the importance of planning pregnancy is presented in Section 3.2.

Evidence statement

The following barriers to preconception care were identified.

Pregnancy planning
Most pregnancies in women with diabetes are unplanned. The evidence suggests that pregnancy planning should be considered a continuous rather than a dichotomous variable – only a minority of unplanned pregnancies are due to contraceptive failure. For example, one study found that the majority of women with unplanned pregnancy were not using contraception and said they were very happy when they found out they were pregnant. That some 'unplanned' pregnancies may not have been unexpected or unwanted, reflects 'conflicting or ambivalent emotions' towards motherhood[112] or an underlying desire to bring about change in other areas of life.

Sociocultural factors
Women with unplanned pregnancies are more likely to be from a lower socio-economic group or a minority ethnic group. This reflects complex social and cultural differences in knowledge, attitudes, motivation and support with regard to diabetes self-management and pregnancy planning. Nonetheless, in one study more than half of unplanned pregnancies were in white women with tertiary education.

Knowledge
Common misconceptions are that diabetes decreases fertility and that oral contraceptives have a detrimental effect on diabetes. One study found that 16% of women with an unplanned pregnancy could not recall hearing any information before pregnancy about diabetes and pregnancy. Knowledge of the effects of the benefits of good glycaemic control prior to pregnancy does not guarantee pregnancy planning. One study found nearly half of the women with unplanned pregnancy had a previous pregnancy with diabetes.

Relationship with healthcare professionals
Feeling judged and being discouraged from becoming pregnant is associated with unplanned pregnancy.

Social support
A lack of social support, in particular, an unsupportive partner, is associated with unplanned pregnancy.

Appropriateness and availability of services

Only a minority of maternity units provide a preconception clinic and services currently provided may not be effective in addressing the barriers to uptake of preconception care identified above. In particular, a service that is provided only after women indicate that they are planning to become pregnant will have limited uptake.

Young women

A case–control study and a qualitative study have investigated attitudes to pregnancy in young women with diabetes. Having diabetes did not reduce risk-taking behaviour in young women and, as for other women with diabetes, they lacked awareness of the importance of planning pregnancy.

From evidence to recommendations

Evidence shows that women with diabetes (including young women) lack awareness of the importance of planning pregnancy and the role and purpose of preconception care. To overcome barriers to preconception care information about the importance of planning pregnancy and achieving good glycaemic control in the periconceptional period should be reinforced at every contact between women with diabetes who are of childbearing age and their healthcare professionals, including the diabetes care team, and the woman's intentions regarding pregnancy in the immediate future or longer term should be discussed.

> **Recommendations for removing barriers to the uptake of preconception care and when to offer information**
>
> Women with diabetes should be informed about the benefits of preconception glycaemic control at each contact with healthcare professionals, including their diabetes care team, from adolescence.
>
> The intentions of women with diabetes regarding pregnancy and contraceptive use should be documented at each contact with their diabetes care team from adolescence.
>
> Preconception care for women with diabetes should be given in a supportive environment and the woman's partner or other family member should be encouraged to attend.

There were no research recommendations relating to the barriers to uptake of preconception care and the information that should be offered to all women of childbearing age with diabetes and/or women with diabetes who are planning a pregnancy.

3.9 Cost-effectiveness of self-management programmes

The effectiveness of self-management of diabetes in pregnancy was identified by the GDG as a priority for health economic analysis. The GDG approached the analysis by considering the cost-effectiveness of preconception care and advice for women with diabetes. The methods and results from the health economic modelling are summarised here; further details are provided in Appendix C.

A retrospective cohort study[120] examined the effect of an intensive diabetes management programme during pregnancy on women's long-term self-management behaviours and glycaemic control. The study showed that there was a significant improvement in all diabetes self-management behaviours including frequency of self-monitoring of blood glucose, frequency of insulin injections and frequency and complexity of insulin dose adjustment from entry to the programme to birth of the baby. There was also a significant improvement in HbA_{1c} from entry to birth of the baby. [EL = 2–]

An economic model constructed for the purposes of this guideline suggested that some form of preconception care and advice was likely to be cost-effective. Due to data limitations and uncertainty about the effectiveness of different forms of preconception care and advice, the robustness of baseline results were assessed using threshold analyses. These showed that the reduction in major congenital malformations needed for preconception care and advice to be considered cost-effective was much lower than reported in a meta-analysis of cohort studies of preconception care and advice,[121] [EL = 2++] and that cost-effectiveness of preconception care and advice relative to no preconception care and advice was not very sensitive to the costs of preconception care and advice or the 'downstream' costs associated with major congenital malformations.

From evidence to recommendations

NICE recommends that structured education programmes are made available to people with type 1 and type 2 diabetes.[18] The benefits of such programmes, which include DAFNE[69] for type 1 diabetes, and Diabetes Education and Self Management for Ongoing and Newly Diagnosed type 2 diabetes (DESMOND) and X-PERT for people with type 2 diabetes, are likely to be even greater for women planning a pregnancy because good glycaemic control improves pregnancy outcomes. The GDG considers, therefore, that it is particularly important that women with diabetes do not forego the benefits of such programmes.

A meta-analysis of preconception care and advice found that it conferred a statistically significant reduction in the rate of major congenital malformations in offspring born to women with diabetes.[62] There is some concern that confounding may explain at least some of the observed effect and that the potential benefits in term of improved glycaemic control may be lessened in settings where structured education programmes are offered more generally to women with diabetes. However, the economic model demonstrated that a much smaller effect size than reported in the meta-analysis would still be considered cost-effective and the GDG considered that preconception care and advice would meet the threshold for cost-effectiveness.

Preconception care and advice can take many different forms and some of this heterogeneity was reflected in the meta-analysis.[121] However, the different methods of delivering preconception care and advice vary enormously in terms of their resource use and ideally the incremental cost-effectiveness ratios (ICERs) of these alternative methods should be compared. However, such an analysis is not really possible using existing data and their inherent limitations. Therefore, the GDG did not recommend a specific form of preconception care and advice.

The GDG has used the phrase 'preconception care and advice' (rather than 'preconception counselling') in the recommendations to emphasise that this is care and advice provided by members of the multidisciplinary diabetes and antenatal care team (see Section 5.8) during the preconception period, rather than services provided by trained counsellors.

Recommendations for self-management programmes

Women with diabetes who are planning to become pregnant should be offered a structured education programme as soon as possible if they have not already attended one (see 'Guidance on the use of patient-education models for diabetes' [NICE technology appraisal guidance 60], available from www.nice.org.uk/TA060*.

Women with diabetes who are planning to become pregnant should be offered preconception care and advice before discontinuing contraception.

Research recommendations for self-management programmes

What is the most clinically and cost-effective form of preconception care and advice for women with diabetes?

Why this is important
Preconception care and advice for women with pre-existing diabetes is recommended because a health economic analysis has demonstrated cost-effectiveness of attendance at a preconception clinic. Due to limitations in the clinical evidence available to inform the health economic modelling it was not possible to establish the optimal form of preconception care and advice for this group of women. Future research should seek to establish the clinical and cost-effectiveness of different models of preconception care and advice for women with pre-existing

---

* The clinical guideline 'Type 2 diabetes: the management of type 2 diabetes' will update the information on type 2 diabetes in this technology appraisal. It is currently in development and is expected to be published in April 2008.

diabetes. Specifically it should evaluate different forms of content (i.e. what topics are covered), frequency and timing of contact with healthcare professionals (for example, whether one long session is more clinically and cost-effective than a series of shorter sessions), which healthcare professionals should be involved (for example, whether preconception care and advice provided by a multidisciplinary team is more clinically and cost-effective than contact with one healthcare professional), and format (for example, whether group sessions are more clinically and cost-effective than providing care and advice for each woman separately). The research should also seek to establish whether women with type 1 and type 2 diabetes have different needs in terms of preconception care and advice, and how different models of care and advice compare to structured education programmes already offered to women with type 1 and type 2 diabetes.

3.10 Retinal assessment in the preconception period

The evidence in relation to retinal assessment in the preconception period and the GDG's interpretation of the evidence are presented in Section 5.4.

Recommendations for retinal assessment in the preconception period

Women with diabetes seeking preconception care should be offered retinal assessment at their first appointment (unless an annual retinal assessment has occurred within the previous 6 months) and annually thereafter if no diabetic retinopathy is found.

Retinal assessment should be carried out by digital imaging with mydriasis using tropicamide*, in line with the UK National Screening Committee's recommendations for annual mydriatic two-field digital photographic screening as part of a systematic screening programme.

Women with diabetes who are planning to become pregnant should be advised to defer rapid optimisation of glycaemic control until after retinal assessment and treatment have been completed.

There were no research recommendations in relation to retinal assessment in the preconception period.

3.11 Renal assessment in the preconception period

The evidence in relation to renal assessment in the preconception period and the GDG's interpretation of the evidence are presented in Section 5.5.

Recommendations for renal assessment in the preconception period

Women with diabetes should be offered a renal assessment, including a measure of microalbuminuria, before discontinuing contraception. If serum creatinine is abnormal (120 micromol/litre or more), or the estimated glomerular filtration rate (eGFR) is less than 45 ml/minute/1.73 m², referral to a nephrologist should be considered before discontinuing contraception.

There were no research recommendations in relation to renal assessment in the preconception period.

---

* This drug does not have UK marketing authorisation specifically for pregnant and breastfeeding women at the time of publication (March 2008). Informed consent should be obtained and documented.

4 Gestational diabetes

4.1 Risk factors for gestational diabetes

Gestational diabetes is defined by the World Health Organization (WHO) as 'carbohydrate intolerance resulting in hyperglycaemia of variable severity with onset or first recognition during pregnancy'.[31] According to the Pedersen hypothesis,[122] maternal hyperglycaemia results in excess transfer of glucose to the fetus resulting in fetal hyperinsulinaemia. The effects of fetal hyperinsulinaemia include:

- an overgrowth of insulin-sensitive tissues such as adipose tissues, especially around the chest, shoulders and abdomen, which increases the risk of shoulder dystocia, perinatal death, birth trauma and the need for caesarean section
- neonatal metabolic complications such as hypoglycaemia
- a hypoxaemic state in utero which may increase the risk of intrauterine fetal death, fetal polycythaemia, hyperbilirubinaemia and renal vein thrombosis[123]
- an increased long-term risk of obesity and diabetes in the child.

The potential benefits of recognising and treating gestational diabetes include reductions in ill health in the woman and/or the baby during or immediately after pregnancy, as well as the benefits of reducing the risk of progression to type 2 diabetes in the longer term and/or future pregnancies being complicated by pre-existing or gestational diabetes.[124]

The 'gold standard' diagnostic test for gestational diabetes is the 75 g oral glucose tolerance test (OGTT) conducted at 24–28 weeks of gestation. The WHO definition of gestational diabetes encompasses both impaired glucose tolerance (IGT) (fasting blood glucose (FBG) less than 7.0 mmol/litre and a 2 hour blood glucose 7.8 mmol/litre or more) and diabetes (FBG 7.0 mmol/litre or more or 2 hour blood glucose 11.1 mmol/litre or more).[31]

Description of the evidence

A systematic review of screening for gestational diabetes was undertaken for a health technology assessment (HTA),[124] which included one UK study.[125] An additional study was identified that was published after the systematic review was published.[126]

The systematic review included 135 studies, although in only 16 studies were all women given a diagnostic OGTT regardless of screening result.[124] The review found risk factors for gestational diabetes were obesity, advanced maternal age, family history of diabetes, minority ethnic background, increased weight gain in early adulthood and current smoker. [EL = 2++] Ethnic groups with increased risk of developing gestational diabetes are South Asian (specifically women whose country of family origin is India, Pakistan or Bangladesh) and black Carribean.[127]

In the one UK study included in the HTA systematic review,[125] 1.5% (170/11205) of women were diagnosed with gestational diabetes. Women with gestational diabetes were significantly older (32.3 versus 28.3 years, $P < 0.001$), had higher BMI (27.7 kg/m² versus 23.8 kg/m², $P < 0.001$) and were more likely to be from a minority ethnic group (55.4% versus 15.3%, $P < 0.0001$). Rates of gestational diabetes by ethnicity were: white 0.4% (26/6135), black 1.5% (29/1977), south-east Asian 3.5% (20/572) and Indian 4.4% (54/1218). After adjusting for age, BMI and parity, the relative risks (RRs) (with white ethnicity as the reference category) were as follows: black 3.1 (95% CI 1.8 to 5.5), south-east Asian 7.6 (95% CI 4.1 to 14.1) and Indian 11.3 (95% CI 6.8 to 18.8).

The HTA systematic review found that using risk factors alone as a screening test produced low sensitivities (50–69%) and specificities (58–68%; eight studies). One non-randomised, uncontrolled observational study[128] that gave all women ($n = 1185$) a 75 g OGTT found 39.2% (31) of women with gestational diabetes had no risk factors and would have been missed if only selective testing was used. In this study women with no risk factors had a gestational diabetes prevalence of 4.8%. One study[129] found that four risk factors (age, BMI, ethnic group and family history) gave most of the information and that adding other items added little. [EL = 2++]

One study was identified that had been published since the HTA and had given all women a diagnostic OGTT. This prospective population-based study conducted in Sweden offered all pregnant women without diabetes a 75 g OGTT at 28–32 weeks of gestation.[126] Seventy-four percent (3616/4918) of women agreed to the OGTT. Women who did not take the OGTT were more likely to be multiparous and of non-Nordic origin but were less likely to have a family history of diabetes, previous macrosomic baby or previous gestational diabetes. Of the women who had the OGTT, 1.7% (61) had gestational diabetes. The risk factors with the strongest association were previous gestational diabetes (12/61, OR 23.6, 95% CI 11.6 to 48.0) and previous macrosomic baby (9/61, OR 5.59, 95% CI 2.68 to 11.7). Other risk factors were family history of diabetes (13/61, OR 2.74, CI 1.47 to 5.11), non-Nordic origin (13/61, OR 2.19, 95% CI 1.18 to 4.08), weight 90 kg or more (8/61, OR 3.33, 95% CI 1.56 to 7.13), BMI 30 kg/m² or more (11/61, OR 2.65, 95% CI 1.36 to 5.14) and age 25 years or more (55/61, OR 3.37, 95% CI 1.45 to 7.85). [EL = 2+]

A cohort study[130] examined the effects of pre-pregnancy BMI on antenatal, intrapartum, postnatal and neonatal outcomes. The study showed that women who are obese were more likely to develop gestational diabetes ($P < 0.001$). It was concluded that pre-pregnancy obesity is a risk factor gestational diabetes. [EL = 2+]

A prospective cohort study[131] examined the incidence and outcomes of pregnancy in women with gestational diabetes in an Iranian population. The study compared women with gestational diabetes to women with normal glucose tolerance. The results showed a statistically significant difference in risk factors between the two groups. Women with gestational diabetes had a significantly higher rate of stillbirth, hydramnios, gestational hypertension, macrosomia and caesarean section. [EL = 2+]

An RCT conducted in the USA[132] compared a risk factor-based screening programme for gestational diabetes with universal screening. Women in the risk factor group were given a 3 hour 100 g OGTT at 32 weeks of gestation if any risk factor was present. Women in the universal screening group were given a 50 g GCT followed by a 3 hour 100 g OGTT if the plasma glucose at 1 hour was 7.8 mmol/litre or more. The study reported the following PPVs for risk factors: first-degree relative with type 2 diabetes 6.7%, first-degree relative with type 1 diabetes 15%, previous macosomic baby (more than 4500 g) 12.2%, glycosuria in current pregnancy 50%, macrosomia in current pregnancy 40% and polyhydramnios in current pregnancy 40%. The detection rate for gestational diabetes using universal screening was significantly higher than using risk factor screening (2.7% vs 1.45%). [EL = 2+]

A study conducted in Denmark[133] retrospectively investigated the power of pre-screening based on risk factors to identify gestational diabetes and screening to predict adverse clinical outcomes. Pregnant women with at least one risk factor were offered capillary FBG at 20 and 32 weeks of gestation. If the capillary FBG measurements were 4.1 mmol/litre or more and less than 6.7 mmol/litre, then a 3 hour 75 g OGTT was offered. If capillary FBG values were 6.7 mmol/litre or more, the woman was diagnosed as having gestational diabetes. The most frequent pre-screening risk factors were BMI 27 kg/m² or more (present in 65% of women with gestational diabetes) and age 35 years or older (present in 16% of women with gestational diabetes). No single risk factor seemed the best indicator for gestational diabetes. The strongest predictor of developing gestational diabetes was glycosuria (OR 9.04, 95% CI 2.6 to 63.7). [EL = 2−]

A cross-sectional 5 year investigation conducted in the Netherlands[134] examined the clinical utility of antenatal clinical characteristics and measures of glucose tolerance in multi-ethnic women with gestational diabetes for their ability to predict type 2 diabetes within 6 months of birth (early postpartum diabetes). The following risk factors were assessed for all women: age and gestational age at entry into the study, pre-pregnancy BMI, ethnicity, obstetric and clinical history, including the onset of early postpartum diabetes, and pregnancy outcome. The study showed that apart from family history of diabetes no other risk factor showed an association with the development of early postpartum diabetes. [EL = 2−]

A cohort study[135] of 6214 pregnancies among 6034 women evaluated the sensitivity and cost-effectiveness of various screening schemes for gestational diabetes. Women were tested at 24–28 weeks using 1 hour 59 g GCT without regard to their last meal. Women were also asked for their age and risk factors. Two percent of pregnancies (n = 125) were complicated by gestational diabetes. Gestational diabetes increased with maternal age (P < 0.001). Of women with gestational diabetes, 70 (56%) were younger than 30 years; of these, 58% had one or more risk factors. If a threshold of more than 7.8 mmol/litre had been used, 10% of women with gestational diabetes, who had screening values of 7.2–7.8 mmol/litre, would have been missed. [EL = 2+]

A cross-sectional survey[136] of 14 613 women without previous gestational diabetes or other known diabetes who reported singleton pregnancy between 1990 and 1994 were used to measure risk factors for gestational diabetes. Gestational diabetes developed in 722 women during the study period. Maternal age over 40 years had a two-fold increased risk of gestational diabetes compared with women aged 25–29 years. Crude RR for gestational diabetes increased 4% (95% CI 2% to 6%) with each year over 25. Gestational diabetes risk increased with weight gain between age 18 and the year the study began, 1989 (RR for weight gain 5–9.9 kg 1.67, 95% CI 1.37 to 2.05 compared with stable weight). Risk for gestational diabetes increased directly with greater weight gain (RR 3.56, 95% CI 2.70 to 4.69) for weight gain of 20 kg or more since age 18 years. Family history of diabetes in a first-degree relative increased the risk of gestational diabetes (RR 1.68, 95% CI 1.39 to 2.04). Women of African-American, Hispanic or Asian ethnicity all had significantly increased age-adjusted RRs for gestational diabetes compared with white women. Higher pre-pregnancy (1989) BMI, higher BMI at age 18 years and weight gain between 18 years and 1989 all significantly increased the risk for gestational diabetes. Current smoking increased the risk of gestational diabetes when compared with never smokers (RR 1.43, 95% CI 1.14 to 1.80). Past smokers had no increased risk. Pre-pregnancy physical activity was not associated with risk for gestational diabetes. [EL = 2+]

Additional information about the prevalence of gestational diabetes was obtained using type 2 diabetes as a marker for gestational diabetes. An atlas showing the worldwide prevalence of type 2 diabetes in 2007 indicated that Middle Eastern countries (Saudi Arabia, United Arab Emirates, Iraq, Jordan, Syria, Egypt, Oman, Qatar, Kuwait and the Lebanon) have high prevalence (more than 10% of women; see www.eatlas.idf.org/webdata/docs/Map%201.1_large.jpg). [EL = 3]

A recent systematic review[137] examined the rates and factors associated with recurrence of gestational diabetes among women with a history of gestational diabetes. A total of 13 studies were included. The review showed the recurrence rate of glucose intolerance during subsequent pregnancies varied markedly across studies. The most consistent predictor of future recurrence appeared to be non-white race/ethnicity, although the racial groups were not always clearly described in the original studies. Recurrence rates varied between 30% and 84% after the index pregnancy. Recurrence rates were higher in the minority ethnic populations (52–69%) compared with lower rates found in non-Hispanic white populations (30–37%). No other risk factors were consistently associated with recurrence of gestational diabetes across studies. Other risk factors, such as maternal age, parity, BMI, OGTT results and insulin use, inconsistently predicted recurrence of gestational diabetes across studies. However, the systematic review included two studies[138,139] that reported the probability of gestational diabetes given insulin-treated gestational diabetes in a previous pregnancy to be 75–77%. [EL = 2++]

An audit conducted in the UK in 2002 assessed whether the introduction of an appointment form for administering an OGTT had improved the understanding of antenatal care staff.[140] The audit showed that 89% of healthcare professionals were aware of the scheduled time for OGTT administration (26–28 weeks of gestation) in 2002, whereas a similar audit conducted in 2001 showed that only 69% of healthcare professionals knew when to screen. The following risk factors and clinical measurements were listed on the appointment form as indications for OGTT: [EL = 3]

- glycosuria ≥ 1+ on more than one occasion or ≥ 2+ on one occasion
- macrosomia in current pregnancy
- previous large infant (more than 4.5 kg, or above the 95th centile for gestational age)
- previous gestational diabetes
- first-degree relative with diabetes
- previous unexpected perinatal death
- history of polycystic ovary syndrome
- obesity (BMI more than 30 kg/m²) or booking weight more than 100 kg
- polyhydramnios
- Asian ethnic background
- FBG more than 6.0 mmol/litre, or random blood glucose more than 7.0 mmol/litre.

Evidence statement

Evidence shows that risk factors for developing gestational diabetes are: pre-pregnancy obesity, advanced maternal age, previous gestational diabetes, family history of diabetes, minority ethnic background, previous macrosomic baby (4500 g or more for white and black women), increased maternal weight gain in early adulthood, and current smoker. Family origins with a high prevalence of gestational diabetes are South Asian (specifically women whose country of family origin is India, Pakistan or Bangladesh), black Carribean and Middle Eastern (specifically women whose country of family origin is Saudi Arabia, United Arab Emirates, Iraq, Jordan, Syria, Oman, Qatar, Kuwait, Lebanon or Egypt)

Recurrence rates for gestational diabetes varied from 30% to 84% after the index pregnancy. The probability of gestational diabetes given insulin-treated gestational diabetes in a previous pregnancy is approximately 75%.

From evidence to recommendations

The following have been shown to be independent risk factors for gestational diabetes and should be recognised as such by healthcare professionals:

- BMI more than 30 kg/m²
- previous macrosomic baby weighing 4.5 kg or more
- previous gestational diabetes
- family history of diabetes (first-degree relative with diabetes)
- family origin with a high prevalence of diabetes:
  - South Asian (specifically women whose country of family origin is India, Pakistan or Bangladesh)
  - black Caribbean
  - Middle Eastern (specifically women whose country of family origin is Saudi Arabia, United Arab Emirates, Iraq, Jordan, Syria, Oman, Qatar, Kuwait, Lebanon or Egypt).

The consensus view of the combined GDGs for antenatal care and diabetes in pregnancy is that advanced maternal age should not be used as a risk factor for gestational diabetes because this would result in most pregnant women receiving an OGTT (see Section 4.3).

The probability of gestational diabetes for a woman who has had gestational diabetes in a previous pregnancy is 30–84%, and so it is straightforward to demonstrate the cost-effectiveness of offering a diagnostic test for gestational diabetes to women who have had gestational diabetes in a previous pregnancy. Moreover, the probability of gestational diabetes given insulin-treated gestational diabetes in a previous pregnancy is approximately 75%. In its discussions, the GDG also noted that there is a strong possibility of developing frank type 1 diabetes or type 2 diabetes given gestational diabetes in a previous pregnancy (see Section 8.2). Recommendations relating to recurrence of gestational diabetes and the need for early testing for gestational diabetes in future pregnancies are presented in Section 8.2.

Recommendations for risk factors for gestational diabetes

Healthcare professionals should be aware that the following have been shown to be independent risk factors for gestational diabetes:

- body mass index above 30 kg/m²
- previous macrosomic baby weighing 4.5 kg or above
- previous gestational diabetes
- family history of diabetes (first-degree relative with diabetes)
- family origin with a high prevalence of diabetes:
  - South Asian (specifically women whose country of family origin is India, Pakistan or Bangladesh)
  - black Caribbean
  - Middle Eastern (specifically women whose country of family origin is Saudi Arabia, United Arab Emirates, Iraq, Jordan, Syria, Oman, Qatar, Kuwait, Lebanon or Egypt).

There were no research recommendations relating to which women are at high risk of gestational diabetes.

4.2 Diagnosis of gestational diabetes

Internationally there are at least six different criteria for the diagnosis of gestational diabetes.[141] Diagnostic tests vary in the glucose load to be used, the timing and the type of blood sample. The most commonly used tests are the 2 hour 75 g OGTT used by the WHO (Table 4.1)[31] and the 3 hour 100 g OGTT as recommended by the American Diabetes Association (Table 4.2).[142]

Table 4.1   World Health Organization criteria for the 75 g OGTT[31]

	Whole blood venous	Whole blood capillary	Plasma venous	Plasma capillary
Fasting	≥ 6.1 mmol/litre	≥ 6.1 mmol/litre	≥ 7.0 mmol/litre	≥ 7.0 mmol/litre
2 hours	≥ 6.7 mmol/litre	≥ 7.8 mmol/litre	≥ 7.8 mmol/litre	≥ 8.9 mmol/litre

Table 4.2   Criteria for the 100 g OGTT (gestational diabetes is diagnosed if two or more measurements in one column are abnormal, i.e. if they exceed the levels indicated)[142]

Time	O'Sullivan and Mahan (whole blood)	National Diabetes Data Group (NDDG) recommendations (plasma glucose)	Carpenter and Coustan adaptation (plasma glucose)
Fasting	≥ 5.0 mmol/litre	≥ 5.8 mmol/litre	≥ 5.3 mmol/litre
1 hour	≥ 9.1 mmol/litre	≥ 10.0 mmol/litre	≥ 10.0 mmol/litre
2 hours	≥ 8.0 mmol/litre	≥ 9.1 mmol/litre	≥ 8.6 mmol/litre
3 hours	≥ 6.9 mmol/litre	≥ 8.0 mmol/litre	≥ 7.8 mmol/litre

Description of the evidence

Levels of glucose intolerance and adverse pregnancy outcomes
Three cohort studies found adverse pregnancy outcomes increased with increasing gradients of glucose intolerance. In all three studies the glucose intolerance was previously undiagnosed and untreated and the confounding effects of obesity and maternal age were controlled.

The first study[143] divided women with normal results on a 100 g OGTT (O'Sullivan and Mahan criteria) into three groups: group A ($n = 151$) had 2 hour glucose levels below 5.6 mmol/litre, group B ($n = 58$) had 2 hour levels of 5.6–6.6 mmol/litre and group C ($n = 40$) had 2 hour values of 6.6–9.1 mmol/litre. The study found a positive correlation between the 2 hour glucose level and macrosomia and maternal complications (pre-eclampsia and/or caesarean section; test for linear trend, $P < 0.01$). [EL = 2++]

The second study was of 3352 women with 75 g OGTT FBG less than 5.8 mmol/litre and 2 hour values less than 11.0 mmol/litre.[144] This study found a progressive increase in the prevalence of macrosomia with incremental fasting, 1 hour and 2 hour values. Receiver operating characteristic (ROC) curves were constructed but no inflexion point could be identified. [EL = 2++]

The third study was of 3352 women who did not fulfil the National Diabetes Data Group (NDDG) criteria for gestational diabetes. It found progressively increasing plasma glucose associated with increased incidence of macrosomia and caesarean section.[145] [EL = 2++]

A cohort study considered the association between glucose tolerance and the ratio of fetal cranial : thoracic circumference in 829 women who had been diagnosed with gestational diabetes (Carpenter and Coustan criteria).[146] The study found the 1 hour value on a 75 g glucose load was significantly associated with a cranial : thoracic ratio of ≤ 10th percentile. This was apparent as early as 16–20 weeks of gestation (adjusted OR 1.81, 95% CI 1.15 to 2.83). ROC curves for the prediction of neonatal cranial : thoracic ratio ≤ 10th percentile identified a threshold 1 hour value of 8.3 mmol/litre at 16–20 weeks of gestation and 8.8 mmol/litre at 26–30 weeks of gestation. [EL = 2++]

A case–control study considered the association between glucose tolerance and elevated insulin levels in amniotic fluid.[147] The study included 220 women with elevated amniotic fluid insulin levels (42 pmol/litre or more) who had an OGTT at 28 weeks of gestation (161 had a glucose load of 1 g/kg and 59 had 75 g). The control group was 220 women without diabetes and with amniotic fluid insulin levels less than 42 pmol/litre. The 1 hour OGTT value had the highest sensitivity for raised insulin concentration (97% of women with elevated amniotic fluid insulin concentration had 1 hour levels more than 8.9%). A fasting level of 5.0 mmol/litre or more had a sensitivity of 58% and a 2 hour level of 7.8 mmol/litre or more had a sensitivity of 54%. [EL = 2++]

Four studies found that women with IGT had more adverse outcomes than women with normal glucose tolerance. In all four studies the IGT was previously undiagnosed and untreated. All four studies controlled for the effect of potential confounders including obesity and age.

The first study was a case–control study which compared 126 women with gestational diabetes diagnosed according to the NDDG criteria (two abnormal values on the 100 g OGTT) to 126 women with one abnormal value and 126 women with normal values.[148] There was no significant difference in mean blood glucose values between the gestational diabetes group before treatment and the group with one abnormal OGTT value. The glucose profiles of the gestational diabetes group before treatment were identical to the profiles of the group with one abnormal value. The profiles of the gestational diabetes group before treatment and the group with one abnormal value were significantly different to the group with normal OGTT values. After the gestational diabetes group underwent treatment there was a significant difference in mean blood glucose levels and blood glucose profiles between the gestational diabetes group and the group with one abnormal value. There was no significant difference between the gestational diabetes group after treatment and the normal group. There was a significant difference in the incidence of LGA and macrosomic babies between the group with one abnormal value and the normal group (34% versus 9%, $P < 0.01$) and the gestational diabetes group (34% versus 12%, $P < 0.01$). There was no significant difference in LGA and macrosomic babies between the gestational diabetes group and the normal group. Neonatal metabolic disorders were significantly higher in the group with one abnormal value (15%) when compared with the gestational diabetes and normal groups (3%, $P < 0.01$). [EL = 2++]

The second study was a cohort study[149] of 3260 women that divided women into four groups based on the results of a 2 hour 75 g OGTT: group 1 had a 2 hour value less than 7.8 mmol/litre ($n = 2596$) and were not treated, group 2 had a 2 hour value of 7.8–8.9 mmol/litre ($n = 289$) and were not treated, group 3 had a 2 hour value of 9.0–11.0 mmol/litre ($n = 278$) and were treated, and group 4 had a 2 hour level more than 11.1 mmol/litre ($n = 97$) and were treated. The frequency of macrosomia increased by more than 50% in women with 2 hour OGTT values between 7.8 and 8.9 mmol/litre compared with women with 2 hour OGTT levels less than 7.8 mmol/litre. [EL = 2++]

The third study was a case–control study that compared 213 women with undiagnosed as well as untreated IGT (2 hour 75 g OGGT fasting level less than 6.7 mmol/litre and 2 hour level of 9.0–11.0 mmol/litre) with 815 controls.[150] The study found that IGT was significantly and independently associated with an increased incidence of caesarean section, preterm birth, LGA and macrosomic babies and admission to neonatal intensive care for 2 days or longer. [EL = 2++]

The fourth study was a cohort study that included 1190 black women and 865 white women at 24–29 weeks of gestation.[151] All women were given a 100 g OGTT (Carpenter and Coustan criteria). Among black women 32 had gestational diabetes, 13 had IGT and 820 had normal glucose tolerance. Among white women 70 had gestational diabetes, 40 had IGT and 1080 had normal glucose tolerance. Logistic regression found a significant increase in birthweight in women with IGT compared with women with normal glucose tolerance, among black women, but not white women. [EL = 2+]

A retrospective cohort study[152] hypothesised that elevated 50 g glucose load test results could be associated with unfavourable perinatal outcomes even in the absence of an actual diagnosis of gestational diabetes. The study found that a glucose load test result of 10.5 mmol/litre or more was associated with unfavourable perinatal outcomes and might warrant further follow-up regardless of the subsequent OGTT results. [EL 2–]

Treating impaired glucose tolerance

An RCT (the Australian Carbohydrate Intolerance Study in Pregnant Women (ACHOIS)) allocated 490 women with IGT (2 hour 75 g OGTT fasting level less than 7.8 mmol/litre and 2 hour level of 7.8–11.0 mmol/litre) to treatment and 510 women with IGT to routine care.[153] The rate of serious perinatal outcomes among babies was significantly lower in the intervention group (1% versus 4%, *P* = 0.01). The number needed to treat to prevent a serious outcome in a baby was 34. There was no significant difference between groups in maternal quality of life (see Section 4.3 for further details). [EL = 1++]

An international multicentre prospective cohort study (the Hyperglycemia and Adverse Pregnancy Outcome (HAPO) study) is due to report soon. The aim of the study is to establish the level of hyperglycaemia that results in a significant risk of adverse pregnancy outcome.

Evidence statement

Three studies were identified that demonstrated that adverse outcomes increased with increasing gradients of glucose intolerance.

Four studies were identified that found that women with levels of glucose tolerance above normal but below the threshold values for gestational diabetes as defined by the NDDG or Carpenter and Coustan criteria have significantly higher risk of adverse maternal and neonatal outcomes. This risk remained even when the woman and physician were blinded to the diagnosis of IGT and after controlling for maternal age and obesity. This supports the inclusion of IGT, as defined by the WHO, in a diagnosis of gestational diabetes. Furthermore, a high-quality RCT has shown that treating gestational diabetes (as defined by the WHO) improves maternal and fetal outcomes.

One study found an independent and significant association between the 1 hour value following a 75 g glucose load and a neonatal cranial : thoracic ratio ≤ 10th percentile. ROC curves identified a threshold value of 8.3 mmol/litre at 16–20 weeks of gestation and 8.8 mmol/litre at 26–30 weeks of gestation. This finding suggests a possibility of using a 1 hour 75 g glucose load as a single test for the diagnosis of gestational diabetes. This is supported by a study that found that 97% of women with elevated amniotic fluid insulin concentration had a 1 hour OGTT value of more than 8.9% at 28 weeks of gestation.

From evidence to recommendations

The evidence shows that when gestational diabetes is diagnosed using the 2 hour 75 g OGTT and the WHO criteria there is an increased incidence of (treatable) maternal and neonatal complications. The GDG has, therefore, adopted the 2 hour 75 g OGTT using the WHO criteria as the diagnostic test for gestational diabetes administered at 24–28 weeks of gestation.

The recommendations in relation to the diagnosis of gestational diabetes are presented in Section 4.3.

4.3 Screening and treatment for gestational diabetes

This section includes work undertaken jointly with the GDG for the NICE antenatal care guideline update on the cost-effectiveness of screening, diagnosis and treatment for gestational diabetes. The clinical evidence in relation to screening methods is presented in the antenatal care guideline.[9] The clinical evidence in relation to treating gestational diabetes is presented in this section. The cost-effectiveness of screening, diagnosis and treatment was addressed through a single health economics model which is described below.

Description of the evidence

The ACHOIS trial has shown that treating gestational diabetes as defined by the WHO improves outcomes for women and babies (see Section 4.2).[153] Treatments for gestational diabetes include lifestyle interventions, such as diet and exercise and self-monitoring of blood glucose, and hypoglycaemic therapy, using hypoglycaemic agents (metformin and glibenclamide), regular insulin and/or rapid-acting insulin analogues (lispro and aspart).

The primary goal of interventions for gestational diabetes is to maintain near normal glycaemic control in order to reduce morbidity and mortality in women and babies.

Diet

The goals of dietary interventions in pregnancies complicated by diabetes are the optimisation of glycaemic control while avoiding ketoacidosis and minimising the risk of hypoglycaemia in women taking insulin.[154] In women with gestational diabetes adverse outcomes have been associated with postprandial hyperglycaemia,[155] therefore an important aim of dietary therapy is reducing postprandial glucose levels.

Seven studies were identified that considered the influence of a diet based on carbohydrates of low glycaemic index on postprandial glucose levels.

A study in an African population compared blood glucose values in women during pregnancy with those in non-pregnant women.[156] All women consumed a diet high in carbohydrates of low glycaemic index. Pregnant women demonstrated improved glucose homeostasis with advancing pregnancy. For example, the mean (SD) 1 hour postprandial value was 6 (1.5) mmol/litre in women in the 13th week of gestation and 5.9 (1.4) mmol/litre in women at 37–40 weeks of gestation. In non-pregnant women the mean (SD) 1 hour postprandial value was 7 (1.3) mmol/litre. [EL = 2++]

In a crossover study[157] 15 women without diabetes were evaluated following three diets. Diet 1 reflected a typical 'Western' diet and consisted of 1830 kcal, 20 g protein, 39 g fat, 41 g carbohydrate and 10 g dietary fibre. Diet 2 consisted of 1820 kcal, 22 g protein, 38 g fat, 40 g carbohydrate and 52 g dietary fibre. Diet 3 consisted of 1850 kcal, 17 g protein, 16 g fat, 60 g carbohydrate and 84 g dietary fibre. The study revealed a loss of insulin sensitivity on diet 1 but not on diets 2 or 3. [EL = 1++]

A crossover study of 14 non-pregnant women without diabetes compared low glycaemic index (GI) diets with high GI diets.[158] After 7–10 days on the diet postprandial glucose was measured after a 540 kcal test meal. Each meal contained 17% protein, 28% fat and 55% carbohydrate but differed in the GI of the carbohydrates (54 versus 92). The average increase in blood sugar was significantly lower on the low GI diet ($P < 0.001$). Insulin response was also significantly lower ($P < 0.01$) on the low GI diet. [EL = 1+]

An RCT compared ten pregnant women on a low GI diet with ten pregnant women on a high GI diet (none of the women had diabetes).[159] The low GI group had significantly lower FBG (3.78 versus 4.28 mmol/litre, $P < 0.05$), fasting insulin levels (63 nmol/litre versus 131 nmol/litre, $P < 0.05$), average postprandial glucose increase (0.60 mmol/litre per minute versus 1.56 mmol/litre per minute, $P < 0.05$) and average insulin increase (186 nmol/litre per minute versus 324 nmol/litre per minute, $P < 0.05$). Birthweight, ponderal index, fat mass and maternal weight gain were all significantly lower in the low GI group ($P < 0.01$). [EL = 1+]

A case–control study compared the diets of 16 women with newly diagnosed gestational diabetes with those of 24 healthy pregnant women.[160] The women with gestational diabetes consumed significantly fewer carbohydrate foods with low GI values ($P < 0.05$). [EL = 2+]

A small crossover study in five women with gestational diabetes compared a diet that was low in fat and high in carbohydrates of low glycaemic index with a low carbohydrate diet.[161] The highly unrefined carbohydrate diet was made up of 70% carbohydrate, 10% fat, 20% protein and 70 g fibre each day. The low carbohydrate diet was made up of 35% carbohydrate, 45% fat, 20% protein and 70 g fibre each day. Unrefined carbohydrate sources (mostly complex) were used in both diets. Glucose tolerance was assessed by measuring plasma glucose and insulin response to a 50 g glucose load. There was a significant improvement in glucose tolerance on the highly unrefined carbohydrate diet ($P < 0.05$). Fasting plasma cholesterol concentrations on the highly unrefined carbohydrate diet were 6% lower than on the low carbohydrate diet ($P < 0.01$). Fasting free fatty acids levels were 14% lower than on the low carbohydrate diet ($P < 0.02$). [EL = 1+]

A randomised crossover study in seven women with IGT and previous gestational diabetes compared the effect on insulin secretion and insulin sensitivity of low GI/high dietary fibre bread with high GI/low dietary fibre bread.[162] The study comprised two 3 week study periods separated by a 3 week wash-out period. Following inclusion of low GI/high dietary fibre bread all women lowered their insulin response to the intravenous glucose challenge (mean 35%). No changes were found in fasting levels of glucose, insulin, high-density lipoprotein cholesterol or triglycerides. [EL = 1+]

A cohort study[163] compared glucose measurements for women with diet-controlled gestational diabetes during two 9 hour fasts, one during the day and one overnight, and analysed hormones and metabolites involved in intermediary metabolism. The study showed that glucose concentrations in women with diet-treated gestational diabetes were significantly higher 3–9 hours after an evening meal. [EL = 2–]

Calorie restriction
Three observational studies were identified that considered calorie restriction in women with gestational diabetes.

An observational study included 35 women with gestational diabetes on a calorie-restricted diet.[164] The study used three control groups: (i) 2337 healthy pregnant women (general antenatal population); (ii) a group of 35 women matched on ethnic background, age, BMI and parity with a negative GCT result (screen negative); and (iii) a matched group of 35 women with a positive screening test result but a negative diagnostic test result (screen positive). Women with gestational diabetes were prescribed a calorie-restricted diet with complex carbohydrates replacing refined carbohydrates and fats. The total calorie intake was prescribed to be 30% less than consumed before pregnancy. The composition of the diet was 50% carbohydrate, 15% protein and 35% fat, with most carbohydrate taken as unrefined carbohydrate, protein as fish, white meat, beans and dairy products, and fat as polyunsaturated fat. The criterion for remaining on dietary treatment alone was a diurnal glucose profile averaged over six measurements of 6 mmol/litre or less. The women in the gestational diabetes group had significantly less weight gain during pregnancy than the control groups ($P < 0.005$). Incidence of macrosomia was similar to that of the general antenatal population. In contrast, the screen positive group had a significantly higher incidence of macrosomia than the women with gestational diabetes and the general antenatal population ($P < 0.005$). [EL = 2++]

An RCT was designed to compare the effect of a moderate reduction in energy intake (30%) in women with gestational diabetes who were obese on requirement for insulin therapy and incidence of macrosomia.[165] The control group was contaminated, but women in the intervention group reduced their pregnancy weight gain without significant ketonuria or fetal or maternal compromise. Glycaemic control was good; 17.5% of the intervention group required insulin and 28.8% of babies were LGA. [EL = 2+]

A cohort study compared 22 women with gestational diabetes who were obese (BMI 27 kg/m² or more) to 31 women with gestational diabetes who were lean (BMI less than 27 kg/m²). A control group consisted of ten women who were not obese (BMI 24 kg/m² or less) and with normal glucose tolerance.[166] The women who were obese were prescribed a diet of 1700–1800 kcal/ day (two women received small amounts of regular insulin before each meal). The women who were lean were prescribed 2000–3000 kcal/day and the women with normal glucose tolerance were prescribed a diet appropriate for pregnancy. Mean birthweight was significantly higher in women with gestational diabetes who were obese than in the other two groups despite a lower caloric intake and a smaller weight gain during pregnancy. Ketonuria was not observed in any woman even when reported caloric intakes were as low as 1500–1600 kcal/day. All women had excellent glycaemic control (2 hour post-breakfast plasma glucose levels less than 7 mmol/litre). HbA_{1c} at 35 weeks of gestation was 6.8 ± 0.4% in the women who were obese, 6.7 ± 0.7% in the women who were lean and 6.4 ± 1.2% in the control group. [EL = 2+]

A prospective randomised crossover study[167] studied 40% versus 55% carbohydrate calorically restricted diets to compare weight loss and metabolic response. Two groups were compared: group 1 consisted of women who were obese with previous gestational diabetes and group 2 consisted of women who were obese with no previous history of gestational diabetes. The study showed that a weight-loss regimen consisting of 40% carbohydrate resulted in lower triglyceride levels than was achieved with a 55% carbohydrate content diet in women who were obese. [EL = 1+]

Exercise
Three RCTs and a retrospective study were identified that compared diet with diet plus exercise in women with gestational diabetes.

In the first RCT 20 women with gestational diabetes were randomised to diet or diet plus 20 minutes of supervised exercise three times a week.[168] Exercise consisted of arm movements while seated in a chair. By the 6th week women in the diet plus exercise group had mean HbA_{1c} of 4.2 ± 0.2% compared with 4.7 ± 0.2% in the diet-only group ($P < 0.001$). The glucose challenge fasting value was 3.9 ± 0.4 mmol/litre versus 4.8 ± 0.3 mmol/litre ($P < 0.001$). The 1 hour postprandial value was 5.9 ± 1.0 mmol/litre versus 10.4 ± 0.16 mmol/litre, $P < 0.001$. [EL = 1++]

The second RCT compared 16 women with gestational diabetes treated with diet alone to 16 women treated with diet plus resistance exercise three times a week.[169] The number of women who required insulin treatment was not significantly different between the two groups. However, a subgroup analysis that looked only at women with a pre-pregnancy BMI more than 25 kg/m² found that women in the diet plus exercise group had a significantly lower incidence of insulin use (3/10 versus 8/10, $P < 0.05$). Within the intervention group, 30% of the women who exercised two to three times per week were prescribed insulin therapy compared with 67% of those who exercised less than twice per week. The amount of insulin that was prescribed was significantly lower in the diet plus exercise group as was the latency period between the first clinic visit and the initiation of insulin. There were no differences in self-monitored blood glucose values; however, when all postprandial results were pooled, women in the diet plus exercise group had significantly lower values ($P < 0.05$). There were no significant differences in gestational age at birth, rate of caesarean section or birthweight. [EL = 1++]

The third RCT was a randomised crossover study[170] which compared fasting glucose and insulin levels, peak glucose and insulin levels, and incremental area of the glycaemic and insulin curves following a mixed nutrient meal with or without an exercise stress in women with normal glucose levels and women with gestational diabetes. They found that a single bout of exercise did not blunt the glycaemic response observed following a mixed nutrient meal. [EL 1+]

A retrospective study[171] sought to examine the postnatal exercise beliefs and behaviours of women who had been diagnosed with gestational diabetes in a recent pregnancy. The study showed that the perceived advantage of exercise during pregnancy was controlling blood glucose and during that postnatal period it was controlling weight. The most common barrier to exercise was lack of time, although women exercised more during the postnatal period than before or during pregnancy. The women's husbands/partners strongly influenced their levels of exercise during pregnancy and in the postnatal period. [EL = 2−]

Blood glucose monitoring

Blood glucose targets during pregnancy for women with diabetes (including gestational diabetes) are a preprandial value of 3.5–5.9 mmol and a 1 hour postprandial value of less than 7.8 mmol/litre (see Section 5.1). The recommendations for self-monitoring of blood glucose during pregnancy are to test FBG levels and to test blood glucose 1 hour after eating (see Section 5.2).

When to initiate insulin

Insulin therapy is needed when near-normal blood glucose control cannot be achieved by diet alone. The duration of dietary treatment prior to initiation of insulin will depend on gestational age at diagnosis and the level of glycaemic control.

An RCT randomised 202 women with IGT to treatment with diet or diet plus insulin.[172] Self-monitoring of blood glucose was performed six times per day three times per week. Insulin doses were adjusted according to blood glucose values, aiming at fasting and postprandial values below 5 and 6.5 mmol/litre, respectively. Women in the diet-only group were switched to diet plus insulin if fasting and postprandial values exceeded 7 and 9 mmol/litre, respectively. In the diet-only group, 15 women (14%) were switched to diet plus insulin. Otherwise there were no differences between the two groups in maternal blood glucose control, HbA_1 at birth, obstetric or neonatal complications, birthweight, skinfold thickness or C-peptide concentration in cord serum. [EL = 1++]

Another RCT randomised 108 women with gestational diabetes to receive either diet alone or diet plus insulin for glycaemic control.[173] Blood glucose levels were evaluated weekly in a high-risk clinic where medical and nutritional support and counselling were provided. Among 68 women successfully treated for a minimum of 6 weeks, the mean birthweight and macrosomia rate were reduced significantly in the insulin-treated group. Insulin reduced birthweights significantly in women receiving insulin. Women with poor glycaemic control were at greatest risk (30%) for fetal overgrowth whether initially receiving insulin or not. [EL = 1+]

A cohort study included 153 women with gestational diabetes treated with diet and intensive self-monitoring of blood glucose.[174] A group of 2153 healthy pregnant women served as controls. During the first 1–2 weeks following diagnosis, women with gestational diabetes used monitors to measure fasting and 2 hour postprandial levels three to five times per week. If the fasting and postprandial levels were persistently less than 5.8 mmol/litre and 7.7 mmol/litre, respectively, women continued with the diet and reduced monitoring to 1 day per week. If self-monitored blood glucose was consistently equal to or higher than these values, adjustments were made to the diet. If, after dietary adjustments, blood glucose could not be controlled below these levels insulin therapy was started. Eleven women (7.2%) required insulin. There were no differences between the study and reference populations in mean birthweight or incidence of macrosomia. [EL = 2++]

A cohort study compared 52 women with gestational diabetes who were treated with diet alone with 23 who required insulin.[175] The aim of the study was to identify which factors predicted insulin treatment. Women in this study consumed a diet containing 25 kcal/kg/day and started insulin when fasting and 2 hour postprandial blood glucose levels were higher than 5.2 mmol/litre and 6.9 mmol/litre, respectively. Pre-pregnancy BMI more than 28 kg/m², early diagnosis of gestational diabetes, early rise in triglyceride levels and elevated 3 hour OGTT levels were predictive of insulin treatment. [EL = 2+]

Ultrasound measurement of abdominal circumference
A cohort study included 201 women with gestational diabetes who underwent ultrasound at 30–33 weeks of gestation.[176] Women with a fetal abdominal circumference > 90th percentile had a significantly higher incidence of caesarean section for failure to progress in labour (41.7% versus 14.3%, $P < 0.001$), shoulder dystocia (16.7% versus 0.7%, $P < 0.001$) and birth trauma (20.8% versus 3.6%, $P < 0.001$) compared with women with a fetal abdominal circumference ≤ 90th percentile. The sensitivity of an abdominal circumference measurement at 30–33 weeks of gestation for detecting macrosomia was 88%, the specificity was 83%, the PPV was 56% and the NPV was 96%. [EL = 2+]

An RCT involved 303 women with gestational diabetes.[177] All women had an ultrasound scan at 29–33 weeks of gestation. Sixty-eight percent (205/303) had abdominal circumference < 75th percentile. Of these, 7.3% (15) were placed on insulin therapy because of persistent fasting glycaemia 5.8 mol/litre or more. The women with an abdominal circumference ≥ 75th percentile were randomised to diet ($n = 29$) or diet plus insulin ($n = 30$). Women in the two treatment groups underwent breakfast tests at baseline and at 36–37 weeks of gestation. Glucose levels in both groups were lower at the follow-up breakfast test than at baseline ($P < 0.01$ for diet only, $P < 0.0001$ for insulin group). Weekly capillary blood glucose (CBG) readings also reduced significantly in both treatment groups, although they were 0.3–0.6 mmol/litre lower in the insulin group throughout the treatment period ($P < 0.005$). Birthweights (3647 ± 67 g versus 3878 ± 84 g, $P < 0.02$) and the incidence of LGA babies (13% versus 45%, $P < 0.02$) were lower in the insulin group, as were neonatal skinfold measurements ($P < 0.005$). The insulin-treated group had much higher caesarean section rates (43%, $P < 0.05$ versus other groups). The frequency of symptomatic hypoglycaemia (less than 3.3 mmol/litre) in the insulin group was 0.3 episodes per week. There were no episodes requiring assistance. [EL = 1+]

An RCT compared a management strategy based on glycaemic targets (control group, $n = 48$) with one based on ultrasound evaluation (intervention group, $n = 48$) for women with gestational diabetes.[178] Women in the control group were prescribed insulin immediately, the dose being adjusted to achieve preprandial CBG concentrations 4.95 mmol/litre or less and 2 hour postprandial values 6.6 mmol/litre or less. Women in the intervention group were prescribed insulin if fetal abdominal circumference was ≥ 70th percentile or fasting plasma glucose (FPG) more than 6.6 mmol/litre. Insulin dose was adjusted to achieve preprandial CBG 4.4 mmol/litre or less and 2 hour postprandial values of 6.05 mmol/litre or less. In the intervention group, 45% (22) of women had a fetal abdominal circumference of ≥ 70th percentile at enrolment. Of these, 21 were immediately started on insulin. An additional nine women in the intervention group began insulin subsequently because of an abdominal circumference ≥ 70th percentile ($n = 6$) or FPG more than 6.6 mmol/litre ($n = 2$) or because of inadequate self-monitoring of blood glucose

($n = 1$). Birthweights (3271 ± 458 g versus 3369 ± 461 g), LGA babies (6.3% versus 8.3%) and neonatal morbidity (25% versus 25%) did not differ between groups. The caesarean section rate was significantly lower in the control group. In the intervention group, babies of women who did not receive insulin had lower birthweights than babies of women treated using insulin (3180 ± 425 versus 3482 ± 451, $P = 0.03$). [EL = 1+]

An RCT compared 99 women with gestational diabetes managed according to ultrasound assessment of abdominal circumference (intervention group) to 100 women with gestational diabetes managed according to glycaemic levels (control group).[179] In the intervention group insulin was started when fetal abdominal circumference was > 75th percentile (before 36 completed weeks of gestation). Glucose targets were not discussed with the women and glucose values were not used as a guide to management unless any fasting value was more than 6.6 mmol/litre or any 2 hour value was more than 11.0 mmol/litre. Insulin was not prescribed, regardless of abdominal circumference, when fasting capillary glucose (FCG) less than 4.4 mmol/litre and 2 hour value was less than 5.5 mmol/litre. Ultrasound was performed at entry and then at 4 week intervals. Insulin dose was adjusted to achieve FCG less than 4.4 mmol/litre and 2 hour less than 6.05 mmol/litre. In the control group insulin was prescribed if two glucose profiles had two or more elevated values (FCG more than 4.95 mmol/litre, 2 hour more than 6.6 mmol/litre) or if four profiles had at least one elevated value during a 2 week period. Insulin dose was adjusted to achieve FCG less than 4.95 mmol/litre and 2 hour postprandial less than 6.6 mmol/litre. In the intervention group 40% (40) of women met the criteria for insulin. In the control group 30% (30) met the criteria for insulin. There was no difference between the intervention and control groups in rates of caesarean section (18% versus 19%), LGA babies (12% versus 10%), SGA babies (12% versus 13%) or any other neonatal outcome. [EL = 1+]

An RCT compared 151 women with gestational diabetes managed according to ultrasound assessment of abdominal circumference with 78 women in a control group who were conventionally managed (self-monitoring of blood glucose plus diet or self-monitoring plus diet and insulin).[180] Ultrasound examinations were scheduled every 2 weeks in the intervention group and at 34–38 weeks of gestation in the control group. Blood glucose targets for the control group were 5 mmol/litre fasting and 6.6 mmol/litre postprandial. Blood glucose targets for the intervention group were 4.4 mmol/litre fasting and 5.5 mmol/litre postprandial if ≥ 75th abdominal circumference centile, and 5.5 mmol/litre fasting and 7.7 mmol/litre postprandial if < 75th abdominal circumference centile. Insulin treatment was required in 16.7% of the control group and 30.5% of the intervention group ($P = 0.024$). The intervention group had significantly lower incidence of macrosomia (3.3% versus 11.5%, $P < 0.05$) and babies who were LGA (7.9% versus 17.9%, $P < 0.05$). [EL = 1+]

An RCT involving 141 women with gestational diabetes investigated the gestational age considered adequate for ultrasound assessment of abdominal circumference to prevent fetal overgrowth.[181] Seventy-three of the women were evaluated at both 28 weeks of and 32 weeks of gestation and 68 women at 32 weeks of gestation only. In both groups, insulin therapy was started when abdominal circumference of the baby exceeded the 75th percentile. Babies of women who had ultrasound assessment only at 32 weeks of gestation had a significantly higher percentage of macrosomic babies compared with women evaluated at 28 weeks of and 32 weeks of gestation (71.43% versus 33.33%, $P < 0.05$). The findings suggest that fetal ultrasound assessment at 28 weeks of gestation and early introduction of insulin therapy should be encouraged since insulin administration after 32 weeks of gestation is less effective in lowering the rate of macrosomic babies. [EL = 1++]

Oral hypoglycaemic agents

Two RCTs and four cohort studies were identified that considered the use of glibenclamide in women with gestational diabetes.

One RCT[74] enrolled 404 women with gestational diabetes. Approximately 83% were Hispanic, 12% were white and 5% were black. All women were Medicaid recipients. Women were randomly assigned at 11–33 weeks of gestation to receive either glibenclamide ($n = 201$) or insulin ($n = 203$). The mean blood glucose concentrations during treatment were 5.9 ± 0.9 mmol/litre in the glibenclamide group and 5.9 ± 1.0 mmol/litre in the insulin group ($P = 0.99$). Eight women (4%) in the glibenclamide group required insulin treatment. There were no significant differences between the glibenclamide and insulin groups in the percentage of babies who were LGA (12%

versus 13%), macrosomic (7% versus 4%), had lung complications (8% versus 6%), neonatal hypoglycaemia (9% versus 6%), admission to NICU (6% versus 7%) or fetal anomalies (2% and 2%). Cord-serum insulin concentrations were similar in the two groups and glibenclamide was not detected in the cord serum of any baby in the glibenclamide group. Four women in the glibenclamide group and 41 women in the insulin group had blood glucose concentrations less than 2.2 mmol/litre ($P = 0.03$). [EL = 1++]

The other RCT compared 27 women with gestational diabetes assigned to insulin therapy, 24 women assigned to glibenclamide therapy and 19 assigned to acarbose therapy.[182] Whenever maximum dose of oral hypoglycaemic agents was reached without reaching glucose control, this therapy was replaced by insulin therapy. Glucose control was not achieved in five women in the glibenclamide group (20.8%) and eight women in the acarbose group (42.1%). No maternal hypoglycaemia requiring hospital admission was reported. There were no significant differences in fasting or postprandial glucose levels or in mean birthweights in the three groups. The rate of LGA was 3.7% in the insulin group, 25% in the glibenclamide group and 10.5% in the acarbose group ($P = 0.073$). Neonatal hypoglycaemia was observed in one baby in the insulin group, one baby in the acarbose group and six babies in the glibenclamide group ($P = 0.006$). [EL = 1+]

A cohort study compared 236 women treated using glibenclamide with 268 historical controls treated using insulin.[183] The study population was a large US managed care organisation in which the extremes of socio-economic distribution were excluded. In the glibenclamide group, 28 women (12%) switched to insulin: eight for side effects primarily attributed to hypoglycaemia and 14 for poor control (for six the reason was not clear). For these women the mean BMI was 31.6 kg/m², mean fasting level on OGTT 5.7 mmol/litre and mean pregnancy weight gain 11.6 kg. Only three women who switched for poor control were on the maximum dose of 20 mg/day. An additional 11 (5%) discontinued glibenclamide (most for side effects attributed to hypoglycaemia) and never started insulin. There were no significant differences between the two groups in birthweight, macrosomia or caesarean section rates. After logistic regression (adjusting for BMI, ethnicity, gestational age at diagnosis, FPG on OGTT) glibenclamide treatment was significantly more likely to be associated with achieving mean glucose goals (adjusted OR 0.27, 95% CI 0.13 to 0.52). Women in the glibenclamide group were more likely to have pre-eclampsia (adjusted OR 2.32, 95% CI 1.17 to 4.63), but their babies were less likely to be admitted to a NICU (adjusted OR 0.7, 95% CI 0.34 to 0.93). Three babies in the insulin group had birth injuries (one clavicle fracture, one brachial plexus injury and one bone injury). Eight babies in the glibenclamide group had birth injuries (four clavicle fractures, one brachial plexus injury and three bone injuries). [EL = 2++]

A cohort study reported on 75 women with gestational diabetes treated using glibenclamide.[184] In the study institution, targets for blood glucose for women with gestational diabetes were mean level 5.8 mmol/litre or less, fasting 5.2 mmol/litre or less and 2 hour postprandial 6.3 mmol/litre or less. If good control was not achieved within 2 weeks of diet women were offered glibenclamide as an alternative to insulin. Eighty-four percent (63/75) of women treated using glibenclamide achieved good glycaemic control, 16% (12) switched to insulin prior to birth. The two groups were similar in terms of baseline characteristics and diabetes risk factors but women who were successfully treated using glibenclamide had significantly lower values on the OGTT. Fasting levels of 5.2 mmol/litre or more detected 92% of women who converted to insulin but had a false-positive rate of 70%. [EL = 2+]

A cohort study reported outcomes for 197 women with gestational diabetes.[185] Eighty-two percent of women had a BMI more than 30 kg/m² and 33% had BMI more than 40 kg/m². The targets for blood glucose control were mean plasma fasting glucose 5 mmol/litre or less and mean 1 hour value 7.4 mmol/litre or less. Sixty-three percent (124) of women achieved satisfactory blood glucose control with diet alone and 37% (73) required glibenclamide. Women in the glibenclamide group were significantly more likely to be morbidly obese than the group controlled by diet ($P < 0.05$). Of the 73 women treated using glibenclamide, 59 (81%, 95% CI 76.4% to 86.6%) had acceptable glucose control on medical therapy. Nine women experienced side effects (four malaise and weakness, two nausea, one light headedness, two symptoms of hypoglycaemia), of which one woman discontinued the therapy. In the 59 women whose gestational diabetes was controlled with glibenclamide, 11 (19%) had babies who weighed more than 4000 g. Forty-nine percent (36/73) required caesarean section; 9% had caesarean sections because of labour abnormalities or suspected macrosomia (compared with 14–17% primary caesarean section rate in the general obstetric population). [EL = 2+]

A cohort study compared 27 women with gestational diabetes managed with diet to 30 women treated using insulin and 25 women treated using glibenclamide.[186] The aim of the study was to assess the prevalence of hypoglycaemia by 72 hour continuous glucose monitoring. There were no symptomatic or significant hypoglycaemic episodes in any group. Overall asymptomatic hypoglycaemic episodes were recorded in 26/82 (31%) of women with gestational diabetes in comparison with 0/35 non-diabetic controls. Asymptomatic hypoglycaemic events were identified in 19 out of 30 (63%) insulin-treated women and 7/25 (28%) glibenclamide-treated women ($P = 0.009$, OR 4.4, 95% CI 1.4–13.9). No hypoglycaemic events were identified in women with gestational diabetes treated by diet alone. [EL = 2++]

An RCT of metformin for the treatment of gestational diabetes (the MIG trial) is due to report soon. A pilot study randomised 14 women to insulin and 16 to metformin. There were no differences in perinatal outcomes.[75]

Insulin analogues
An RCT randomly allocated 42 women with insulin-requiring gestational diabetes to either insulin lispro or regular insulin.[187] The women receiving insulin lispro had significantly lower glucose excursions after a test meal and experienced fewer episodes of hypoglycaemia. There was no difference in obstetric or fetal outcomes. [EL = 1++]

A further RCT evaluated pregnancy outcomes in 23 women with gestational diabetes who used rapid- or long-acting insulin.[188] Insulin dose was raised in six of the 11 pregnant women on rapid-acting insulin and birthweight was higher in the long-acting insulin group (3943 g ± 492 g versus 3079 g ± 722 g, $P = 0.005$). There were no differences in the mode of birth, neonatal complications, malformations, number of babies with Apgar score less than 7 at 1 minute or maternal HbA$_{1c}$ between the groups. The study suggests that gestational diabetes can be treated using rapid-acting insulin. [EL = 1+]

An RCT compared 24 women with gestational diabetes treated using insulin lispro to 24 women with gestational diabetes treated using regular human insulin and 50 women with a normal GCT.[85] The 1 hour postprandial blood glucose values were significantly higher in the regular insulin group than in the lispro or control groups. The rate of babies with a cranial : thoracic circumference ratio between the 10th and 25th percentile was significantly higher in the group treated using regular insulin compared with the lispro and control groups. There were no other differences in neonatal outcomes between the three groups. [EL = 1+]

An RCT allocated 35 women to either insulin lispro or regular human insulin.[4] Glucose response to a test meal was significantly lower in the lispro group. Occurrence of hypoglycaemia during a 6 week period was 25% lower in the lispro group. There was no difference between groups in glycosylated protein levels or anti-insulin antibodies.

A small RCT randomised 27 women with gestational diabetes to either insulin aspart or regular human insulin.[80] The trial period extended from the diagnosis of gestational diabetes (18–28 weeks) to 6 weeks postpartum. There was no significant difference in mean reduction in HbA$_{1c}$ over the trial period (0.3 ± 0.5% for insulin aspart versus 0.1 ± 0.4% for human insulin). The safety profile for both groups was similar. [EL = 1+]

A crossover study randomised 15 women with gestational diabetes to no insulin, insulin aspart or regular human insulin.[189] The glucose areas under the curve following a test meal were significantly lower with insulin aspart compared with no insulin, but not with regular human insulin. [EL = 1+]

A prospective paired study[190] tested two insulin-meal intervals to evaluate their effects on short-term glucose fluctuations in women with tightly controlled gestational diabetes. Insulin-meal intervals of 15 minutes avoided preprandial hypoglycaemia without increasing 2 hour postprandial hyperglycaemia and so were beneficial compared with 30 minute intervals. [EL = 2–]

Education
A descriptive study[191] compared a hospital outpatient-based nursing intervention and traditional office-based care provided by obstetricians using a research model involving three types of

variables: input variables (risk factors before pregnancy), moderating variables (conditions that occur during pregnancy) and outcome variables (normal versus abnormal outcomes for women and babies). The nurse-led education did not reduce the risk of abnormal outcomes for women or babies, but there was a significantly greater risk of having a baby with one or more abnormal outcomes in first-time mothers, women with gestational diabetes treated pharmacologically and women with gestational diabetes experiencing complications. [EL = 3]

Outcomes and risks for the woman and baby
No specific searches were undertaken to identify the outcomes and risks for women with gestational diabetes and their babies. Publications identified in searches for other sections of the guideline show that women with gestational diabetes are at increased risk of having a macrosomic baby, trauma during birth to themselves and the baby, neonatal hypoglycaemia, perinatal death, induction of labour and caesarean section (see Sections 4.2, 5.4, 5.5, 6.1 and 8.2). [EL = 2–3]

Evidence statement

A high-quality RCT has shown that diagnosis and intervention for gestational diabetes (as defined by the WHO) improves maternal and fetal outcomes.

A diet that is high in carbohydrates of low glycaemic index improves overall glucose control and reduces postprandial glucose excursions. In women who are obese, moderate calorie restriction improves glycaemic control without resulting in ketonaemia. Exercise in conjunction with diet improves blood glucose control over and above the improvement achieved by diet alone, and may reduce the need for insulin.

Between 82% and 93% of women with gestational diabetes will achieve blood glucose targets on diet alone. In women requiring hypoglycaemic therapy (those in whom ultrasound investigation suggests incipient fetal macrosomia (abdominal circumference above the 70th percentile) at diagnosis), between 79% and 96% of women will achieve blood glucose targets on glibenclamide. The relative prevalence of maternal hypoglycaemia and LGA babies compared with insulin therapy differs between studies. Insulin lispro reduces postprandial glucose excursions and hypoglycaemic episodes compared with regular insulin, with no difference in other maternal or fetal outcomes. Insulin aspart may reduce postprandial excursions in women with gestational diabetes compared with regular insulin, with no difference in other maternal or fetal outcomes.

Women with gestational diabetes are at increased risk of having a macrosomic baby, trauma during birth to themselves and the baby, neonatal hypoglycaemia, perinatal death, induction of labour and caesarean section.

Two studies that may inform future NICE guidelines on the management of diabetes in pregnancy are the HAPO study (an international multicentre prospective cohort study designed to establish the level of hyperglycaemia that results in a significant risk of adverse pregnancy outcome) and the MIG trial (an RCT of metformin for treatment of gestational diabetes). Neither study has reported in time for inclusion in this guideline.

Cost-effectiveness

The effectiveness of screening, diagnosis and treatment (including monitoring) for gestational diabetes was identified by the GDG as a priority for health economic analysis. The analysis of cost-effectiveness was addressed through joint work with the GDG for the NICE antenatal care guideline update. The methods and results from the health economic modelling are summarised here; further details are provided in Appendix D.

Eight publications were identified in the health economics literature in relation to cost-effectiveness of screening and/or treatment for gestational diabetes. None of the published studies answered the specific cost-effectiveness question addressed by the combined GDGs.

The ACHOIS trial demonstrated potential benefit of treatment for (mild) gestational diabetes.[153] Evidence of clinical effectiveness is not always sufficient for a treatment to be cost-effective. Often the people who would benefit from treatment must be identified from among a larger group of people, some of whom do not require treatment. This is the case with gestational diabetes; the cost-effectiveness of screening and treatment for gestational diabetes are highly interdependent. As a result, a single decision-analytic health economic model was developed to help the combined GDGs make recommendations in relation to screening and treatment for gestational diabetes (see Appendix D).

The health economic model considered screening based on risk factors (age, ethnicity, BMI and family history of gestational diabetes) and/or blood tests (random blood glucose, FPG and a 1 hour 50 g GCT) followed by a diagnostic test (2 hour 75 g OGTT). The possibility of universal diagnostic testing was also considered. The treatment alternatives considered in the model were diet, oral hypoglycaemic agents (glibenclamide and metformin) and insulin. All women diagnosed with gestational diabetes were assumed to undertake self monitoring of blood glucose, regardless of which form of treatment they were using.

Under the baseline assumptions of the health economic model, two screening stategies were not dominated by other strategies. A strategy of offering an OGTT to women from high-risk ethnic backgrounds had an ICER of £3,678 compared with no screening or treatment. A strategy of offering an OGTT to all women defined by the American Diabetes Association as being at high risk of gestational diabetes (i.e. women older than 25 years or BMI above 27 kg/m² or family history of diabetes or high-risk ethnic background) had an ICER of £21,739 compared with screening based on ethnicity alone. However, the combined GDGs expressed concern over the number of women that would undergo an OGTT if the American Diabetes Association screening strategy were recommended because a large proportion of women would be tested based on age criteria alone. Using age as a risk factor for screening has a high sensitivity (i.e. it will identify the majority of women with gestational diabetes). Due to data limitations it was not possible to evaluate the cost-effectiveness of using a combination of the individual risk factors considered in the model (see Appendix D). In the absence of this possibility, an analysis of the cost-effectiveness of each individual risk factor followed by an OGTT was conducted, with each strategy being compared with a strategy of no screening or treatment. The ICERs for ethnicity, BMI and family history were £6,936, £12,737 and £5,209, respectively. All of these are below the £20,000 per quality-adjusted life year (QALY) threshold used by NICE as a willingness to pay for cost-effectiveness and so each one could be regarded as being cost-effective.

Given that some form of screening followed by treatment as outlined in the ACHOIS trial is cost-effective, the cost-effectiveness of different treatment options can be considered separately. An RCT has shown that insulin and glibenclamide are equally effective and, since glibenclamide is cheaper than insulin, it is straightforward to show that glibenclamide is cost-effective. There are currently no data available for comparing the clinical effectiveness of metformin to insulin for the treatment of gestational diabetes. However, the MIG trial currently in progress should provide data on the effectiveness of metformin compared with insulin. Given that metformin is even cheaper than glibenclamide, metformin would be cost-effective if its clinical effectiveness were equal to or greater than that of insulin.

From evidence to recommendations

Currently an unselected pregnant population will have the risk of gestational diabetes assessed using the risk factors identified in Section 4.1, namely:

* BMI more than 30 kg/m²
* previous macrosomic baby weighing 4.5 kg or more
* previous gestational diabetes
* family history of diabetes (first-degree relative with diabetes)
* family origin with a high prevalence of diabetes:
  – South Asian (specifically women whose country of family origin is India, Pakistan or Bangladesh)
  – black Caribbean
  – Middle Eastern (specifically women whose country of family origin is Saudi Arabia, United Arab Emirates, Iraq, Jordan, Syria, Oman, Qatar, Kuwait, Lebanon or Egypt).

Approximately 20–50% of women will have a positive screening result using these risk factors with proportions varying considerably from one geographical area to another.

According to a 1999 survey,[192] 67% of UK maternity service providers currently screen using a combination of these factors.

Whilst screening using risk factors is less sensitive than performing a GCT or OGTT, it is more practical and less disruptive for women. The biochemical tests considered (GCT, FPG, random blood glucose and urine testing) perform only moderately well in terms of diagnostic value.

Given that screening, diagnosis and treatment for gestational diabetes has been shown to be cost-effective, the GDG for the diabetes in pregnancy guideline is of the opinion that gestational diabetes should be treated initially with diet and exercise. If near-normal blood glucose is not achieved by diet and exercise alone, or if ultrasound scans suggest fetal macrosomia, hypoglycaemic therapy should be considered. Clinically effective hypoglycaemic therapy includes oral hypoglycaemic agents (metformin and glibenclamide) and insulin therapy using regular human insulin or rapid-acting insulin analogues. Health economic analysis has demonstrated that glibenclamide is cost-effective, but the clinical evidence comes from a healthcare setting outside the UK and the GDG's view is that the acceptability to women of treating gestational diabetes with glibenclamide has not been demonstrated in the NHS healthcare setting. An RCT investigating the effectiveness of metformin as a treatment for gestational diabetes is due to report imminently. If treatment with metformin is shown to be as effective as treatment with insulin then it is likely to be cost-effective because metformin is considerably cheaper than glibenclamide. The GDG has, therefore, recommended that hypoglycaemic therapy for women with gestational diabetes be tailored to the glycaemic profile of the individual and acceptability to the woman.

Women with gestational diabetes should be informed that they are at increased risk of having a macrosomic baby, trauma during birth to themselves and the baby, neonatal hypoglycaemia, perinatal death, induction of labour and caesarean section. They should also be informed about the role of diet, body weight and exercise, the importance of maternal glycaemic control during labour and birth and early feeding of the baby in order to reduce the risk of neonatal hypoglycaemia, and the risk of the baby developing obesity and/or diabetes in later life.

Recommendations for screening, diagnosis and treatment for gestational diabetes

Screening for gestational diabetes using risk factors is recommended in a healthy population. At the booking appointment, the following risk factors for gestational diabetes should be determined:[*]

- body mass index above 30 kg/m²
- previous macrosomic baby weighing 4.5 kg or above
- previous gestational diabetes
- family history of diabetes (first-degree relative with diabetes)
- family origin with a high prevalence of diabetes:
  - South Asian (specifically women whose country of family origin is India, Pakistan or Bangladesh)
  - black Caribbean
  - Middle Eastern (specifically women whose country of family origin is Saudi Arabia, United Arab Emirates, Iraq, Jordan, Syria, Oman, Qatar, Kuwait, Lebanon or Egypt).

Women with any one of these risk factors should be offered testing for gestational diabetes.

In order to make an informed decision about screening and testing for gestational diabetes, women should be informed that:[*]

- in most women, gestational diabetes will respond to changes in diet and exercise
- some women (between 10% and 20%) will need oral hypoglycaemic agents or insulin therapy if diet and exercise are not effective in controlling gestational diabetes
- if gestational diabetes is not detected and controlled there is a small risk of birth complications such as shoulder dystocia
- a diagnosis of gestational diabetes may lead to increased monitoring and interventions during both pregnancy and labour.

Screening for gestational diabetes using fasting plasma glucose, random blood glucose, glucose challenge test and urinalysis for glucose should not be undertaken.[*]

---

[*] This recommendation is taken from 'Antenatal care: routine care for the healthy pregnant woman' (NICE clinical guideline 62), available from www.nice.org.uk/CG062.

The 2 hour 75 g oral glucose tolerance test (OGTT) should be used to test for gestational diabetes and diagnosis made using the criteria defined by the World Health Organization*. Women who have had gestational diabetes in a previous pregnancy should be offered early self-monitoring of blood glucose or OGTT at 16–18 weeks, and a further OGTT at 28 weeks if the results are normal. Women with any of the other risk factors for gestational diabetes should be offered an OGTT at 24–28 weeks.

Women with gestational diabetes should be instructed in self-monitoring of blood glucose. Targets for blood glucose control should be determined in the same way as for women with pre-existing diabetes.

Women with gestational diabetes should be informed that good glycaemic control throughout pregnancy will reduce the risk of fetal macrosomia, trauma during birth (to themselves and the baby), induction of labour or caesarean section, neonatal hypoglycaemia and perinatal death.

Women with gestational diabetes should be offered information covering:

- the role of diet, body weight and exercise
- the increased risk of having a baby who is large for gestational age, which increases the likelihood of birth trauma, induction of labour and caesarean section
- the importance of maternal glycaemic control during labour and birth and early feeding of the baby in order to reduce the risk of neonatal hypoglycaemia
- the possibility of transient morbidity in the baby during the neonatal period, which may require admission to the neonatal unit
- the risk of the baby developing obesity and/or diabetes in later life.

Women with gestational diabetes should be advised to choose, where possible, carbohydrates from low glycaemic index sources, lean proteins including oily fish and a balance of polyunsaturated fats and monounsaturated fats.

Women with gestational diabetes whose pre-pregnancy body mass index was above 27 kg/m² should be advised to restrict calorie intake (to 25 kcal/kg/day or less) and to take moderate exercise (of at least 30 minutes daily).

Hypoglycaemic therapy should be considered for women with gestational diabetes if diet and exercise fail to maintain blood glucose targets during a period of 1–2 weeks.

Hypoglycaemic therapy should be considered for women with gestational diabetes if ultrasound investigation suggests incipient fetal macrosomia (abdominal circumference above the 70th percentile) at diagnosis.

Hypoglycaemic therapy for women with gestational diabetes (which may include regular insulin,[†] rapid-acting insulin analogues [aspart and lispro[†]] and/or hypoglycaemic agents [metformin[†] and glibenclamide[†]] should be tailored to the glycaemic profile of, and acceptability to, the individual woman.

Research recommendations for screening, diagnosis and treatment for gestational diabetes

What is the clinical and cost-effectiveness of the three main available screening techniques for gestational diabetes: risk factors, two-stage screening by the glucose challenge test and OGTT, and universal OGTT (with or without fasting)?

Why this is important
Following the Australian carbohydrate intolerance study in pregnant women (ACHOIS) it seems that systematic screening for gestational diabetes may be beneficial to the UK population. A multicentre randomised controlled trial is required to test the existing screening techniques, which have not been systematically evaluated for clinical and cost-effectiveness (including acceptability) within the UK.

---

* Fasting plasma venous glucose concentration greater than or equal to 7.0 mmol/litre or 2 hour plasma venous glucose concentration greater than or equal to 7.8 mmol/litre. World Health Organization Department of Noncommunicable Disease Surveillance (1999) *Definition, diagnosis and classification of diabetes mellitus and its complications. Report of a WHO consultation. Part 1: diagnosis and classification of diabetes mellitus.* Geneva: World Health Organization.

† This drug does not have UK marketing authorisation specifically for pregnant and breastfeeding women at the time of publication (March 2008). Informed consent should be obtained and documented.

5 Antenatal care

5.1 Target ranges for blood glucose during pregnancy

Description of the evidence

Fetal macrosomia

The term macrosomia is often used to describe birthweight more than 4000 g. It is also sometimes used to refer to birthweight ≥ 90th percentile for gestational age, which is also referred to as LGA. There are two types of macrosomia: symmetric and asymmetric. Symmetric macrosomia accounts for about 70% of cases. In symmetric macrosomia the baby is big but the only potential problem is trauma during birth. Symmetric macrosomia may also occur in women without diabetes. Asymmetric macrosomia is characterised by thoracic and abdominal circumference that is relatively larger than the head circumference. The baby is at risk of shoulder dystocia, clavicular fracture and brachial palsy and, as a consequence, the woman is more likely to undergo caesarean section. It has also been suggested that babies with asymmetric macrosomia may be at increased risk of obesity, coronary heart disease, hypertension and type 2 diabetes later in life.[193] [EL = 3]

Eleven studies were identified that examined the relationship between birthweight and blood glucose control during pregnancy.

A non-randomised intervention study in women with gestational diabetes[194] compared intensive ($n = 1316$) and conventional ($n = 1145$) management. All women were diagnosed by a 1 hour glucose challenge test (GCT) followed by a 100 g OGTT if plasma glucose was 7.2 mmol/litre or more. In the intensive management group women were assigned memory reflectance meters and were instructed by nurses in self-monitoring of blood glucose (seven times a day: fasting, preprandial, 2 hour postprandial and at bedtime). In the conventional management group women were instructed by a nurse and were assessed weekly for fasting and 3 hour postprandial venous plasma glucose during clinic visits. The women performed four daily self-monitored blood glucose determinations with glucose strips (fasting and 2 hours after breakfast, lunch and dinner). Assignment to groups depended on the availability of reflectance meters. There were no significant differences between groups with regard to parity, ethnicity, obesity, obstetric history or family history. Women in the intensive group had a mean blood glucose of 5 ± 2 mmol/litre. Women in the conventional group were significantly more likely to have a macrosomic baby (13.6% versus 7.1%, RR 2.07, 95% CI 1.6 to 2.8, $P < 0.0001$), caesarean section (19% versus 13%, $P < 0.01$), augmentation of labour (28% versus 15%, $P < 0.01$), induction of labour (27% versus 22%, $P < 0.01$), a longer hospital stay (mean 4.3 days versus 3.7 days, $P < 0.01$) and a baby admitted to intensive care (25% versus 6.3%, $P < 0.0001$). [EL = 2++]

A cohort study of 75 women with type 1 diabetes[195] compared women with mean capillary blood glucose (CBG) less than 6.0 mmol/litre during the second and third trimesters ($n = 43$) to women with mean CBG more than 6.0 mmol/litre ($n = 32$). Women with mean CBG more than 6.0 mmol/litre during the second and third trimesters were significantly more likely to have a macrosomic baby (28% versus 17%, $P < 0.05$). [EL = 2++]

In a cohort study of 66 women with diabetes (22 with type 1 diabetes, four with type 2 diabetes, 41 with gestational diabetes) 13 (20%) had at least one of the following ultrasound markers for macrosomia: estimated fetal weight > 90th percentile for gestational age using the Williams growth curve; polyhydramnios (amniotic fluid index 25 cm or more or one fluid pocket 8 cm or more) or fat line (5 mm or more subcutaneous tissue near the level of the umbilical vein insertion).[196] Of these 13, ten had HbA_{1c} more than 6.3% and also had birthweight macrosomia. There was a significant difference in HbA_{1c} between those with markers and those without ($P < 0.03$). [EL = 2++]

A cohort study of 127 women with type 1 diabetes[197] found 43% of babies were LGA. The HbA_1 at birth was significantly higher in women whose babies who were LGA than those who had appropriate-for-gestational-age (AGA) babies (8.4 ± 0.3% versus 7. 6 ± 0.2%, $P < 0.05$). Insulin dose, maternal weight gain and glucose control during the first two trimesters did not influence the incidence of LGA. [EL = 2++]

A cohort study compared 52 women with type 1 diabetes to 52 women without diabetes.[198] The women with diabetes maintained 'normal' blood glucose levels from the 12 weeks of gestation (defined as a fasting level of 3.0–3.6 mmol/litre, a mean blood glucose level of 4.4–4.8 mmol/litre and postprandial level not exceeding 7 7 mmol/litre). The mean infant body weight was 2910 g with no babies above the 75th percentile. [EL = 2+]

HbA_{1c} or postprandial peaks

A cohort study of 289 women with type 1 diabetes[199] found high rates of macrosomia (48.8%) despite good glycaemic control, as measured by HbA_{1c}. HbA_{1c} in the third trimester was the most powerful predictor of macrosomia, but it explained less than 5% of the variance. A possible explanation for the finding is that HbA_{1c} is not predictive of macrosomia as it fails to detect the more relevant postprandial peaks in blood glucose. [EL = 2++]

A cohort study compared 323 women with type 1 diabetes and 361 women without diabetes.[200] Women with diabetes were significantly more likely to have an LGA baby (> 90th percentile) than women without diabetes (18.5% versus 13.1%, $P < 0.001$). The strongest predictor of birthweight was third-trimester non-fasting glucose levels ($P = 0.001$). [EL = 2++]

A cohort study of 111 women with type 1 diabetes[201] found macrosomia in 32 (29%) babies. In logistic regression the only variable that was associated with macrosomia was postprandial glucose between 29 and 32 weeks of gestation ($P < 0.05$). Postprandial values less than 7.3 mmol/litre were associated with an increased risk of SGA babies (18%) compared with values above this level (1%). [EL = 2++]

An RCT involving 66 women with gestational diabetes[155] who required insulin therapy at 30 weeks of gestation or earlier randomly assigned women to monitor either preprandial or 1 hour postprandial blood glucose levels.[155] The goal of insulin therapy was a preprandial value of 3.3–5.9 mmol/litre or a postprandial value less than 7.8 mmol/litre. The pre-pregnancy weight, weight gain during pregnancy, gestational age at diagnosis of gestational diabetes and at birth, degree of adherence to therapy and degree of achievement of target blood glucose concentrations were similar in both groups. There were 3/33 (9%) macrosomic babies in the postprandial monitoring group compared with 12/33 (36%) in the preprandial monitoring group ($P = 0.01$). Women in the postprandial group were significantly less likely to have a caesarean section for cephalopelvic disproportion (12% versus 36%, $P = 0.04$) and a baby with neonatal hypoglycaemia (3% versus 21%, $P = 0.05$). There were also fewer instances of shoulder dystocia (3% versus 18%) and third or fourth degree perineal laceration (9% versus 24%). [EL = 1+]

An RCT of 61 women with type 1 diabetes[202] randomly assigned women at 16 weeks of gestation to preprandial or postprandial blood glucose monitoring. Maternal age, parity, age at onset of diabetes, number of prior miscarriages, smoking status, social class, weight gain in pregnancy and adherence to therapy were similar in the two groups. The postprandial monitoring group had a significantly reduced incidence of pre-eclampsia (3% versus 21%, $P < 0.05$), a greater success in achieving glycaemic control targets (55% versus 30%, $P < 0.001$) and smaller neonatal triceps skinfold thickness (4.5 ± 0.9 versus 5.1 ± 1.3, $P = 0.05$). [EL = 1+]

A study of 51 pregnant women without diabetes[203] who monitored their blood glucose from 28–38 weeks found overall mean blood glucose during the third trimester to be 3.11 mmol/litre. The mean peak postprandial response occurred 1 hour postprandially and never exceeded 5.84 mmol/litre. There was a significant association between fetal abdominal circumference and 1 hour postprandial glucose values ($P < 0.0003$) and a significant negative relationship between head : abdominal circumference ratio ($P = 0.001$). The findings from this study indicate that there is a continuum, even in the normal range, of degrees of hyperglycaemia and overgrowth. [EL = 2++]

Respiratory distress

In a study of 180 babies in 179 women (20 with gestational diabetes and 160 with type 1 diabetes) mean blood glucose was calculated for the period from gestational week 30–32 until birth.[204]

Respiratory distress was significantly more frequent in women with mean blood glucose more than 5.5 mmol/litre. [EL = 2+]

A cohort study of 75 women with type 1 diabetes[195] compared women with mean CBG less than 6.0 mmol/litre ($n = 43$) to women with mean capillary glucose more than 6.0 mmol/litre ($n = 32$). Respiratory distress was significantly more frequent in babies of women with mean CBG above 6.0 mmol/litre (21.8% versus 2.3%, $P < 0.01$). [EL = 2++]

A cohort study compared 52 women with type 1 diabetes to 52 women without diabetes.[198] The women with diabetes maintained 'normal' blood glucose levels (defined as a fasting level of 3.0–3.6 mmol/litre, a mean blood glucose level of 4.4–4.8 mmol/litre and postprandial level not exceeding 7.7 mmol/litre) from 12 weeks of gestation. There were no cases of respiratory distress in babies of women with type 1 diabetes compared to five cases in women without diabetes ($P < 0.03$). [EL = 2+]

Preterm labour
A cohort study of 145 women with type 1 diabetes recruited during the first trimester considered the relationship between glycaemic control and preterm labour.[205] Logistic regression found HbA$_{1c}$ at 26 weeks of gestation and urogenital infection to predict the onset of preterm labour. [EL = 2++]

Congenital malformations, stillbirth and neonatal death
A cohort study of women with type 1 diabetes considered the relationship between glycaemic control during pregnancy and the incidence of minor congenital malformations.[206] Thirty-nine minor congenital malformations were diagnosed in 32 babies (18.7%). There were significant differences in HbA$_{1c}$ between the group with minor malformations and the group without malformations at 12, 16 and 20 weeks of gestation, but not at 8 or 24 weeks of gestation. [EL = 2+]

In a cohort study of 180 babies in 179 women (20 with gestational diabetes and 160 with type 1 diabetes) mean blood glucose was calculated for the period from gestational week 30–32 until birth.[204] Malformations and perinatal death were more frequent in women with mean blood glucose more than 5.5 mmol/litre ($P < 0.05$). [EL = 2+]

The association between first-trimester HbA$_{1c}$ levels and risk of adverse pregnancy outcomes of women with type 1 diabetes was evaluated in a cohort study[207] involving 573 pregnant women with type 1 diabetes. One hundred and sixty-five (29%) of the pregnancies terminated with adverse outcomes (congenital anomaly, morbidity of the baby diagnosed within the first month of life and mortality). HbA$_{1c}$ levels above 7% showed almost linear association with risk of adverse outcome, with every 1% increase in HbA$_{1c}$ corresponding to 5.5% increased risk of adverse outcome. The prevalence of adverse outcomes varied six-fold, from 12% (95% CI 7.2% to 17%) in the lowest quintile of HbA$_{1c}$ measurements to 79% (95% CI 60% to 91%) in the highest quintile. The data show a dose-dependent association between HbA$_{1c}$ levels above 7% in the first trimester and risk of adverse pregnancy outcome. [EL = 2++]

Tight versus very tight control
A systematic review and meta-analysis of tight versus very tight control for diabetes in pregnancy identified two small RCTs involving 182 women. In one study the aim was to keep all blood glucose levels less than 5.6 mmol/litre in the very tight group. In the other study the aim for the very tight group were fasting values less than 4.4 mmol/litre and postprandial values less than 6.7 mmol/litre. Maternal hypoglycaemia was common among women whose diabetic control was very tight (1 trial, 45 women, OR 25.96 95% CI 4.91–137.26). There were no detected differences in perinatal outcome.[208] [EL = 1+]

Current practice
A CEMACH audit[2] of 3733 women in England, Wales and Northern Ireland with pre-existing type 1 or type 2 diabetes who gave birth between March 2002 and February 2003 (3808 pregnancies) reported that women who had babies with malformations, stillbirth or neonatal death had worse glycaemic control before and during pregnancy. [EL = 3] The proportion of women with HbA$_{1c}$ less than 7% in each trimester is shown in Table 5.1.

Table 5.1 Proportion of women with HbA_{1c} less than 7% in each trimester and birth outcomes[2]

	Pre-pregnancy	< 13 weeks of gestation	18–23 weeks of gestation	27 weeks of gestation
Malformations	22.0%	25.7%	57.3%	58%
Normally formed stillbirths or neonatal deaths	12.9%	19.4%	39.7%	40.0%
Normally formed and alive at 28 days	28.5%	40.3%	70.9%	66.9%

The CEMACH enquiry found 38% of the women who had an HbA_{1c} measurement had a recorded a value of less that 7%.[2] The CEMACH case–control study found sub-optimal glycaemic control was associated with poor pregnancy outcome. Of the women with poor pregnancy outcome 84% (171/204) were documented as having sub-optimal control in the first trimester compared with 61% (117/192) of the women with good pregnancy outcome (OR 3.4, 95% CI 2.1 to 5.7).[33] Of the women with poor pregnancy outcome 71% (146/205) were documented as having sub-optimal control after the first trimester compared with 37% (77/209) of the women with good pregnancy outcome (OR 5.2, 95% CI 3.3 to 8.2). The enquiry panels identified that there were incidents of failure to change insulin regimens, non-responsive local strategy of diabetes antenatal care and problems within the diabetes multidisciplinary team in both groups of women. No local targets were set for glycaemic control during pregnancy for more women who had a poor pregnancy outcome than for women who had a good pregnancy outcome (49% [44/90] versus 33% [28/86], OR 2.0 95% CI 1.1 to 3.8). [EL = 3–4]

The CEMACH enquiry (comparison of women with type 1 and type 2 diabetes) reported that 65% of women with type 1 diabetes and 54% of women with type 2 diabetes had sub-optimal glycaemic control in the first trimester ($P = 0.064$). After the first trimester 41% of women with type 1 diabetes and 35% of women with type 2 diabetes had sub-optimal glycaemic control.[33] [EL = 3–4]

Existing guidance

The NSF for diabetes[20] recommends regular blood glucose monitoring with the aim of maintaining blood glucose within the normal non-diabetic range.

Evidence statement

There is evidence that high blood glucose levels during pregnancy are associated with fetal macrosomia (and associated birth injury and caesarean sections) and fetal morbidity. Postprandial blood glucose levels have a stronger association with incidence of macrosomia than HbA_{1c}. Two RCTs found that monitoring of postprandial blood glucose produced better outcomes than preprandial monitoring. There is evidence that in women without diabetes blood glucose levels in the third trimester of pregnancy are lower than in non-pregnant women.

No evidence was identified to support the clinical utility of HbA_{1c} measurements in the second and third trimesters of pregnancy.

From evidence to recommendations

The evidence suggests that the important intervention for preventing fetal macrosomia is blunting postprandial blood glucose peaks and, therefore, the postprandial blood glucose target for women during pregnancy should be lower than when not pregnant. As in the preconception period, the targets for blood glucose control during pregnancy should be agreed with the individual woman, taking into account the risk of hypoglycaemia. If it is safely achievable, women with diabetes should aim to keep fasting blood glucose between 3.5 and 5.9 mmol/litre and 1 hour postprandial blood glucose below 7.8 mmol/litre during pregnancy.

The GDG's view is that HbA_{1c} is not a reliable indicator of glycaemic control in the second and third trimesters of pregnancy because of physiological changes that occur in all pregnant women and lead to reduced HbA_{1c} in women without diabetes, meaning that any apparent reduction in HbA$_{1c}$ in women with diabetes during the second and third trimesters of pregnancy does not necessarily indicate improved glycaemic control. HbA$_{1c}$ should, therefore, not be used routinely for assessing glycaemic control in the second and third trimesters of pregnancy. This represents a change in clinical practice to avoid unnecessary and misleading HbA$_{1c}$ measurements.

> **Recommendations for target ranges for blood glucose during pregnancy**
>
> Individualised targets for self-monitoring of blood glucose should be agreed with women with diabetes in pregnancy, taking into account the risk of hypoglycaemia.
>
> If it is safely achievable, women with diabetes should aim to keep fasting blood glucose between 3.5 and 5.9 mmol/litre and 1 hour postprandial blood glucose below 7.8 mmol/litre during pregnancy.
>
> HbA$_{1c}$ should not be used routinely for assessing glycaemic control in the second and third trimesters of pregnancy.

There were no research recommendations relating to the target ranges for blood glucose during pregnancy.

5.2 Monitoring blood glucose and ketones during pregnancy

Description of the evidence

Two RCTs were identified that investigated preprandial versus postprandial monitoring of blood glucose during pregnancy.

The first study consisted of 61 women with type 1 diabetes who were randomly assigned at 16 weeks of gestation to either preprandial or postprandial blood glucose monitoring.[202] All women were on a four-times-daily basal bolus insulin regimen. The preprandial group was asked to monitor before breakfast and preprandially. The postprandial group was asked to monitor before breakfast and 1 hour after meals. CBG readings were measured by using a memory-based glucose reflectance meter. Insulin doses and glucose readings were also recorded by diary and brought to the clinic. The postprandial monitoring group had a significantly reduced incidence of pre-eclampsia (3% versus 21%, $P < 0.05$), greater success in achieving glycaemic control targets (55% versus 30%, $P < 0.001$) and smaller neonatal triceps skinfold thickness (4.5 ± 0.9 versus 5.1 ± 1.3, $P = 0.05$). [EL = 1++]

The second study consisted of 66 women with gestational diabetes who required insulin therapy.[155] The ethnic background of the sample was 85% Hispanic, 11% white and 4% black or Asian. Women were randomly assigned to monitor either preprandial or 1 hour postprandial blood glucose levels. The preprandial monitoring protocol required daily monitoring of fasting, preprandial and bedtime CBG concentrations. The postprandial protocol required daily monitoring of blood glucose concentrations before breakfast (fasting) and 1 hour after each meal. The women measured their blood glucose concentration using memory-based reflectance glucometers. All blood glucose values as well as insulin doses and dietary intake were recorded. There were 3/33 (9%) macrosomic babies in the postprandial monitoring group compared with 12/33 (36%) in the preprandial monitoring group ($P = 0.01$). Women in the postprandial group were significantly less likely to have a caesarean section for cephalopelvic disproportion (12% versus 36%, $P = 0.04$) or a baby with neonatal hypoglycaemia (3% versus 21%, $P = 0.05$). There were also fewer instances of shoulder dystocia (3% versus 18%) and third- or fourth-degree perineal laceration (9% versus 24%). [EL = 1++]

The ACHOIS trial randomly assigned 1000 women with gestational diabetes to either an intervention group or routine care.[153] The intervention was a package of care that included instructions on self-monitoring of blood glucose four times daily until blood glucose levels had been in the recommended range for 2 weeks (fasting glucose levels more than 3.5 mmol/litre and 5.5 mmol/litre or less, preprandial levels 5.5 mmol/litre or less and 2 hour postprandial levels 7.0 mmol/litre or less) followed by daily monitoring at rotating times. The package of care also included insulin therapy with the dose adjusted on the basis of glucose levels and individualised dietary advice from a qualified dietitian. The rate of serious perinatal outcomes among babies was significantly lower in the intervention group (1% versus 4%, $P = 0.01$). The number needed to treat to prevent a serious outcome in a baby was 34. There was no significant difference between groups in maternal quality of life. [EL = 1++]

Three studies were identified that reported on the use of continuous blood glucose monitoring in women with diabetes. Two cohort studies were in women with type 1 diabetes[209,210] [EL = 2+] and one case series was in women with gestational diabetes.[211] [EL = 3] All three studies reported hyperglycaemic episodes undetected by self-monitoring of blood glucose. These episodes were usually due to the consumption of high carbohydrate food between meals and were undetected by self-monitoring protocols that required testing only after main meals. The three studies showed that examining 72 hour glucose profiles can help to identify patterns of glucose control, better target insulin treatment, assist in patient education and improve dietary adherence.

A retrospective study[120] examined the effect of an intensive diabetes management programme during pregnancy on women's long-term self-management behaviours and glycaemic control. There was a significant improvement in all diabetes self-management behaviours, including frequency of self-monitoring of blood glucose, frequency of insulin injections, and frequency and complexity of insulin dose adjustment from entry to the programme to the baby's birth. There was also a significant improvement in HbA_{1c} from entry to the baby's birth. [EL = 2−]

An RCT[212] investigated whether glycaemic control achieved by women using telephone modems for the transmission of self-monitored blood glucose data was better than that achieved by women managed in a similar fashion without modem connection. The study showed that telemedicine is a practical way of providing specialist care to pregnant women. [EL = 1+]

A systematic review of observational studies[213] investigated the risk of adverse pregnancy outcomes in pregnant women with diabetes in relation to glycaemic control. The review showed that an increase in adverse pregnancy outcomes in women with diabetes who had poor glycaemic control (congenital malformations, pooled OR 3.44, 95% CI 2.30 to 5.15; risk reduction of congenital malformation 0.39–0.59 for each 1% decrease in HbA_{1c}; miscarriage, pooled OR 3.23, 95% CI 1.64 to 6.36; perinatal mortality, pooled OR 3.03, 95% CI 1.87 to 4.92). [EL = 3]

No studies were identified that assessed how ketones should be monitored during pregnancy.

Existing guidance

The NSF for diabetes[20] recommends that 'women should be supported and encouraged to monitor their blood glucose regularly'.

Evidence statement

Two high quality RCTs have found better pregnancy outcomes for women with diabetes when blood glucose is monitored 1 hour after meals than when it is monitored before meals. One RCT found that a treatment package that included self-monitoring of blood glucose improved outcomes in women with gestational diabetes compared with routine obstetric care. Two cohort studies and a case series showed that self-monitoring of blood glucose undertaken only after main meals may not detect hyperglycaemia following the consumption of food between meals.

No studies were found on monitoring for ketones during pregnancy.

From evidence to recommendations

The evidence regarding the effectiveness of self-monitoring of blood glucose 1 hour after meals for improving pregnancy outcomes suggests that postprandial monitoring should not be restricted to main meals. The effectiveness of monitoring using meters supports the provision of such meters (see Section 3.5).

The GDG's view is that women with insulin-treated diabetes are vulnerable to nocturnal hypoglycaemia during pregnancy and that it is good clinical practice to undertake an additional test before going to bed at night.

As no evidence was identified in relation to monitoring for ketones during pregnancy, the GDG's consensus recommendation based on current best practice is to provide urine and blood ketone testing strips and to advise women to test ketone levels if they are hyperglycaemic or unwell.

Recommendations for monitoring blood glucose and ketones during pregnancy

Women with diabetes should be advised to test fasting blood glucose levels and blood glucose levels 1 hour after every meal during pregnancy.

Women with insulin-treated diabetes should be advised to test blood glucose levels before going to bed at night during pregnancy.

Women with type 1 diabetes who are pregnant should be offered ketone testing strips and advised to test for ketonuria or ketonaemia if they become hyperglycaemic or unwell.

Research recommendations for monitoring blood glucose and ketones during pregnancy

How effective is ambulatory continuous blood glucose monitoring in pregnancies complicated by diabetes?

Why this is important
The technology for performing ambulatory continuous blood glucose monitoring is only just becoming available, so there is currently no evidence to assess its effectiveness outside the laboratory situation. Research is needed to determine whether the technology is likely to have a place in the clinical management of diabetes in pregnancy. The new technology may identify women in whom short-term postprandial peaks of glycaemia are not detected by intermittent blood glucose testing. The aim of monitoring is to adjust insulin regimens to reduce the incidence of adverse outcomes of pregnancy (for example, fetal macrosomia, caesarean section and neonatal hypoglycaemia), so these outcomes should be assessed as part of the research.

5.3   Management of diabetes during pregnancy

Description of the evidence

Hypoglycaemia
Hypoglycaemia significantly affects maternal quality of life and increases the risk of physical injury. During pregnancy the frequency of hypoglycaemia may increase due to intensification of treatment, an impairment of counter-regulatory hormonal responses and an increased risk of hypoglycaemia unawareness.[214,215] Pregnancy nausea and vomiting can also contribute to hypoglycaemia due to fluctuations in carbohydrate ingestion. [EL = 2+]

A cohort study of 84 pregnant women with type 1 diabetes undergoing intensified treatment[68] found hypoglycaemia requiring third-party assistance occurred in 71% of women, with a peak incidence between 10–15 weeks of gestation. Consequences of maternal hypoglycaemia included several grand mal seizures, five episodes of cerebral oedema, and two road traffic accidents and comminuted fracture of the tibia and fibula. [EL = 2++]

Hyperemesis gravidarum
Severe nausea and vomiting in pregnant women with diabetes can lead to ketoacidosis, and DKA during pregnancy carries a risk of fetal death.

Two case studies were identified that reported healthy live births to women with diabetes and hyperemesis gravidarum following treatment with parenteral nutrition.[216,217] One case study reported a fetal death in a woman with hyperemesis gravidarum and DKA following a delay in treatment.[218] [EL = 3]

Diabetic ketoacidosis
A case series of 37 women admitted with DKA[219] concluded that vomiting and the use of betamimetic drugs were the primary cause in 57% of cases. Non-adherence to treatment and physician management errors were the primary cause in 24% of cases and contributory in 16%.

Common physician management errors included the use of urine instead of blood to monitor maternal glucose control, failure to adhere to pregnancy standards of glucose control and failure to employ home blood glucose monitoring. [EL = 3]

A cohort study of 257 people[220] with DKA admitted to a large urban teaching hospital compared outcomes in people treated by a general physician (n = 224) with those in people treated by a physician with subspecialty training in diabetes (n = 33). People treated by a diabetes specialist had shorter length of stay (3.3 versus 4.9 days, P < 0.0043) and incurred lower hospital charges ($5,463 versus $10,109, P < 0.0001). Plasma glucose in generalist-treated people took longer to fall to less than 11.1 mmol/litre and they had a higher rate of readmission for DKA than the specialist-treated people (6% versus 2%, P = 0.03). [EL = 2+]

Rapid-acting insulin analogues
Rapid-acting insulin analogues (aspart and lispro) confer the following benefits compared with regular insulin outside pregnancy:[221]

- fewer episodes of hypoglycaemia
- a reduction in postprandial glucose excursions
- an improvement in overall glycaemic control
- an improvement in patient satisfaction.

These benefits have also been demonstrated in the pregnant population (see Section 3.6).

Long-acting insulin analogues
The NICE guideline for the management of type 1 diabetes recommends the long-acting insulin analogue glargine for use outside of pregnancy.[221] However, no clinical trials have as yet been published for their use in pregnancy (see Section 3.6).

Four-times-daily versus twice-daily insulin regimens
An open label RCT compared glycaemic control and perinatal outcomes in pregnant women with diabetes using two different insulin regimens.[222] One hundred and thirty-eight women with gestational diabetes and 58 with pre-existing diabetes received insulin four times daily, and 136 women with gestational diabetes and 60 with pre-existing diabetes received insulin twice daily. Glycaemic control was better with the four-times-daily regimen than with the twice-daily regimen. In women with gestational diabetes the four-times-daily regimen resulted in a lower rate of overall neonatal morbidity than the twice-daily regimen. Four-times-daily rather than twice-daily insulin improved glycaemic control and perinatal outcomes without increasing the risks of maternal hypoglycaemia and caesarean section. [EL = 1++]

Continuous subcutaneous insulin infusion (insulin pump therapy)
The most widespread method of administering insulin is via subcutaneous insulin injections using a basal/bolus regimen consisting of a basal dose of long-acting insulin, usually administered with a pen before bed, and bolus of rapid-acting insulin given before meals. This is often referred to as a multiple daily injection (MDI) regimen. Insulin can also be administered using CSII (also known as insulin pump therapy). Both regular insulin and rapid-acting insulin can be administered by pump. The potential benefits of CSII are reduced risk of hypoglycaemia, decreased risk of fasting hyperglycaemia and improved adherence as the woman does not have to constantly inject insulin.[223]

NICE guidance for the non-pregnant population concluded that, compared with MDI regimens, CSII results in a modest but worthwhile improvement in blood glucose control and quality of life.[14]

A systematic review[224] investigated the effectiveness of insulin delivery via CSII as compared with MDI regimens for the treatment of diabetes during pregnancy in women with pre-existing diabetes or gestational diabetes. Only two studies were included in the review, neither included women with gestational diabetes. There was a significant increase in mean birthweight associated with CSII as opposed to MDI (two trials, 61 participants, weighted mean difference (WMD) 220.56, 95% CI −2.09 to 443.20). However, taking into consideration the lack of significant difference in rate of macrosomia (birthweight greater than 4000 g; RR 3.20, 95% CI 0.14 to 72.62), this finding was not viewed by the authors as being clinically significant. There were no significant differences in perinatal outcomes between CSII and MDI (perinatal mortality, including stillbirths from 24 weeks of gestation and neonatal deaths up to 7 days of life, RR 2.00, 95% CI 0.20 to 19.91;

fetal anomaly, RR 1.07, 95% CI 0.07 to 15.54; gestational age at birth, WMD 0.63, 95% CI −4.87 to 6.13; neonatal hypoglycaemia, RR 1.00, 95% CI 0.07 to 14.64; and SGA, RR 1.55, 95% CI 0.27 to 9.00). Neither were there any significant differences in maternal outcomes between CSII and MDI (caesarean section rate, RR 1.03, 95% CI 0.57 to 1.84; mean maternal HbA_{1c}; 24 hour mean blood glucose level in each trimester; hypoglycaemia; or hyperglycaemia). [EL1+]

Three further RCTs of CSII in women with type 1 diabetes during pregnancy were identified.[225–227] The studies included a total of 200 women. There were no significant differences between groups in glycaemic control or in obstetric or neonatal outcomes. There were four cases of ketoacidosis in women using pumps. This was attributed to catheter occlusion (one case), catheter leakage (one case) and pump failure (one case). Another case was reported but without attribution. [EL = 1++]

One RCT was designed to assess the effect of CSII on retinopathy.[226] This study of 40 women with type 1 diabetes reported progression to proliferative retinopathy in two women using CSII. This was attributed to rapid and significant improvement in glycaemic control. [EL = 1+]

Three cohort studies compared outcomes in women using CSII with those in women using MDI regimens. [EL = 2+][228] [EL = 2+][229] [EL = 2++][230] In each study women were offered pump therapy due to difficulties achieving glycaemic control. All studies reported good glycaemic control and obstetric and neonatal outcomes.

Current practice
The CEMACH enquiry (comparison of women with type 1 and type 2 diabetes) reported that women with type 1 diabetes were more likely to experience recurrent episodes of hypoglycaemia than women with type 2 diabetes ($P < 0.001$), with 61% (105/171) of women with type 1 diabetes and 21% (25/121) of the women with type 2 diabetes having recurrent episodes of hypoglycaemia.[33] One or more episodes of hypoglycaemia required help in 25% (33/133) of the women with type 1 diabetes and 4% (4/102) of the women with type 2 diabetes. [EL = 3–4]

Existing guidance

The NICE technology appraisal relating to insulin pump therapy (CSII) for people with type 1 diabetes states that insulin pumps can be used in pregnancy even if there is good glycaemic control on MDI regimens.[14]

The Driver and Vehicle Licensing Agency (DVLA) medical rules for drivers do not include any special considerations for diabetes in pregnancy. Fitness to drive is assessed on the basis of the risk of hypoglycaemia, regardless of whether or not the driver is pregnant (see www.dvla.gov.uk/medical. aspx and www.direct.gov.uk/en/Motoring/DriverLicensing/MedicalRulesForDrivers/index.htm).

Evidence statement

During pregnancy women with diabetes treated using insulin are at an increased risk of hypoglycaemia and hypoglycaemia unawareness.

Rapid-acting insulin analogues (aspart and lispro) are associated with fewer episodes of hypoglycaemia compared with regular human insulin. When compared with regular human insulin the use of rapid-acting insulin analogues during pregnancy has also been associated with a reduction in postprandial glucose excursions, an improvement in overall glycaemic control and an improvement in patient satisfaction.

Ketoacidosis is a complication that can result in fetal death. Outcomes may be improved with prompt assessment and treatment by a health professional with specialist diabetes training.

RCTs have shown similar outcomes in women using CSII and MDI regimens. Ketoacidosis may result from pump failure. Cohort studies have reported good outcomes in women offered pump therapy because of difficulty achieving glycaemic control using MDI regimens.

From evidence to recommendations

Women and their partners should be informed of the increased risk of hypoglycaemia and hypoglycaemia unawareness during pregnancy, and information about prevention, recognition and treatment (including the provision of a concentrated glucose solution and, if they have type 1 diabetes, glucagon, and education in their use) should be reinforced in women with insulin-treated diabetes who are pregnant. Women with insulin-treated diabetes should also be advised of the consequences of hypoglycaemia and the dangers associated with driving during periods of hypoglycaemia unawareness. They should be encouraged to carry something that identifies them as having diabetes so they can be treated promptly if disabling hypoglycaemia occurs.

The evidence supports the use of the rapid-acting insulin analogues aspart and lispro in women with diabetes in pregnancy, and also insulin pump therapy (CSII) in women who have difficulty achieving glycaemic control without disabling hypoglycaemia.

Since DKA can be accelerated in pregnancy and is associated with maternal and fetal adverse outcomes (including fetal death), the GDG's consensus view is that current best practice should be followed, i.e. DKA should be excluded in women with type 1 diabetes who become unwell in pregnancy and pregnant women with DKA should be admitted immediately for level 2 critical care* where they can receive medical and obstetric care.

Recommendations for management of diabetes during pregnancy

Healthcare professionals should be aware that the rapid-acting insulin analogues (aspart and lispro†) have advantages over soluble human insulin† during pregnancy and should consider their use.

Women with insulin-treated diabetes should be advised of the risks of hypoglycaemia and hypoglycaemia unawareness in pregnancy, particularly in the first trimester.

During pregnancy, women with insulin-treated diabetes should be provided with a concentrated glucose solution and women with type 1 diabetes should also be given glucagon; women and their partners or other family members should be instructed in their use.

During pregnancy, women with insulin-treated diabetes should be offered continuous subcutaneous insulin infusion (CSII or insulin pump therapy) if adequate glycaemic control is not obtained by multiple daily injections of insulin without significant disabling hypoglycaemia.‡

During pregnancy, women with type 1 diabetes who become unwell should have diabetic ketoacidosis excluded as a matter of urgency.

During pregnancy, women who are suspected of having diabetic ketoacidosis should be admitted immediately for level 2 critical care*, where they can receive both medical and obstetric care.

Research recommendations for management of diabetes during pregnancy

Do new-generation CSII pumps offer an advantage over traditional intermittent insulin injections in terms of pregnancy outcomes in women with type 1 diabetes?

Why this is important
Randomised controlled trials have shown no advantage or disadvantage of using CSII pumps over intermittent insulin injections in pregnancy. A new generation of CSII pumps may offer technological advantages that would make a randomised controlled trial appropriate, particularly with the availability of insulin analogues (which may have improved the effectiveness of intermittent insulin injections).

---

* Level 2 critical care is defined as care for patients requiring detailed observation or intervention, including support for a single failing organ system or postoperative care and those 'stepping down' from higher levels of care.

† This drug does not have UK marketing authorisation specifically for pregnant and breastfeeding women at the time of publication (March 2008). Informed consent should be obtained and documented.

‡ For the purpose of this guidance, 'disabling hypoglycaemia' means the repeated and unpredicted occurrence of hypoglycaemia requiring third-party assistance that results in continuing anxiety about recurrence and is associated with significant adverse effect on quality of life.

5.4   Retinal assessment during pregnancy

There are two widely used classifications for grading the levels of diabetic retinopathy. The English classification for sight-threatening diabetic retinopathy is used for two-field diabetic retinopathy screening (see the National Screening Committee's diabetic retinopathy screening programme for England and Wales, available at www.retinalscreening.nhs.uk/). The English classification progresses from no diabetic retinopathy, to background diabetic retinopathy, to pre-proliferative diabetic retinopathy, to proliferative diabetic retinopathy (PDR). The Early Treatment Diabetic Retinopathy Study (ETDRS) classification has provided an evidence base for progression of diabetic retinopathy based on grading of seven-field stereo-photographs. The ETDRS classification progresses from no diabetic retinopathy, to mild non-proliferative diabetic retinopathy (NPDR), to moderate NPDR, to moderately severe NPDR, to severe NPDR, to PDR. The lesions found within the two classifications follow a common language: background diabetic retinopathy is equivalent to mild NPDR and is characterised by increased vascular permeability; pre-proliferative diabetic retinopathy is equivalent to moderate NPDR, moderately severe NPDR and severe NPDR; in PDR the development of new blood vessels can significantly reduce vision. The progression from no diabetic retinopathy to PDR normally occurs over a period of years, but sudden worsening may occur in pregnancy.

Duration of diabetes is known to be an important factor in the progression of diabetic retinopathy and in the development of PDR in people with diabetes. Data from an epidemiological study showed that PDR varied from 1.2% to 67% in people who had had diabetes for less than 10 years and more than 35 years, respectively.[231]

Description of the evidence

A cohort study[232] determined the prevalence of retinopathy characteristically seen in people with diabetes and IGT, and in people with new-onset diabetes of known duration in the Diabetes Prevention Program (DPP) cohort. The DPP recruited and followed people with elevated fasting glucose (5.3–6.9 mmol/litre) and IGT with no history of diabetes other than gestational diabetes that did not persist after pregnancy. A random sample of 302 participants who developed diabetes and those who remained free from diabetes after 3 years follow-up was used for the retinopathy study. Retinopathy consistent with diabetic retinopathy was detected in 12.6% of people with diabetes and 7.9% of people without diabetes ($P = 0.03$). The study suggests that retinopathy is present in people with elevated fasting glucose and IGT with no known history of diabetes. [EL = 2+]

Progression of diabetic retinopathy
Three cohort studies were identified that found pregnancy to be independently associated with progression of diabetic retinopathy.

One study compared 180 women who became pregnant during an RCT of intensive versus conventional treatment of type 1 diabetes with women who did not become pregnant.[233] In the intensive treatment group 693/2950 (23%) non-pregnant women had progression of retinopathy compared with 39/124 (31%) pregnant women (OR 1.62, 95% CI 1.01 to 2.59, $P < 0.05$). In the conventional treatment group 1742/5605 (31%) non-pregnant women had progression of retinopathy compared with 37/73 (50.3%) pregnant women (OR 2.54, 95% CI 1.59 to 4.03, $P < 0.0001$). [EL = 2++]

A cohort study compared 60 pregnant women with type 1 diabetes to 80 non-pregnant women with type 1 diabetes.[234] Progression of retinopathy occurred in 10/35 women with pre-existing retinopathy in the pregnant group. There was no progression of retinopathy in the non-pregnant controls (24 had pre-existing retinopathy). [EL = 2+]

A cohort study compared 171 pregnant women with type 1 diabetes to 298 non-pregnant women with type 1 diabetes.[235] A multivariate analysis (pregnancy, HbA$_{1c}$, blood pressure, number of previous pregnancies and duration of diabetes) found pregnancy to be independently associated with progression of retinopathy (OR 1.8, 95% CI 1.1 to 2.8, $P < 0.02$). [EL = 2++]

Severity of retinopathy at conception
Four studies found progression of retinopathy during pregnancy to be associated with severity of retinopathy at conception.

A cohort study of 155 pregnant women with type 1 diabetes found women with more severe retinopathy at conception were more likely to show progression during pregnancy (χ^2 for trend, $P < 0.001$).[236] The study found progression of two steps or more in 4/39 (10.3%) women with no retinopathy, 8/38 (21.1%) women with microaneurysms only, 5/32 (18.8%) women with mild NPDR and 17/31 (54.8%) women with moderate NPDR. Women with no retinopathy or only microaneurysms at conception did not develop PDR. PDR developed in 2/32 (6%) women with mild NPDR and 9/31 (29%) women with moderate NPDR at conception. [EL = 2++]

A cohort study of 35 women with type 1 diabetes found progression during pregnancy in 3/10 women with no retinopathy at baseline and in 3/20 with background retinopathy (2/20 developed proliferative retinopathy).[237] Diabetic retinopathy deteriorated during pregnancy in all five women with proliferative retinopathy at baseline. [EL = 2+]

A cohort study evaluated 65 women with type 1 diabetes before pregnancy, during each trimester and 12 months postpartum.[238] The study found 38 women had no retinopathy at conception, 28 (74%) showed no progression and ten (26%) progressed to mild NPDR. Twenty-two women had NPDR at conception, 5 (22.5%) showed no progression, 12 (55%) had NPDR progression and 5 (22.5%) progressed to PDR necessitating photocoagulation. The difference in progression of retinopathy between these two groups was statistically significant ($P = 0.0001$). [EL = 2+]

A cohort study followed 154 women with type 1 diabetes.[239] Twenty-three percent (18/78) of women with no retinopathy in the first trimester progressed; 28/68 (41%) women with NPDR in the first trimester progressed; and 5/8 (63%) women with PDR in the first trimester progressed ($P = 0.01$). [EL = 2++]

Duration of diabetes
Six cohort studies of women with type 1 diabetes found progression of retinopathy during pregnancy was associated with duration of diabetes.[234,236,238–241]

The effect of duration of diabetes on progression of retinopathy during pregnancy is difficult to separate from the effect of the severity of retinopathy at conception as the two are correlated. A study of 155 pregnant women with type 1 diabetes[236] found that in women with moderate or more severe retinopathy at baseline, retinopathy progressed by two steps or more in 55% of women with 15 years or less of duration of diabetes and 50% of women with more than 15 years of duration of diabetes. However, PDR developed in only 18% of women with 15 years or less of duration of diabetes compared with 39% of women with more than 15 years of duration of diabetes. This suggests that severity of retinopathy at conception is more important than duration of diabetes for the progression of diabetes during pregnancy, but that duration of diabetes may be an important factor in the development of PDR. [EL = 2++]

A recent cohort study of 179 pregnancies in 139 women with type 1 diabetes[241] found progression of retinopathy was significantly increased in women with duration of diabetes of 10–19 years compared with duration less than 10 years (8/80 versus 0/71, $P = 0.007$) and in women with moderate to severe NPDR at booking (6/163 versus 3/10, $P = 0.01$). The study included 20 pregnancies in women with duration of diabetes more than 20 years who had no or mild retinopathy at booking and of these only one progressed. This suggests that severity of retinopathy at conception may be more important than duration of diabetes in the progression of retinopathy during pregnancy. [EL = 2++]

Glycaemic control
Seven studies considered the effect of glycaemic control on the progression of diabetic retinopathy during pregnancy.[233,235–239,242] All studies found poor glycaemic control to be associated with progression of retinopathy during pregnancy.

Magnitude of improvement in glycaemic control:
Three studies[233,237,239] found that a large improvement in glycaemic control in the first trimester was associated with progression of retinopathy. The effect of large improvement of glycaemic control is difficult to separate from poor glycaemic control as women with the largest improvement were those who had poor initial control.[236] [EL = 2++]

Progression of retinopathy following commencement of intensive treatment has also been observed in non-pregnant adults with diabetes.[243–246] In the DCCT study[70,243] involving 1441 people with type 1 diabetes (726 with no retinopathy at baseline) progression of retinopathy was observed at the 6 and/or 12 month visit in 13.1% of people in the intensive group compared with 7.6% in the conventional group ($P < 0.001$). Among people who had experienced early worsening of retinopathy, 69% in the intensive group and 57% in the conventional group had shown complete recovery by the 18 month visit. Overall people with early worsening of retinopathy in the intensive group had a 74% reduction in the risk of subsequent progression as compared with people with early worsening who received conventional treatment ($P < 0.001$). [EL = 1++]

Logistic regression incorporating both initial HbA_{1c} and the change between initial HbA_{1c} and 4 month HbA_{1c} found the latter to be the dominant factor for early worsening of retinopathy. There was no evidence that people with more rapid reduction of HbA_{1c} had a greater risk of early worsening of retinopathy than people with more gradual reduction when the reductions were of similar magnitude.[243] [EL = 1++]

Hypertension
A cohort study of 154 women with type 1 diabetes examined the effect of hypertension on the progression of retinopathy during pregnancy.[239] Multiple regression found pregnancy-induced hypertension ($P = 0.01$) and chronic hypertension ($P = 0.02$) to be associated with progression of retinopathy. [EL = 2++]

A cohort study of 65 pregnant women with type 1 diabetes[238] found systolic blood pressure to be higher in women who showed progression of retinopathy during pregnancy than in those who did not ($P < 0.005$). [EL = 2++]

Postpartum regression
A cohort study followed 154 women with type 1 diabetes through pregnancy to 12 weeks postpartum.[239] Fifty-one women had progression of retinopathy during pregnancy of which seven developed PDR. Thirteen women experienced postpartum regression. None of the women who developed PDR during pregnancy experienced postpartum regression. [EL = 2++]

A cohort study of 65 women with type 1 diabetes were followed until 12 months postpartum.[238] Thirty-eight women had no retinopathy at conception. Of these 28 showed no change during pregnancy. Ten showed mild progression during pregnancy, of which five showed complete postpartum regression. There was no development of PDR in the group with no retinopathy at conception. Twenty-two women had NPDR at conception: five of these women experienced no change during pregnancy; twelve progressed from mild to severe NPDR, of which two showed regression postpartum; five progressed to PDR. [EL = 2+]

Laser treatment for diabetic macular oedema
A large multicentre RCT[247] in which people with macular oedema and mild or moderate diabetic retinopathy in one or both eyes were randomly assigned to focal argon laser photocoagulation (754 eyes) or deferred photocoagulation (1490 eyes) showed that focal photocoagulation substantially reduced the risk of visual loss (12% versus 24% at 3 year follow-up). However this RCT did not mention whether pregnant women were included. [EL = 1+] A further report[248] from the RCT described treatment techniques in detail. It defined the concepts of 'clinically significant macular oedema' and 'treatable lesions'. [EL = 3–4]

A subsequent RCT[249] compared eyes selected for early photocoagulation in the first RCT[247] by treating with one of four combinations of scatter (panretinal) and focal treatment. It was found that for eyes with macular oedema, focal photocoagulation was effective in reducing the risk of moderate visual loss but that scatter photocoagulation was not. Focal treatment also increased the chance of visual improvement, decreased the frequency of persistent macular oedema and caused only minor visual field losses. [EL = 1+]

An audit by the UK National Diabetic Retinopathy Laser Treatment group[250,251] was conducted in 546 people undergoing their first photocoagulation treatment for maculopathy. At 9 month follow-up, the results showed that 9.2% had a deterioration in visual acuity equivalent to a doubling of the visual angle and 3.3% of eyes had a visual acuity less than 6/60. Improvement in the macular oedema occurred in 64.6% and exudates in 77.3%. [EL = 3–4]

Laser treatment for proliferatvie diabetic retinopathy
A study of 55 pregnant women with type 1 diabetes found that progression of retinal disease was arrested with photocoagulation during pregnancy in four women with proliferative retinopathy.[240] [EL = 3]

The Diabetic Retinopathy Study group[252] recommend treatment for control eyes with 'high risk characteristics'. They reported four retinopathy factors that increase the 2 year risk of developing severe visual loss: presence of vitreous or preretinal haemorrhage; presence of new vessels; location of new vessels on or near the optic disc and severity of new vessels. [EL = 3–4]

An RCT[253] that compared photocoagulation with no treatment found that photocoagulation reduced the risk of severe visual loss by 50% or more. The 2 year risk of severe visual loss without treatment outweighed the risk of harmful treatment effects for eyes with new vessels and preretinal or vitreous haemorrhage and for eyes with new vessels on or within one disc diameter of the optic disc (NVD) equalling or exceeding one-quarter to one-third of the disc area, even in the absence of preretinal or vitreous haemorrhage. [EL = 1+]

The UK National Diabetic Retinopathy Laser Treatment audit[251] was conducted on 546 people undergoing their first photocoagulation treatment for maculopathy. At 9 month follow-up neovascularisation had regressed fully in 50.8% of cases with proliferative retinopathy, and there was no change or deterioration in 10.3%. This audit showed that regression of neovascularisation was associated with greater areas of retinal ablation at the initial treatment session. [EL = 3–4]

Effect of blood pressure on macular oedema and diabetic retinopathy
A study[254] investigated the relationship between blood pressure and diabetic retinopathy in 249 young people with type 1 diabetes. Retinopathy was present in 63% of young people and hypertension in 2%. The presence of high-normal blood pressure (> 90th percentile but less than 141/90 mm Hg) resulted in a prospectively higher occurrence of retinopathy and of progression of pre-existing retinopathy. [EL 3–4]

A cross-sectional study[255] in Norway of 600 people with a mean age of 19.8 years evaluated the association of various risk factors with retinopathy. In a multiple logistic regression model, age ($P = 0.0001$), higher mean HbA_{1c} ($P = 0.009$), duration of diabetes ($P = 0.0001$) and mean arterial blood pressure ($P = 0.0001$) were significantly associated with retinopathy. [EL 2++]

A cross-sectional study[256] in the USA of 634 people with type 1 diabetes diagnosed before age 30 years evaluated retinopathy after 14 years. Progression was more likely with higher HbA_{1c} or diastolic blood pressure at baseline, an increase in the HbA_{1c} level and an increase in diastolic blood pressure level from the baseline to the 4 year follow-up. The increased risk of proliferative retinopathy was associated with the presence of hypertension at baseline, whereas the increased risk of a person developing macular oedema was associated with the presence of gross proteinuria at baseline. [EL 2+]

An RCT[257] investigated the effect of tight blood pressure control and risk of microvascular complications in people with type 2 diabetes. After 9 years follow-up the group assigned to tight blood pressure control had a 34% reduction in risk in the proportion of participants with deterioration of retinopathy by two steps (99% CI 11% to 50%, $P = 0.0004$) and a 47% reduced risk (99% CI 7% to 70%, $P = 0.004$) of deterioration in visual acuity by three lines of the ETDRS chart. [EL 1++]

A cross-sectional study[258] investigated risk factors related to the incidence and progression of diabetic retinopathy from diagnosis over 6 years in 1919 people with type 2 diabetes. Development of retinopathy (incidence) was strongly associated with baseline glycaemia, glycaemic exposure over 6 years, higher blood pressure and with not smoking. In those who already had retinopathy, progression was associated with older age, male sex, hyperglycaemia (higher HbA_{1c}) and with not smoking. [EL 2++]

A prospective RCT[259] compared the effects of intensive and moderate blood pressure control on the incidence and progression of type 2 diabetic complications in 470 people. At 5.3 years follow-up no difference was found in the incidence between the intensive and moderate groups with regard to the progression of diabetic retinopathy. [EL 1+]

An RCT[260] compared tight blood pressure control (blood pressure less than 150/85) with less tight blood pressure control (blood pressure less than 180/105) and its relationship with diabetic retinopathy in 1148 people with diabetes. At 4.5 years follow-up people allocated to tight blood pressure control were less likely to undergo photocoagulation (RR 0.65, $P = 0.03$). This difference was driven by a difference in photocoagulation due to maculopathy (RR 0.58, $P = 0.02$). [EL = 1+]

Current practice

The CEMACH enquiry reported that a detailed retinal assessment was recorded in the woman's notes at least once during pregnancy in 79.9% of women with pre-existing diabetes.[2] The CEMACH case–control study reported that women with poor pregnancy outcome were as likely not to have a retinal assessment during the first trimester or at booking if later (36% [70/194]) than women who had a good pregnancy outcome (27% [49/183], OR 1.4, 95% CI 0.9 to 2.2, adjusted for maternal age and deprivation).[33] Only 55% of the 258 assessments were recorded to have been done through dilated pupils and for 40% of women details about the retinal assessment procedure were not documented. The most common concern noted by the CEMACH enquiry panels over sub-optimal diabetes care in pregnancy was sub-optimal retinal function monitoring and management. [EL = 3–4]

The CEMACH enquiry (comparison of women with type 1 and type 2 diabetes) reported that women with type 1 diabetes were more likely to have retinopathy than women with type 2 diabetes ($P < 0.001$), with 36% (50/138) of women with type 1 diabetes and 9% (9/96) of the women with type 2 diabetes having retinopathy in pregnancy.[33] This was a new finding in 26% (13/50) of the women with type 1 diabetes and 56% (5/9) of the women with type 2 diabetes. Of the women with pre-existing retinopathy there was evidence of deterioration in 18% of the women with type 1 diabetes and 11% of the women with type 2 diabetes. Women with type 1 diabetes were more likely to have a retinal assessment compared to women with type 2 diabetes (78% versus 64%, $P = 0.02$). Where retinopathy was found both groups of women were as likely to be referred to an ophthalmologist (35% versus 44%, $P = 0.62$). [EL = 3–4]

Existing guidance

The NSF for diabetes recommends full retinal assessment in all women with pre-existing diabetes during the first trimester (or at booking if this is later).[20]

Evidence statement

In some women pregnancy may accelerate progression of diabetic retinopathy. This is more likely in women with more severe diabetic retinopathy, poor glycaemic control and hypertension. Some diabetic retinopathy may regress spontaneously after the woman has given birth.

It is difficult to separate the influence of different factors which have been found to be associated with progression of retinopathy during pregnancy. The magnitude of improvement in glycaemic control is associated with glycaemic control prior to conception (which in turn is associated with duration of diabetes and severity of diabetes at conception). The DCCT found the magnitude, but not the rapidity, of the reduction in HbA$_{1c}$ during the first 6 months of intensive treatment to be an important risk factor for early worsening of diabetic retinopathy. Whether or not the risk of retinopathy progression can be reduced by more gradual reduction in glycaemic control can be resolved only by an RCT.

Evidence supports the use of laser treatment in diabetic macular oedema. Further evidence shows that control of blood pressure has a positive effect on macular oedema and progression of diabetic retinopathy.

From evidence to recommendations

Given the evidence of a rapid change in diabetic retinopathy during pregnancy (because of persistent hyperglycaemia) the GDG's view is that healthcare professionals should err on the side of caution by offering increased frequency of surveillance in the preconception period and throughout pregnancy to women with long-standing poor glycaemic control and pre-proliferative diabetic retinopathy or PDR, and by treating pre-existing diabetic retinopathy before conception.

There is evidence that rapid optimisation of glycaemic control can worsen diabetic retinopathy. However, it is the GDG's view that the benefits to the fetus of good glycaemic control outweigh the risks to the woman (early worsening of diabetic retinopathy). Healthcare professionals should, therefore, encourage improvement in glycaemic control in pregnancy and address ophthalmological complications of diabetes during pregnancy if they occur. In most women, laser treatment can be performed during pregnancy and will reduce the risks of sight loss as a result of progression of diabetic retinopathy. Careful control of blood pressure will also have a positive effect on sight-threatening diabetic retinopathy. Only in very rare circumstances might early birth be considered to reduce the risks of vision loss in pregnancy.

The GDG's view is that retinal assessment during pregnancy for women with diabetes should be conducted in accordance with the recommendations of the National Screening Committee's diabetic retinopathy screening programme (that is, retinal assessment should be performed using digital imaging with mydriasis (dilation of the pupils) using tropicamide). In making its recommendations, the GDG has also noted the report of the CEMACH diabetes in pregnancy audit, which highlighted that only 55% of women with pre-existing diabetes were documented to have received retinal assessment through dilated pupils.

If diabetic retinopathy is found to be present in early pregnancy, referral should usually be guided by the standard referral criteria (see the National Screening Committee's website), and women should be seen by an ophthalmologist within 4 weeks, except for PDR when urgent referral is required. As with preconception care, if there are concerns in relation to the possible worsening of diabetic retinopathy with imminent improvement of very poor blood glucose control then referral with lesser degrees of retinopathy may be considered.

The recommendations in relation to retinal assessment in the preconception period are presented in Section 3.10.

Recommendations for retinal assessment during pregnancy

Pregnant women with pre-existing diabetes should be offered retinal assessment by digital imaging with mydriasis using tropicamide* following their first antenatal clinic appointment and again at 28 weeks if the first assessment is normal. If any diabetic retinopathy is present, an additional retinal assessment should be performed at 16–20 weeks.

If retinal assessment has not been performed in the preceding 12 months, it should be offered as soon as possible after the first contact in pregnancy in women with pre-existing diabetes.

Diabetic retinopathy should not be considered a contraindication to rapid optimisation of glycaemic control in women who present with a high HbA$_{1c}$ in early pregnancy.

Women who have preproliferative diabetic retinopathy diagnosed during pregnancy should have ophthalmological follow-up for at least 6 months following the birth of the baby.

Diabetic retinopathy should not be considered a contraindication to vaginal birth.

Research recommendations for retinal assessment during pregnancy

Should retinal assessment during pregnancy be offered to women diagnosed with gestational diabetes who are suspected of having pre-existing diabetes?

Why this is important
Women with gestational diabetes may have previously unrecognised type 2 diabetes with retinopathy. At present this is not screened for because of the difficulty in identifying these women amongst the larger group who have reversible gestational diabetes. The benefit of recognising such women is that treatment for diabetic retinopathy is available and could prevent short- or long-term deterioration of visual acuity. The research needed would be an observational study of retinal assessment in women newly diagnosed with gestational diabetes to determine whether there is a significant amount of retinal disease present. The severity of any abnormality detected might identify women most at risk for appropriate retinal assessment.

---

* This drug does not have UK marketing authorisation specifically for pregnant and breastfeeding women at the time of publication (March 2008). Informed consent should be obtained and documented.

5.5   Renal assessment during pregnancy

Diabetic nephropathy is a progressive disease that can be divided into the following stages:[261] [EL = 4]

- microalbuminuria (incipient nephropathy) – small amounts of albumin are excreted in the urine
- macroalbuminuria or proteinuria (overt nephropathy) – widespread glomerular sclerosis resulting in progressively larger amounts of protein excreted in the urine
- end-stage renal disease – decreasing creatinine clearance, increasing serum creatinine and uraemia.

Description of the evidence

Effect of pregnancy on progression of nephropathy
A systematic review[262] considered the effects of pregnancy on diabetic nephropathy. The review included 11 longitudinal studies involving a total of 201 people. Only one study had a non-pregnant control group. The other studies compared the average rate of decline in renal function with the expected rate of decline in the general non-pregnant population of people with diabetic nephropathy. The review found that most studies suggest that pregnancy is not associated with development of nephropathy or with accelerated progression of pre-existing nephropathy, with the exception of women with moderate to advanced disease where pregnancy may accelerate progression to end-stage renal disease. [EL = 2++]

Effect of nephropathy on pregnancy outcome
A systematic review[262] which included 11 studies and 681 people found that women with diabetic nephropathy were at increased risk of adverse pregnancy outcomes, in particular IUGR, chronic hypertension, pre-eclampsia and preterm birth (see Table 5.2). Pre-eclampsia and preterm birth were associated with incipient nephropathy (microalbuminuria) as well as overt nephropathy. [EL = 1++]

Table 5.2   Outcome of pregnancy in women with diabetic nephropathy[262]

Outcome	Occurrence (%)
Chronic hypertension	23–77
Pre-eclampsia	15–64
Caesarean section	63–86
Intrauterine growth restriction	9–45
Birth before 34 weeks	16–45

A cohort study was identified that had been published since the systematic review. The cohort study considered pregnancy outcome in women with type 1 diabetes and microalbuminuria.[263] Of 240 consecutive pregnancies, 203 women (85%) had normal urinary albumin excretion, 26 (11%) had microalbuminuria and 11 (5%) had diabetic nephropathy. In this study normal urinary albumin excretion was defined as less than 30 mg/24 hours, microalbuminuria was defined as urinary albumin excretion 30–300 mg/24 hours and diabetic nephropathy was defined as urinary albumin excretion more than 300 mg/24 hours. The incidence of pre-eclampsia was 6% in women with normal urinary albumin excretion, 42% in women with microalbuminuria and 64% in women with nephropathy ($P < 0.001$). The incidence of preterm birth (before 34 weeks) was 6% in women with normal urinary albumin excretion, 23% in women with microalbuminuria and 45% in women with diabetic nephropathy ($P < 0.001$). The incidence of SGA babies was 2% in women with normal urinary albumin excretion, 4% in women with microalbuminuria and 45% in women with diabetic nephropathy ($P < 0.001$). [EL = 2++]

Antihypertensive treatment for microalbuminuria
A cohort study involving 46 women evaluated the impact of antihypertensive treatment with methyldopa in normotensive pregnant women with type 1 diabetes and microalbuminuria.[264] The women were similar in terms of age, diabetes duration, pre-pregnancy BMI, HbA$_{1c}$ and blood

pressure, and all were referred before 17 weeks of gestation. The prevalence of preterm birth before 34 weeks of gestation was reduced from 23% to 0% ($P = 0.02$); the prevalence of preterm birth before 37 weeks of gestation was reduced from 62% to 40% ($P = 0.15$); and the prevalence of pre-eclampsia was reduced from 42% to 20% ($P = 0.11$). Perinatal mortality occurred in 4% versus 0%. [EL = 2++]

Current practice
The CEMACH enquiry reported that women who had a poor pregnancy outcome were more likely not to have monitoring for nephropathy (22% [46/209]) than women who had a good pregnancy outcome (13% [26/206], OR 1.9, 95% CI 1.1 to 3.3, adjusted for maternal age and deprivation). In an additional case–control analysis lack of monitoring for nephropathy was associated only with fetal congenital anomaly and not with fetal or neonatal death after 20 weeks of gestation; it is therefore unlikely to have been causative for poor pregnancy outcome. Nephropathy itself was not associated with poor pregnancy outcome. One of the most common concerns noted by the CEMACH enquiry panels over sub-optimal diabetes care in pregnancy was sub-optimal renal function monitoring and management.[33] [EL = 3–4]

The CEMACH enquiry (comparison of women with type 1 and type 2 diabetes) reported that there was no significant difference in the rate on nephropathy in pregnancy in women with type 1 or type 2 diabetes, with 8% (12/148) of women with type 1 diabetes and 5% (6/119) of the women with type 2 diabetes having nephropathy during their pregnancy.[33] Women with type 1 diabetes were as likely to have monitoring for nephropathy as women with type 2 diabetes (86% versus 79%, $P = 0.60$). Where nephropathy was found both groups of women were as likely to have a test of renal function (75% versus 50%, $P = 0.29$). [EL = 3–4]

The CEMACH enquiry did not state an explicit standard of monitoring for nephropathy, but it recommended that appropriate monitoring included testing for microalbuminuria (incipient nephropathy) via protein dipstick testing of urine or serum creatinine.[33] [EL = 3–4]

Existing guidance

The NICE guideline for type 2 diabetes defines microalbuminuria as albumin : creatinine ratio 3.5 mg/mmol or more (for women) or albumin concentration 20 mg/litre or more. Macroalbuminuria is defined as albumin : creatinine ratio 30 mg/mmol or more or albumin concentration 200 mg/litre or more.[8]

The NICE guidelines for type 1 and type 2 diabetes in adults recommend annual testing for nephropathy using urine albumin : creatinine ratio and serum creatinine. It is recommended that people with nephropathy have measurements of urine albumin and serum creatinine levels at each visit.[7,8]

Evidence statement

In the majority of studies pregnancy has not been associated with the development of nephropathy or with accelerated progression of pre-existing nephropathy. Data from three studies suggest that in women with moderate to advanced disease pregnancy may accelerate progression to end-stage renal disease.

All stages of nephropathy, including microalbuminuria, are associated with adverse pregnancy outcomes, especially IUGR, pre-eclampsia and preterm birth.

A small cohort study suggested that antihypertensive treatment with methyldopa in women with type 1 diabetes and microalbuminuria reduced the risk of preterm birth (before 34 weeks of gestation).

No evidence was identified in relation to thromboprophylaxis in the presence of macro-albuminuria.

From evidence to recommendations

NICE recommends that renal assessment outside pregnancy should use urine albumin : creatinine ratio and serum creatinine. Estimated glomerular filtration rate (eGFR) should not be used during pregnancy as it underestimates the glomerular filtration rate.[439] There is no evidence on the optimal assessment schedule during pregnancy. As both microalbuminuria and macroalbuminuria are associated with adverse outcomes the GDG recommends assessment in the preconception period or at the first presentation after conception. All pregnant women should have their urine tested for proteinuria as part of routine antenatal care (see the NICE antenatal care guideline).[9] If serum creatinine is abnormal (120 micromol/litre or more) or if total protein excretion exceeds 2 g/day, referral to a nephrologist should be considered.

No evidence was identified in relation to thromboprophylaxis in the presence of macroalbuminuria. The GDG's consensus view is that healthcare professionals should follow best current practice in terms of thromboprophylaxis for women with diabetes and macroalbuminuria (antenatal administration of aspirin for proteinuria less than 5 mg/day and heparin for proteinuria more than 5 mg/day; planned early birth may need to be considered because of the risk of developing pre-eclampsia).

The recommendations in relation to renal assessment in the preconception period are presented in Section 3.11.

Recommendations for renal assessment during pregnancy

If renal assessment has not been undertaken in the preceding 12 months in women with pre-existing diabetes, it should be arranged at the first contact in pregnancy. If serum creatinine is abnormal (120 micromol/litre or more) or if total protein excretion exceeds 2 g/day, referral to a nephrologist should be considered (eGFR should not be used during pregnancy). Thromboprophylaxis should be considered for women with proteinuria above 5 g/day (macroalbuminuria).

Research recommendations for renal assessment during pregnancy

Does identification of microalbuminuria during pregnancy offer the opportunity for appropriate pharmacological treatment to prevent progression to pre-eclampsia in women with pre-existing diabetes?

Why this is important
Microalbuminuria testing is available, but it is not performed routinely in antenatal clinics for women with pre-existing diabetes because a place for prophylactic treatment of pre-eclampsia in microalbuminuria-positive women has not been investigated. The benefit of clinically and cost-effective prophylactic treatment would be to significantly improve pregnancy outcomes in this group of women.

5.6 Screening for congenital malformations

Description of the evidence

Women with diabetes have an increased risk of having a baby with a congenital malformation. Major congenital malformations affecting babies of women with diabetes include cardiac, neural tube and genitourinary anomalies. Table 5.3 lists anomalies associated with diabetes as well as the estimated prevalence and RR compared to women without diabetes, as reported in published studies.[265]

More recent data from the CEMACH enquiry found the prevalence of confirmed major anomalies to be 41.8 per 1000 total births (live and stillborn).[2] Separate rates for babies of women with type 1 diabetes (n = 1707) and type 2 diabetes (n = 652) born between 1 March 2002 and 28 February 2003 are summarised in Table 5.4.[266] Women with type 2 diabetes were more likely to come from a Black, Asian or Other Minority Ethnic group (type 1 diabetes 9.1%, type 2 diabetes 48.8%). Perinatal mortality in babies of women with diabetes was 31.8 per 1000 births, nearly four times higher than the general maternity population. One hundred and ninety-seven major congenital anomalies were confirmed in 148 babies. The prevalence of major congenital anomaly

Table 5.3 Detectable major congenital malformations in babies of women with pre-existing diabetes[265]

Group of malformations	Specific malformations	Prevalence per 100 births	Relative risk compared to women without diabetes
Cardiac	Transposition of the great arteries Ventricular septal defect Coarctation of the aorta Atrial septal defect Asymmetric septal hypertrophy	3.0–10.0	3–5
Caudal regression syndrome		0.2–0.5	200
Central nervous system	Neural tube defects (including anencephaly) Microcephaly Isolated hydrocephlus	2.1	2–10
Gastrointestinal	Duodenal atresia Anorectal atresia Hypoplastic left colon	1.0	3
Musculoskeletal system	Talipes Arthrogryposis	0.8–2.4	2–20
Orofacial cleft		1.8	1.5
Urinary tract	Uretal duplication Cystic kidney Renal dysgenesis Hydronephrosis	1.7–3.0	5–2

Table 5.4 Observed and expected prevalence of congenital malformations in babies of women with type 1 and type 2 diabetes (from CEMACH)[266]

Type of malformation	Babies of women with type 1 diabetes, observed (expected)a	Babies of women with type 2 diabetes, observed (expected)[a]	Standardised prevalence ratio for babies of women with both type1 and type 2 diabetes (95% CI)
One or more malformations	81 (37)	28 (12.8)	2.2 (1.8 to 2.6)
Neural tube defects	6 (2.4)	4 (0.9)	4.2 (2.0 to 7.8)
Other central nervous system	5 (1.7)	0 (0.6)	1.5 (0.3 to 3.6)
Eye	1 (2.4)	0 (0.9)	1.0 (0.1 to 7.0)
Ear	0 (0.7)	0 (0.3)	–
Congenital heart disease	33 (8.9)	9(3.4)	3.4 (2.5 to 4.6)
Cleft lip and palate	0 (1.3)	0 (0.5)	–
Cleft palate	2 (0.9)	0 (0.3)	1.6 (0.2 to 5.9)
Digestive system	1 (2.6)	2 (1.0)	0.8 (0.2 to 2.5)
Internal urogenital system	9 (6.1)	1 (2.3)	1.2 (0.6 to 2.2)
External genital system	3 (2.5)	2 (0.9)	1.5 (0.5 to 3.4)
Limb	15 (10.2)	4 (3.7)	1.4 (0.8 to 2.1)
Other (non-chromosomal)	6	4	–
Trisomy 21	2	0	–
Other chromosomal	2	2	–

[a] Expected rates are based on European Surveillance of Congenital Anomalies (EUROCAT) 2002.[267]

was 46 per 1000 births in women with diabetes (48 per 1000 births for type 1 diabetes, 43 per 1000 births for type 2 diabetes), more than twice the expected rate. The increase was mainly due to an increase in neural tube defects (4.2-fold) and congenital heart disease (3.4-fold). Anomalies in 65% (71/109) of babies were diagnosed antenatally. Congenital heart disease was diagnosed antenatally in 54.8% (23/42) of babies. Anomalies other than congenital heart disease were diagnosed antenatally in 71.6% (48/67) of babies. [EL = 3–4]

The benefits of screening for congenital malformations include the opportunity for counselling, enabling families time to prepare, allowing antenatal treatment, and ensuring appropriate obstetric management.

According to the NICE antenatal care guideline,[9] all pregnant women should be offered screening for congenital malformations at 18–20 weeks of gestation as part of routine antenatal care. This section considers what additional screening should be offered to women with diabetes.

First-trimester screening for chromosomal anomalies
The NICE antenatal care guideline[9] recommends that all pregnant women should be offered screening for Down's syndrome. Women should understand that it is their choice to embark on screening for Down's syndrome. Screening should be performed by the end of the first trimester (14 weeks of gestation), but provision should be made to allow later screening (up to 20 weeks of gestation) for women booking later in pregnancy. The screening test offered should be the 'combined test' (nuchal translucency (NT), beta human chorionic gonadotropin [β-hCG] and pregnancy-associated plasma protein-A (PAPP-A)) at 11–14 weeks of gestation. At 15–20 weeks of gestation the most clinically effective and cost-effective serum screening test should be offered, namely the 'triple test' or 'quadruple test' (hCG, alpha fetoprotein (AFP), unconjugated estriol (uE3) and inhibin A). The integrated test should not be routinely used as a screening test for Down's syndrome. Information about screening options for Down's syndrome that can be understood by all women, including those whose first language is not English, should be given to women as early as possible and ideally before the booking visit, allowing the opportunity for further discussion before embarking on screening. If a woman receives a screen-positive result, she should have rapid access to appropriate counselling by trained staff. The second-trimester ultrasound scan (at 18–20 weeks of) should not be routinely used for Down's syndrome screening using soft markers. The presence of an isolated soft marker with an exception of increased nuchal fold noted on the routine anomaly scan (at 18–20 weeks of gestation) should not be used to adjust the *a priori* risk for Down's syndrome. The presence of an increased nuchal fold or two or more soft markers should prompt the offer of fetal medicine referral.

Women with diabetes do not have an increased risk of chromosomal anomalies, however published studies have shown that some biochemical markers tend to be lower in women with type 1 diabetes than in women without diabetes. Therefore, clinical practice has been to make adjustments when calculating the risk of anomalies for women with type 1 diabetes to take account of these differences.

A meta-analysis[268] included published studies of differences in AFP (14 studies, 253 women with type 1 diabetes), uE3 (six studies, 687 women with type 1 diabetes), total hCG (nine studies, 1350 women with type 1 diabetes), free β-hCG (one study, 251 women) and inhibin (three studies, 445 women). The weight-corrected median multiple-of-median (MoM) was 0.92 for AFP, 0.94 for uE3, 0.96 for total hCG, 0.96 for free β-hCG and 1.03 for inhibin (MoM values are ratios of median MoM in women with type 1 diabetes to median MoM in women without diabetes). No CIs or tests of statistical significance were presented in the meta-analysis. [EL = 2+]

Since publication of the meta-analysis, one study has been published on free β-hCG.[269] The study compared 79 women with type 1 diabetes to 16366 women without diabetes. There were no significant differences in weight-corrected free β-hCG (type 1 diabetes MoM 0.87, 95% CI 0.75 to 1.16, women without diabetes MoM 1.00, $P = 0.52$). [EL = 2+]

Two studies were identified that compared levels of PAPP-A in women with and without diabetes during pregnancy. One study compared 79 women with type 1 diabetes to 93 pregnant women without diabetes.[270] Levels of PAPP-A were significantly lower in women with type 1 diabetes ($P = 0.024$). [EL = 2+]

The second study compared PAPP-A levels in 79 women with type 1 diabetes to those in 16366 women without diabetes.[269] There was no significant difference in PAPP-A levels (type 1 diabetes MoM 1.02, 95% CI 0.83 to 1.05, women without diabetes MoM 1.01, $P = 0.36$). [EL = 2+]

One study was identified that compared NT results in 195 women with type 1 diabetes to those in 33301 women without diabetes.[269] There was no difference in mean NT between the two groups (0.0358 mm versus 0.0002 mm, $P = 0.418$). [EL = 2++]

Second-trimester ultrasound screening for structural anomalies

The NICE antenatal care guideline[9] recommends that 'ultrasound screening for fetal anomalies should be routinely offered, normally between 18 weeks 0 days and 20 weeks 6 days.'

A cohort study compared 130 women with diabetes (85 type 1 diabetes, 45 type 2 diabetes) with 12169 low-risk pregnant women for the same period.[271] All women had routine ultrasound at 16–24 weeks of gestation. A total of ten major anomalies (7.7%) and three minor anomalies (2.3%) were present in the fetuses of women with diabetes. The incidence of major congenital malformations was greater in the women with diabetes than in the low-risk control group (8% versus 1.4%, $P < 0.001$). The detection rate was significantly lower in the women with diabetes (30% versus 73%, $P < 0.01$) and the mean BMI was significantly higher (29 kg/m² versus 23 kg/m²). Thirty-seven percent (48/130) of scans undertaken in women with diabetes were judged to be unsatisfactory, mainly because of maternal obesity (45/48). The majority (86% [19/22]) of repeat scans were also unsatisfactory. Of the 82 women with diabetes who had satisfactory images, two had congenital malformations. Both were detected antenatally (detection rate 100%). Of the 48 whose image quality was judged to be unsatisfactory there were eight major congenital anomalies. Only one was detected antenatally (detection rate 12.5%). [EL = 2++]

A cohort study considered 432 women with type 1 diabetes who underwent ultrasound screening between 12 and 23 weeks of gestation.[272] The ultrasound included four chambers of the heart and the great vessels. At birth 32 babies had 38 major congenital malformations, 52% (18/32) of which were detected antenatally. There were eight heart anomalies of which five were detected antenatally. All six CNS abnormalities were detected antenatally. The lesions most commonly missed by sonography were ventricular septal defect, abnormal hand or foot, unilateral renal abnormality, and cleft palate without cleft lip. The test performance was: sensitivity 56%, specificity 99.5%, PPV 90%, NPV 97%. [EL = 2++]

In a study of 289 women with diabetes[273] comprehensive ultrasound including a four chamber view undertaken at 18 weeks of gestation by a perinatologist had a test performance for detection of non-cardiac anomalies as follows: sensitivity 59%, specificity 100%, PPV 100%, NPV 98%. The test performance of the standard four chamber view was: sensitivity 33%, specificity 100%, PPV 100%, NPV 97%. In comparison the test performance for echocardiogram was: sensitivity 92%, specificity 99%, PPV 92%, NPV 99%. [EL = 2++]

A cohort study reported on 250 women[274] with pre-existing diabetes who underwent fetal echocardiogram at 20–22 weeks of gestation. Views included the four chamber view, the left ventricular long-axis view with visualisation of the aortic outflow tract, the short-axis view with visualisation of the pulmonary outflow tract and ductus arteriosus, and longitudinal view of the aortic arch. All examinations were undertaken by three experienced ultrasonographers. There were eight cardiac anomalies (3.2%), six of which were detected antenatally by echocardiogram. There was one false-negative result and one false-positive result. One fetus had an apparently normal heart at 21 weeks of gestation but was found to have a small atrial-septal defect at birth. The false positive was a case of perimembranous ventricular-septal defect. The test sensitivity was 85.7% and specificity was 99.5%. [EL = 2++]

A study of 223 women with insulin-requiring diabetes (128 type 1 diabetes, 47 type 2 diabetes, 48 gestational diabetes) considered the utility of different echocardiogram views.[275] There were 11 heart defects, nine of which were detected antenatally. The two missed cases were in women who were obese. Seven defects occurred in women with type 1 diabetes, three in women with type 2 diabetes and one in a woman with insulin-requiring gestational diabetes. The sensitivity of the four chamber view was 73% (8/11) and specificity was 100%. The sensitivity of the four chamber view and aortic outflow tract was 82% (9/11) and the specificity was 100%. Other views did not contribute to detection of a defect. The two missed cases (pulmonary atresia with a ventricular septal defect and an isolated ventricular septal defect) could theoretically have been detected on the four chamber view. [EL = 2++]

One study[276] examined 725 women (with or without diabetes) who had been referred for echocardiogram following a comprehensive anatomy ultrasound that included a four chamber/left ventricular outflow tract view. The indications for referral included pre-existing diabetes (without additional indication, $n = 226$), fetal anomaly seen on anatomy ultrasound ($n = 130$) and family history of congenital heart disease ($n = 133$). Twenty-nine echocardiograms were reported as abnormal (4%). The indications for referral in these cases were an abnormal four chamber/left ventricular outflow tract view at ultrasound (66%), aneuploidy (14%) other fetal anomaly (17%) and fetal arrhythmia (3%). No abnormal fetal echocardiograms were reported in women with isolated pre-existing diabetes (i.e. with a normal four chamber/left ventricular outflow tract view at ultrasound). [EL = 2++]

Evidence statement

A number of studies have found no significant differences between women with type 1 diabetes and women without diabetes in terms of NT and weight-corrected total hCG, β-hCG and inhibin. On this basis it can be advised that no adjustment is required in these biochemical markers when calculating risks for congenital abnormalities in the fetuses of women with diabetes. A meta-analysis found weight-corrected AFP to be approximately 8% lower in women with type 1 diabetes and weight-corrected uE3 to be 6% lower in women with type 1 diabetes and therefore adjustments should be applied accordingly. Two studies have found conflicting results with regard to levels of PAPP-A. Therefore, until further evidence is available, adjustments should continue to be applied.

A number of well-designed observational studies have found more congenital anomalies are detected antenatally in women with diabetes when antenatal examination includes views of the four chambers of the fetal heart and outflow tracts. No more anomalies are detected with additional views. One study found detection rates were significantly worse in women with diabetes compared with low-risk women. This was largely attributed to obesity in women with diabetes resulting in unsatisfactory images.

Cost-effectiveness

The effectiveness of methods of screening for congenital cardiac malformations in women with diabetes was identified by the GDG as a priority for health economic analysis. The methods and results from the health economic modelling are summarised here; further details are provided in Appendix E.

Women with diabetes are at increased risk of having a baby with a cardiac malformation (the risk being approximately five times that of the general maternity population). Therefore, the GDG considered that this was an area where a different screening programme from that used in routine antenatal care might be justified on health economic grounds. An economic model was used to compare the cost-effectiveness of screening for congenital cardiac malformations using the four chamber plus outflow tracts view versus the four chamber view alone, which represents current practice. The baseline model suggested that the four chamber plus outflow tracts view was highly cost-effective in pregnant women with diabetes with a cost per QALY of approximately £4,000. One-way sensitivity analysis showed that four chamber plus outflow tracts view continued to be cost-effective when parameter values were varied within plausible ranges.

Existing guidance

As noted above, the NICE antenatal care guideline[9] recommends that all pregnant women should be offered ultrasound screening for congenital malformations (ideally at 18–20 weeks of gestation) using the four chamber plus outflow tracts view as part of routine antenatal care. Women should be given information regarding the purpose and implications of the anomaly scan in order to enable them make an informed choice as to whether or not to have the scan. The guideline recommends that all pregnant women should be offered screening for Down's syndrome and that women should understand that it is their choice to embark on screening for

Down's syndrome. If a woman receives a screen positive result, she should have rapid access to appropriate counselling by trained staff.

From evidence to recommendations

A health economic model demonstrated the cost-effectiveness of screening for congenital cardiac malformations based on the four chamber view of the fetal heart and outflow tracts relative to current practice of screening using the four chamber view alone. Data from European Surveillance of Congenital Anomalies (EUROCAT) and published literature (see Appendix D) suggest that an antenatal diagnosis of TGA may reduce neonatal mortality. These data, together with the higher prevalence of cardiac malformations in pregnant women with diabetes compared to pregnant women without diabetes underpin this result. For this reason the GDG identified screening for congenital cardiac malformations using the four chamber plus outflow tracts view as a key priority for implementation for women with diabetes (this form of screening is recommended as part of routine antenatal care but it does not form a key priority for implementation in the NICE antenatal care guideline[9]). There may be additional benefits of screening not taken into account in the model, the existence of which would tend to further improve the relative cost-effectiveness of screening based on the four chamber plus outflow tracts view.

The GDG's view is that a specialist cardiac scan should be offered at 22 weeks of gestation only if the results of the four chamber plus outflow tracts view are abnormal or if there is a relevant history of cardiac malformations. This is likely to bring a cost saving to the NHS because there is currently a tendency to offer a specialist cardiac scan to many women with diabetes.

Recommendations for screening for congenital malformations

Women with diabetes should be offered antenatal examination of the four chamber view of the fetal heart and outflow tracts at 18–20 weeks.

Research recommendations for screening for congenital malformations

How reliable is first-trimester screening for Down's syndrome incorporating levels of pregnancy-associated plasma protein (PAPP-A) in women with pre-existing diabetes?

Why this is important
Several screening tests for Down's syndrome incorporate measurements of PAPP-A. However, two clinical studies have reported conflicting results in terms of whether levels of PAPP-A in women with type 1 diabetes are lower than those in other women. Current practice is to adjust PAPP-A measurements in women with diabetes on the assumption that their PAPP-A levels are indeed lower than those of other women. Further research is, therefore, needed to evaluate the diagnostic accuracy and effect on pregnancy outcomes of screening tests for Down's syndrome incorporating measurements of PAPP-A in women with pre-existing diabetes.

How effective is transvaginal ultrasound for the detection of congenital malformations in women with diabetes and coexisting obesity?

Why this is important
Obstetric ultrasound signals are attenuated by the woman's abdominal wall fat. Many women with diabetes (and particularly women with type 2 diabetes) are obese, and this may limit the sensitivity of abdominal ultrasound screening for congenital malformations. Vaginal ultrasound does not have this difficulty, but there is currently no evidence that it is more effective than abdominal ultrasound. Research studies are, therefore, needed to evaluate the diagnostic accuracy and affect on pregnancy outcomes of vaginal ultrasound in women with diabetes and coexisting obesity. This is important because women with diabetes are at increased risk of having a baby with a congenital malformation.

5.7 Monitoring fetal growth and wellbeing

Description of the evidence

Fetal growth

Women with gestational diabetes and pre-existing diabetes are at increased risk of having a baby with macrosomia (see Sections 4.1 and 5.1). Macrosomia is defined in terms of absolute birthweight (usually more than 4000 g) or birthweight percentile for gestational age (usually ≥ 90th percentile), also referred to as LGA. Macrosomia is a risk factor for shoulder dystocia, brachial plexus injury, asphyxia or prolonged labour, operative delivery and postpartum haemorrhage (see Section 6.1 and Chapter 7).

Women with diabetes are also at risk of having a baby that is SGA. The risks associated with a baby that is SGA are not as well documented as for macrosomia, but at least one study was identified that suggested that babies who were SGA (< 10th percentile for gestational age) have an increased risk of perinatal morbidity and mortality.[277]

There is no clear consensus for monitoring fetal size in pregnant women with diabetes.[278] Clinical assessment of fetal size is by measurement of the symphysis–fundal height. Fetal size can also be measured by sonography. The two main ultrasonic methods for predicting birthweight are estimated fetal weight (EFW) and abdominal circumference of the fetus. EFW uses a combination of parameters, for example, the Hadlock formula[279] uses femur length, biparietal diameter, head circumference and abdominal circumference. Mean errors in estimating fetal weight are between 8% and 15% of actual birthweight.[279] EFW increases the rate of caesarean section in false positives (AGA babies incorrectly diagnosed as LGA).[280,281] Accuracy of estimated fetal weight is worse in women with diabetes[282] and for macrosomic babies.[283]

Compared with babies of women with diabetes who are AGA, LGA babies have accelerated growth of insulin-sensitive tissue such as abdominal wall fat.[284] Abdominal circumference is therefore considered to be a more relevant measure of diabetes-related macrosomia and the risk of shoulder dystocia. Abdominal circumference also has the advantage of being a single measure that is accessible even when the head is engaged in the pelvis.

A systematic review of 63 studies (51 evaluating the accuracy of estimated fetal weight and 12 the accuracy of fetal abdominal circumference) involving 19 117 women pooled data to produce summary receiver operating characteristic (sROC) curves for studies with various test thresholds.[278] Summary likelihood ratios (LRs) for positive and negative test results were generated for an estimated fetal weight of 4000 g and an abdominal circumference of 36 cm for predicting birthweight over 4000 g. The sROC curve area for estimated fetal weight was not different from the area for fetal abdominal circumference (0.87 versus 0.85, $P = 0.91$). For predicting a birthweight of over 4000 g the summary LR was 5.7 (95% CI 4.3 to 7.6) for a positive test and 0.48 (95% CI 0.38 to 0.60) for a negative test. For ultrasound fetal abdominal circumference of 36 cm the LR for a positive test for predicting birthweight over 4000 g was 6.9 (95% CI 5.2 to 9.0) and the LR for a negative test was 0.37 (95% CI 0.30 to 0.45). There was no difference in accuracy between estimated fetal weight and abdominal circumference in the prediction of macrosomia at birth. The LRs suggest that both tests are only moderately useful at best. A positive test result is more accurate for ruling in macrosomia than is a negative test for ruling it out. [EL = 1++]

A diagnostic accuracy study compared 31 published formulas for estimated fetal weight in predicting macrosomia (birthweight 4000 g or more) in babies of women with diabetes.[285] One hundred and sixty-five women with pre-existing diabetes or gestational diabetes who had sonograms to estimate fetal weight after 36 weeks of gestation and within 2 weeks of birth were included in the study. Three measures of accuracy were compared: area under the ROC curve relating estimated fetal weight to macrosomia; systematic error; and absolute error. All 31 formulas for estimating fetal weight had similarly poor accuracy for prediction of macrosomia. [EL = 2+]

A cohort study evaluated the reliability of ultrasound estimation of fetal weight in 1117 women (48 with gestational diabetes) with a singleton pregnancy who had undergone ultrasound estimation of fetal weight less than 7 days before a term birth (at or later than 37 weeks of gestation).[286] Both large and normal weight babies of women with diabetes tended to have their weight underestimated. Given that reliability of ultrasound estimation of fetal weight to detect larger babies was poor, the study suggests that ultrasound use in the management of suspected macrosomia should be discouraged. [EL = 2+]

A retrospective cohort study investigated the association between ultrasound fetal biometry and amniotic fluid insulin levels at birth in 93 pregnant women with pre-existing diabetes or IGT.[287] Babies of women with pre-existing diabetes had significantly greater mean growth velocity (1.39, 95% CI 0.43 to 2.23 versus 0.39, 95% CI −01.7 to 0.95, $P = 0.04$), significantly greater mean estimated fetal weight and greater mean birthweight centile than those with gestational diabetes or IGT. Amniotic fluid insulin levels demonstrated a similar significant difference between women with pre-existing diabetes and those with gestational diabetes or IGT. The study demonstrated that ultrasound measures of fetal size and growth are not sufficiently accurate to predict those babies likely to be at risk from the effects of fetal hyperinsulinaemia. [EL = 2+]

A retrospective cohort study involving 242 pregnant women with IGT evaluated the performance of estimated fetal weight and fetal growth velocity in the prediction of birthweight.[288] The study showed that estimated fetal weight and fetal growth velocity have limited utility in predicting LGA babies. Estimated fetal weight and fetal growth velocity did not predict neonatal hypoglycaemia. [EL = 2+]

A prospective study of 181 women with diabetes (133 pre-existing type 1 diabetes, 48 gestational diabetes) compared the prediction power, at different gestational ages, of clinical and ultrasound measurements for fetal size.[289] Clinical and ultrasound estimates were made at 28, 34 and 38 weeks of gestation or before birth. The study found all measurements were poor predictors of eventual standardised birthweight. Prediction improved with closeness to birth. Adding ultrasound to clinical information improved prediction, but only to a small extent. There was no difference in the prediction power for macrosomia between clinical and ultrasound measurements. [EL = 2++]

Fetal wellbeing
Three main tests are used by obstetricians to monitor fetal wellbeing. These are umbilical artery Doppler ultrasound velocimetry, fetal cardiotocography (non-stress test) and the biophysical profile. Monitoring for fetal wellbeing assumes that fetal compromise can be identified and that appropriately timed intervention (induction of labour or caesarean section) may reduce the risk of perinatal morbidity, admission to neonatal intensive care, asphyxia and fetal death.[290]

Doppler ultrasound:
Doppler ultrasound uses sound waves to detect the movement of blood in the umbilical artery. It is used during pregnancy to assess fetus–placenta and/or uterus–placenta circulation.

A systematic review considered the effectiveness of Doppler ultrasound in high-risk pregnancies.[291] The review included 11 studies involving 7000 women. Compared with no Doppler ultrasound, Doppler ultrasound in high-risk pregnancies (especially those complicated by hypertension or presumed impaired fetal growth) was associated with fewer perinatal deaths, fewer inductions of labour (OR 0.83, 95% CI 0.74 to 0.93) and fewer admissions to hospital (OR 0.56, 95% CI 0.43 to 0.72) without adverse effects. [EL = 1++] However, Doppler ultrasound offers no benefits to the low-risk population.[292] [EL = 1++]

Abnormal umbilical Doppler ultrasound results are associated with chronic placental insufficiency, as occurs in pregnancies complicated by pre-eclampsia and IUGR. Although women with diabetes are at increased risk for these conditions, the majority of adverse outcomes in pregnancies complicated by diabetes are not associated with placental insufficiency.[293] Small studies of women with gestational diabetes or pre-existing diabetes with good glycaemic control have considered the performance of Doppler ultrasound in predicting any adverse pregnancy outcome and have reported low sensitivities[294–297] [EL = 2++ to 2+]

Nonetheless a study has reported that Doppler ultrasound is better than fetal cardiotocography or biophysical profile in pregnant women with diabetes.[298] In this study involving 207 women with diabetes, all three tests were performed concurrently within 1 week of birth. An adverse pregnancy outcome was defined as a pregnancy in which the baby was born before 37 weeks of gestation or had at least one of the following: growth restriction, hypocalcaemia, hypoglycaemia, hyperbilirubinaemia, respiratory distress syndrome or fetal risk requiring caesarean section. There were no perinatal deaths in this series. The performance of the three tests is summarised in Table 5.5. [EL = 2++]

Table 5.5 Performance of umbilical artery Doppler ultrasound, fetal cardiotocography and biophysical profile in predicting overall adverse pregnancy outcome; data from Bracero *et al.* (1996)[298]

| | Cardiotocography non-reactive | Biophysical profile ≤ 6 | Umbilical artery Doppler ultrasound | |
			systolic : diastolic ratio ≥ 3	systolic : diastolic ratio ≥ 2.5
Sensitivity	25.3%	8.0%	25.3%	65.3%
Specificity	88.6%	97.0%	96.2%	61.4%
PPV	55.9%	60.0%	79.2%	49.0%
NPV	67.6%	65.0%	69.4%	75.7%
RR	1.7	1.7	2.6	2.0
95% CI	1.2 to 2.5	0.9 to 2.9	1.9 to 3.5	1.4 to 3.0
P value	0.009	0.109	< 0.001	< 0.001

A prospective double-blind randomised study was performed between 28 and 40 weeks of gestation in 92 pregnant women with diabetes to evaluate a random single Doppler ultrasound measurement of the systolic : diastolic ratio of the umbilical artery as a predictor of perinatal outcome in pregnancies complicated by diabetes.[299] The performance of the Doppler ultrasound measurement as a predictor of poor perinatal outcome was: sensitivity 39%, specificity 92%, PPV 54%, NPV 86%. The data suggest that the systolic : diastolic ratio of the umbilical artery offers no advantage over other well-established tests in the management of pregnancy in women with diabetes. [EL = 1+]

Sixty-five pregnant women with diabetes were examined in a cohort study to evaluate the clinical usefulness of Doppler ultrasound flow velocity waveform analysis in such pregnancies.[300] Umbilical and uterine artery flow velocity waveforms were obtained during the third trimester with a continuous wave Doppler ultrasound device. There was no difference in various clinical and Doppler ultrasound parameters between women with good glycaemic control and those with poor control. In contrast, the clinical and Doppler parameters were significantly different in women with pre-eclampsia than in those without pre-eclampsia, regardless of glycaemic control. There was a weak positive linear correlation ($r = 0.30$, $P < 0.02$) between maternal HbA$_{1c}$ and umbilical artery flow velocity waveforms (systolic : diastolic ratio). Proteinuria correlated better with umbilical artery systolic : diastolic ratio ($r = 0.49$, $P < 0.001$). The study suggests that Doppler ultrasound flow velocity waveform analysis may be clinically useful only in pregnancies complicated by diabetes and coexisting pre-eclampsia. [EL = 2+]

A prospective cohort study investigated Doppler ultrasound measurement of the fetal umbilical artery velocimetry in 56 women with diabetes, of whom 14 had varying degrees of vascular complications.[301] The mean Doppler ultrasound values were higher in women with diabetes and vasculopathy than in women without diabetes and women with diabetes but no vasculopathy. The third-trimester systolic : diastolic ratio was greater than 3 in almost 50% of women with vasculopathy. A tendency towards adverse outcomes was observed at systolic : diastolic ratios approaching 4. Statistically significant correlations were found between elevated Doppler indices and maternal vasculopathy associated with hypertension and worsening renal insufficiency. IUGR and neonatal metabolic complications were also significantly correlated with elevated Doppler indices. The data indicate an increased resistance circuit among women with diabetes and vasculopathy, which may reflect a relative reduction in basal uteroplacental blood flow and the need for cautious interpretation of Doppler indices in these women. [EL = 2+]

Another prospective cohort study was conducted to determine whether fetal aortic velocity waveforms were correlated with fetal outcome in pregnancies complicated by type 1 diabetes.[302] Fetal aortic blood flow was assessed in 30 pregnant women with type 1 diabetes. The babies demonstrated no evidence of fetal distress at birth and there was no relationship between the mean third-trimester fetal aortic systolic : diastolic ratios and perinatal death, preterm deliveries, birthweight, Apgar scores at 1 minute and 5 minutes, or neonatal metabolic abnormalities. The data demonstrate a poor correlation between fetal aortic Doppler waveform analysis and fetal outcome. [EL = 2+]

Current practice
The CEMACH enquiry found that 21% of singleton births with a known birthweight had a birthweight of 4000 g or more in women with poor pregnancy outcomes.[33] This was higher than the national average of 11%. A total of 5.7% births were severely macrosomic singleton births (a birthweight of 4500 g or over). The CEMACH enquiry case–control study reported that antenatal evidence of fetal growth restriction was associated with poor pregnancy outcome (OR 2.9, 95% CI 1.4 to 6.3, adjusted for maternal age and deprivation), but antenatal evidence of fetal macrosomia was not (OR 0.8, 95% CI 0.5 to 1.3, adjusted for maternal age and deprivation).[33] Fetal surveillance was sub-optimal for 20% of 37 babies with antenatal evidence of fetal growth restriction and for 45% of 129 babies with antenatal evidence of macrosomia. For babies with antenatal evidence of macrosomia, sub-optimal fetal surveillance was associated with poor pregnancy outcome (OR 5.3, 95% CI 2.4 to 12.0, adjusted for maternal age and deprivation). Additional case–control analysis showed an association with fetal and neonatal death after 20 weeks of gestation, but not with fetal anomaly. [EL = 3–4]

The CEMACH enquiry found no difference in the proportion of women with type 1 or type 2 diabetes with antenatal evidence of macrosomia (*P* = 0.99) or fetal growth restriction (*P* = 0.31).[33] [EL = 3–4]

The CEMACH enquiry found that shoulder dystocia was documented in 7.9% of vaginal births. The rate of shoulder dystocia was related to birthweight with 0.9% of babies weighting less than 2500 g, 4.7% of babies 2500–3999 g, 22.0% of babies 4000–4249 g, 25% of babies 4250–4499 g and 42.9% of babies 4500 g or more. The CEMACH enquiry found that Erb palsy occurred in 4.5 per 100 births; this is greater than the incidence of 0.42 per 1000 live births reported in the general population.[2] [EL = 3]

The CEMACH enquiry found 0.9% of singleton babies born to women with type 1 diabetes and 1.3% singleton babies born to women with type 2 diabetes were less than 1000 g; this is higher than the national average for England and Wales (0.5%).[2] [EL = 3]

The main concerns of the enquiry panels regarding surveillance of macrosomic and growth-restricted babies was lack of timely follow-up (affecting approximately 80% of babies). For macrosomic babies, there were also concerns about poor interpretation of ultrasound scans and about actions taken in response to tests. [EL = 3–4]

Evidence statement

The main ultrasonic methods for predicting birthweight (EFW and abdominal circumference) perform similarly in terms of diagnostic accuracy in women with diabetes. However, no clinical studies were identified that compared clinical outcomes using the two methods.

Umbilical artery Doppler ultrasound has better diagnostic accuracy as a test of fetal wellbeing in pregnant women with diabetes than has fetal cardiotocography or biophysical profile. Doppler ultrasound is also a better predictor of adverse maternal and neonatal outcomes, but its effectiveness is limited to high-risk pregnancies defined in terms of IUGR and/or pre-eclampsia, rather than diabetes *per se*.

Cost-effectiveness

The effectiveness of methods for monitoring fetal growth and wellbeing in women with diabetes was identified by the GDG as a priority for health economic analysis.

The lack of comparative data in relation to clinical outcomes resulting from ultrasonic methods for assessing fetal growth (for example, fetal abdominal circumference alone versus abdominal circumference plus fetal head circumference) precluded formal cost-effectiveness analysis. The GDG's discussions included consideration of the frequency of ultrasound assessment of fetal growth and the implications for cost-effectiveness. The GDG's view was that three scans should be offered (rather than two): this would allow healthcare professionals to advise women with diabetes on the direction of pregnancy, rather than providing estimates of fetal growth that might be masked by measurement error; it would also allow assessment of the need for, and response to, insulin therapy. Nevertheless, three scans at 4-weekly intervals starting at 28 weeks of gestation was thought to represent a reduction in the frequency of growth scans compared with current clinical practice that would, therefore, bring a cost saving to the NHS.

The clinical evidence in relation to monitoring fetal wellbeing showed that umbilical artery Doppler ultrasound is more effective in predicting adverse outcomes in women with diabetes than fetal cardiotocography or biophysical profile. Given that the clinical effectiveness of Doppler ultrasound is limited to women with other risk factors (notably IUGR and/or pre-eclampsia), and that current practice involves routine use of Doppler ultrasound to monitor fetal wellbeing in women with diabetes, a recommendation not to monitor fetal wellbeing routinely before 38 weeks of gestation was considered likely to be cost-effective.

Existing guidance

The NICE antenatal care guideline[9] recommends that symphysis–fundal height should be measured and recorded for pregnant women at each antenatal appointment from 24 weeks of gestation. A fetal growth scan to detect SGA unborn babies should be offered to women if the symphysis–fundal height measurement is at least 3 cm less than the gestational age in weeks. Ultrasound estimation of fetal size for suspected LGA unborn babies should not be undertaken in a low-risk population. Doppler ultrasound should not be used to monitor fetal growth during pregnancy. Customised fetal growth charts should not be used for screening for SGA babies.

From evidence to recommendations

In the absence of comparative data on the effectiveness of different methods of ultrasound monitoring of fetal growth, the GDG recommended that fetal growth and amniotic fluid volume (to detect polyhydramnios) should be monitored by ultrasound every 4 weeks from 28 weeks of gestation to 36 weeks of gestation. The GDG's view is that this would represent a change in clinical practice which would effect a reduction in the frequency of monitoring for fetal growth and amniotic fluid volume in women with diabetes and would, therefore, bring a cost saving to the NHS. Fetal growth and amniotic fluid volume should be measured in all women with pre-existing diabetes and gestational diabetes (i.e. even in women with gestational diabetes controlled by diet alone) because of the increased risk of macrosomia.

Evidence shows that monitoring for fetal wellbeing using umbilical artery Doppler ultrasound is a better predictor of pregnancy outcome than fetal cardiotocography and biophysical profile in women with diabetes. However, routine monitoring of fetal wellbeing for women with diabetes is not recommended before 38 weeks of gestation because the effectiveness of Doppler ultrasound is limited to women at risk of IUGR and/or pre-eclampsia. In making this recommendation the GDG sought to effect a change in clinical practice that would bring a cost saving to the NHS.

Recommendations for monitoring fetal growth and wellbeing

Pregnant women with diabetes should be offered ultrasound monitoring of fetal growth and amniotic fluid volume every 4 weeks from 28 to 36 weeks.

Routine monitoring of fetal wellbeing before 38 weeks is not recommended in pregnant women with diabetes, unless there is a risk of intrauterine growth restriction.

Women with diabetes and a risk of intrauterine growth restriction (macrovascular disease and/or nephropathy) will require an individualised approach to monitoring fetal growth and wellbeing.

Research recommendations for monitoring fetal growth and wellbeing

How can the fetus at risk of intrauterine death be identified in women with diabetes?

Why this is important
Unheralded intrauterine death remains a significant contributor to perinatal mortality in pregnancies complicated by diabetes. Conventional tests of fetal wellbeing (umbilical artery Doppler ultrasound, cardiotocography and other biophysical tests) have been shown to have poor sensitivity for predicting such events. Alternative approaches that include measurements of liquor erythropoietin and magnetic resonance imaging spectroscopy may be effective, but there is currently insufficient clinical evidence to evaluate them. Well-designed randomised controlled trials that are sufficiently powered are needed to determine whether these approaches are clinically and cost-effective.

5.8 Timetable of antenatal appointments

Description of the evidence

No specific searches were undertaken for this section of the guideline. The evidence is drawn from publications identified in searches for other sections.

Current practice
The CEMACH diabetes in pregnancy programme provides data on current practice in England, Wales and Northern Ireland in relation to antenatal care, including care plans, for women with type 1 and type 2 diabetes. The enquiry panels classified maternity care during pregnancy as sub-optimal for 58% of women who had poor pregnancy outcomes and 44% of women who had good pregnancy outcomes (OR 1.9, 95% CI 1.2 to 2.8, adjusted for maternal age and deprivation). The two most frequently cited categories for sub-optimal antenatal care were fetal surveillance (monitoring fetal growth and wellbeing; see Section 5.7) and management of maternal risks. Other categories cited included problems with the antenatal diabetes multidisciplinary team. There were no significant differences between women with type 1 and type 2 diabetes in terms of sub-optimal antenatal care.[33] [EL = 3–4]

The enquiry reported that 63% of maternity units in England Wales and Northern Ireland had a full multidisciplinary team comprising an obstetrician, a diabetes physician, a diabetes specialist nurse, a diabetes specialist midwife and a dietitian. There had been an increase in provision of staff over the preceding 8 years, with the availability of a diabetes specialist midwife in the antenatal clinic increasing from 25% to 77% of units, and the availability of a dietitian increasing from 40% to 80% of units. Seventy-five percent of women were reported to have maternity and diabetes care provided in a joint clinic, although only 22% of women were reported to have the entire multidisciplinary team involved in their care.[33] [EL = 3–4]

The CEMACH enquiry panels commented that infrequent clinic appointments, lack of multidisciplinary involvement and communication issues were factors in sub-optimal diabetes care in pregnancy in some of the women in the case–control study.[33] [EL = 3–4]

The CEMACH enquiry recommended that an individualised care plan for pregnancy (and the postnatal period) be used and that the care plan should include, as a minimum:[33]
- targets for glycaemic control
- a schedule for retinal screening
- a schedule for renal screening
- a plan for fetal surveillance during birth
- postnatal diabetes care.

It was recommended that the care plan should be implemented from the beginning of pregnancy by a multidisciplinary team present at the same time in the same clinic. [EL = 3–4]

Existing guidance

The NSF for diabetes[20] recommends that antenatal care for women with diabetes should be delivered by a multidisciplinary team consisting of an obstetrician, a diabetes physician, a diabetes specialist nurse, a midwife and a dietitian.

The NICE antenatal care guideline[9] contains recommendations on the schedule of appointments that should be offered as part of routine antenatal care, including recommendations about what should happen at each appointment.

From evidence to recommendations

The GDG's view is that women with diabetes who are pregnant should be offered immediate contact with a joint diabetes and antenatal clinic, and they should have contact with the diabetes care team for assessment of glycaemic control every 1–2 weeks throughout pregnancy.

The timing and content of antenatal care appointments for women with diabetes should follow the schedule for routine antenatal care appointments recommended in the NICE antenatal care guideline,[9] except where specific additions and/or differences are indicated below to support the recommendations made elsewhere in the guideline. The main differences between routine antenatal care (as specified in the NICE antenatal care guideline)[9] and antenatal care for women with diabetes are summarised in Table 5.6. Ongoing opportunites for accessing information, education and advice should be offered to women with diabetes throughout the antenatal period.

Evidence from the CEMACH enquiry shows that many maternity units have not yet implemented the recommendation in the NSF for diabetes to provide diabetes and maternity care in a joint diabetes/antenatal clinic delivered by a multidisciplinary team. In formulating its recommendations the GDG sought to reinforce the recommendation contained in the NSF for diabetes.

First antenatal appointment
The GDG's view is that women with diabetes should be offered confirmation of viability and gestational age at the first antenatal appointment. This is earlier than in routine antenatal care because diabetes is associated with a high rate of miscarriage (see Sections 3.4 and 5.1) and because diabetes can disrupt the menstrual cycle leading to difficulty in determining the timing of ovulation.

Women with pre-existing diabetes may already have attended for preconception care and advice. For these women, the first antenatal appointment provides an opportunity to reinforce information, education and advice in relation to achieving optimal glycaemic control (including dietary advice). Women who have not attended for preconception care and advice should be offered the corresponding information, education and advice for the first time; a clinical history should seek to establish the extent of diabetes-related complications (including neuropathy and vascular disease); medications for diabetes and its complications should also be reviewed at this time.

Women with pre-existing diabetes who have not had a retinal assessment in the previous 12 months should be offered an assessment at the first presentation in pregnancy (see Section 5.4). Women with pre-existing diabetes who have not had a renal assessment in the previous 12 months should be offered an assessment at the first presentation in pregnancy (see Section 5.5).

All women with diabetes should have contact with the diabetes care team for assessment of glycaemic control every 1–2 weeks throughout the antenatal period (this could include telephone contact) and HbA$_{1c}$ should be used to assess long-term glycaemic control in the first trimester of pregnancy (see Section 5.1).

The GDG's discussions included consideration of screening for Down's syndrome. Screening methods for Down's syndrome in women with diabetes are currently no different to those for women without diabetes, and so the GDG made no specific recommendations in relation to the schedule for screening for Down's syndrome.

The GDG's discussions also included consideration of surveillance for pre-eclampsia. Women with diabetes are at increased risk of pre-eclampsia (see Sections 4.3 and 5.5), but methods for surveillance (testing for proteinuria) and management of pre-eclampsia in women with diabetes are no different to those for women without diabetes. The schedule of appointments for routine antenatal care recommended in the NICE antenatal care guideline[9] includes testing urine for proteinuria at every appointment, and so the GDG made no specific recommendations in relation to surveillance for pre-eclampsia.

16 weeks of gestation
If any retinopathy is present at booking an additional assessment should be made at 16–20 weeks of gestation for women with pre-existing diabetes (see Section 5.4).

20 weeks of gestation
Women with diabetes should be offered an ultrasound anatomical examination of the four chamber view of the fetal heart and outflow tracts at 20 weeks of gestation because the diagnostic accuracy is better at 20 weeks of gestation than at 18–19 weeks of gestation (see Section 5.6). The GDG's

view is that the routine ultrasound scan for the detecting structural anomalies, which should be offered to all pregnant women, should also be performed at 20 weeks of gestation in women with diabetes because it is more convenient for the woman to have both scans at one visit.

25 weeks of gestation
No evidence was identified to suggest that antenatal care for women with diabetes should be different to routine antenatal care at 25 weeks of gestation.

28 weeks of gestation
Ultrasound monitoring of fetal growth (to detect LGA or SGA babies) and amniotic fluid volume (to detect polyhydramnios) should start at 28 weeks of gestation and continue at 4-weekly intervals (i.e. 32 weeks and 36 weeks; see Section 5.7). Women with pre-existing diabetes who had no diabetic retinopathy at their first antenatal clinic visit should be offered retinal assessment at 28 weeks of gestation (see Section 5.4). Women who have been diagnosed with gestational diabetes as a result of routine antenatal screening enter the care pathway at 28 weeks of gestation (see Section 4.3 and the NICE antenatal care guideline[9]). They should be offered information about the risks to the woman and the baby that is offered to women with pre-existing diabetes in the preconception period.

32 weeks of gestation
Ultrasound monitoring of fetal growth and amniotic fluid volume should be offered at 32 weeks of gestation as part of 4-weekly monitoring (see Section 5.7). It is the GDG's view that, for women with diabetes, the routine investigations that would normally be offered to nulliparous pregnant women at 31 weeks of gestation should instead be offered at 32 weeks of gestation because it is more convenient for the woman to have all the investigations at one visit.

34 weeks of gestation
No evidence was identified to suggest that antenatal care for women with diabetes should be different to routine antenatal care at 34 weeks of gestation.

36 weeks of gestation
Ultrasound monitoring of fetal growth and amniotic fluid volume should be offered at 36 weeks of gestation as part of 4-weekly monitoring (see Section 5.7). Evidence shows that women with diabetes are likely to give birth soon after 36 weeks of gestation, either through spontaneous labour, elective induction of labour or elective caesarean section to reduce the risk of stillbirth and birth trauma associated with fetal macrosomia (see Section 6.1). Given the evidence, the GDG's view is that women with diabetes should be offered information and advice in relation to intrapartum care and postnatal care at 36 weeks of gestation. The information and advice should cover: timing, mode and management of labour and birth, including options for elective early birth (see Section 6.1); analgesia and anaesthesia (see Section 6.2); changes to hypoglycaemic therapy during and after birth (see Sections 6.3 and 8.2); management of the baby after birth, including early feeding, detection and management of neonatal hypoglycaemia and other diabetes-related complications (see Chapter 7); initiation of breastfeeding and the effect of breastfeeding on glycaemic control (see Section 8.1); and information about contraception and follow-up (see Section 8.2).

38 weeks of gestation
Induction of labour, or caesarean section if indicated, should be offered to women with diabetes at 38 weeks of gestation (see Section 6.1). Monitoring of fetal wellbeing should be offered to women with diabetes who are awaiting spontaneous labour.

39–41 weeks of gestation
No evidence was identified to suggest that antenatal care for women with diabetes who have not given birth by 40 weeks of gestation should be different to routine antenatal care at 40–41 weeks of gestation. However, evidence shows that many women with diabetes give birth before 40 weeks of gestation (see Section 6.1). Monitoring of fetal wellbeing should be offered to women with diabetes who are awaiting spontaneous labour at 39–41 weeks of gestation.

The GDG's discussions also included consideration of thyroid function in women with diabetes. There was no reason to suppose that women with diabetes required testing for thyroid function.

Table 5.6 Timetable for antenatal appointments for women with diabetes

Routine antenatal care (NICE antenatal care guideline)[9]	Additional/different care for women with diabetes
First appointment (booking) • give information, with an opportunity to discuss issues and ask questions; offer verbal information supported by written information (on topics such as diet and lifestyle considerations, pregnancy care services available, maternity benefits and sufficient information to enable informed decision making about screening tests) • identify women who may need additional care and plan pattern of care for the pregnancy • check blood group and RhD status • offer screening for haemoglobinopathies, anaemia, red-cell alloantibodies, hepatitis B virus, HIV, rubella susceptibility and syphilis • offer screening for asymptomatic bacteriuria • offering screening for Down's syndrome • offer early ultrasound scan for gestational age assessment • offer ultrasound screening for structural anomalies (18–20 weeks) • measure BMI, blood pressure and test urine for proteinuria. At the first (and possibly second) appointment, for women who choose to have screening, the following tests should be arranged: • blood tests (for checking blood group and RhD status and screening for haemogloinopathies, anaemia, red-cell alloantibodies, hepatitis B virus, HIV, rubella susceptibility and syphilis) ideally before 10 weeks • urine tests (to check for proteinuria and screen for asymptomatic bacteriuria) • ultrasound scan to determine gestational age using: – crown–rump measurement if performed at 10 weeks 0 days to 13 weeks 6 days – head circumference if crown–rump length is above 84 millimetres • Down's syndrome screening using: – nuchal translucency at 11 weeks 0 days to 13 weeks 6 days – serum screening at 15 weeks 0 days to 20 weeks 0 days.	*First appointment (joint diabetes and antenatal clinic)* • if the woman has been attending for preconception care and advice, continue to provide information, education and advice in relation to achieving optimal glycaemic control (including dietary advice) • if the woman has not attended for preconception care and advice give information, education and advice for the first time, take clinical history to establish extent of diabetes-related complications (including neuropathy and vascular disease), and review medications for diabetes and its complications • retinal assessment and renal assessment for women with pre-existing diabetes if these have not been undertaken in preceding 12 months • contact with the diabetes care team every 1–2 weeks throughout pregnancy for all women with diabetes and assessment of long-term glycaemic control using HbA$_{1c}$ (first trimester only).
16 weeks The next appointment should be scheduled at 16 weeks to: • review, discuss and record the results of all screening tests undertaken; reassess planned pattern of care for the pregnancy and identify women who need additional care • investigate a haemoglobin level of less than 11 g/100 ml and consider iron supplementation if indicated • measure blood pressure and test urine for proteinuria • give information, with an opportunity to discuss issues and ask questions, including discussion of the routine anomaly scan; offer verbal information supported by antenatal classes and written information.	*16 weeks* Retinal assessment for women with pre-existing diabetes if diabetic retinopathy was present at booking (16–20 weeks). Early testing of glood glucose or OGTT for women with a history of gestational diabetes and/or ongoing IGT (18–20 weeks).
18–20 weeks At 18–20 weeks, if the woman chooses, an ultrasound scan should be performed for the detection of structural anomalies. For a woman whose placenta is found to extend across the internal cervical os at this time, another scan at 36 weeks should be offered and the results of this scan reviewed at the 36 week appointment.	*20 weeks* Ultrasound scan for detecting structural anomalies and anatomical examination of the four chamber view of the fetal heart plus outflow tracts.
25 weeks At 25 weeks of gestation, another appointment should be scheduled for nulliparous women. At this appointment: • measure and plot symphysis–fundal height • measure blood pressure and test urine for proteinuria • give information, with an opportunity to discuss issues and ask questions; offer verbal information supported by antenatal classes and written information.	*25 weeks* No additional or different care for women with diabetes.
28 weeks The next appointment for all pregnant women should occur at 28 weeks. At this appointment: • offer a second screening for anaemia and atypical red-cell alloantibodies • investigate a haemoglobin level of less than 10.5 g/100 ml and consider iron supplementation, if indicated • offer anti-D to rhesus-negative women • measure blood pressure and test urine for proteinuria • measure and plot symphysis–fundal height • give information, with an opportunity to discuss issues and ask questions; offer verbal information supported by antenatal classes and written information • screening for gestational diabetes.	*28 weeks* Start ultrasound monitoring of fetal growth and amniotic fluid volume Retinal assessment for women with pre-existing diabetes if no diabetic retinopathy was present at the first antenatal clinic visit. Women diagnosed with gestational diabetes as a result of routine antenatal screening enter the care pathway.

Routine antenatal care (NICE antenatal care guideline)[9]	Additional/different care for women with diabetes
31 weeks Nulliparous women should have an appointment scheduled at 31 weeks to: • measure blood pressure and test urine for proteinuria • measure and plot symphysis–fundal height • give information, with an opportunity to discuss issues and ask questions; offer verbal information supported by antenatal classes and written information • review, discuss and record the results of screening tests undertaken at 28 weeks; reassess planned pattern of care for the pregnancy and identify women who need additional care.	*32 weeks (not 31 weeks)* Ultrasound monitoring of fetal growth and amniotic fluid volume. All routine investigations normally scheduled for 31 weeks should also be conducted at 32 weeks.
34 weeks At 34 weeks, all pregnant women should be seen in order to: • offer a second dose of anti-D to rhesus-negative women • measure blood pressure and test urine for proteinuria • measure and plot symphysis–fundal height • give information, with an opportunity to discuss issues and ask questions; offer verbal information supported by antenatal classes and written information • review, discuss and record the results of screening tests undertaken at 28 weeks; reassess planned pattern of care for the pregnancy and identify women who need additional care.	*34 weeks* No additional or different care for women with diabetes
36 weeks At 36 weeks, all pregnant women should be seen again to: • measure blood pressure and test urine for proteinuria • measure and plot symphysis–fundal height • check position of baby • for women whose babies are in the breech presentation, offer external cephalic version • review ultrasound scan report if placenta extended over the internal cervical os at previous scan • give information, with an opportunity to discuss issues and ask questions; offer verbal information supported by antenatal classes and written information.	*36 weeks* Ultrasound monitoring of fetal growth and amniotic fluid volume. Offer information and advice about timing, mode and management of labour and birth, including anaesthetic review/assessment. Plan postnatal diabetes management, breastfeeding, management of the baby after birth and information about follow-up.
38 weeks Another appointment at 38 weeks will allow for: • measurement of blood pressure and urine testing for proteinuria • measurement and plotting of symphysis–fundal height • information giving, including options for management of prolonged pregnancy, with an opportunity to discuss issues and ask questions; verbal information supported by antenatal classes and written information.	*38 weeks* Induction of labour, or caesarean section if indicated, otherwise await spontaneous labour. Monitoring of fetal wellbeing if baby not yet born. *39 weeks* Monitoring of fetal wellbeing if baby not yet born.
40 weeks For nulliparous women, an appointment at 40 weeks should be scheduled to: • measure blood pressure and test urine for proteinuria • measure and plot symphysis–fundal height • give information, with an opportunity to discuss issues and ask questions; offer verbal information supported by antenatal classes and written information.	*40 weeks* No additional or different care for women with diabetes. Monitoring of fetal wellbeing if baby not yet born.
41 weeks For women who have not given birth by 41 weeks: • a membrane sweep should be offered[a] • induction of labour should be offered[a] • blood pressure should be measured and urine tested for proteinuria • symphysis–fundal height should be measured and plotted • information should be given, with an opportunity to discuss issues and ask questions; verbal information supported by written information.	*41 weeks* No additional or different care for women with diabetes. Monitoring of fetal wellbeing if baby not yet born.

[a] The NICE clinical guideline on induction of labour is being updated and is expected to be published in June 2008.
IGT = impaired glucose tolerance; OGTT = oral glucose tolerance test.

Recommendations for timetable of antenatal appointments

Women with diabetes who are pregnant should be offered immediate contact with a joint diabetes and antenatal clinic.

Women with diabetes should have contact with the diabetes care team for assessment of glycaemic control every 1–2 weeks throughout pregnancy.

Antenatal appointments for women with diabetes should provide care specifically for women with diabetes, in addition to the care provided routinely for healthy pregnant women (see 'Antenatal care: routine care for the healthy pregnant woman' [NICE clinical guideline 62], available from www.nice.org.uk/CG062). Table 5.7 describes where care for women with diabetes differs from routine antenatal care. At each appointment women should be offered ongoing opportunities for information and education.

Table 5.7 Specific antenatal care for women with diabetes

Appointment	Care for women with diabetes during pregnancy[a]
First appointment (joint diabetes and antenatal clinic)	Offer information, advice and support in relation to optimising glycaemic control. Take a clinical history to establish the extent of diabetes-related complications. Review medications for diabetes and its complications. Offer retinal and/or renal assessment if these have not been undertaken in the previous 12 months.
7–9 weeks	Confirm viability of pregnancy and gestational age.
Booking appointment (ideally by 10 weeks)	Discuss information, education and advice about how diabetes will affect the pregnancy, birth and early parenting (such as breastfeeding and initial care of the baby).
16 weeks	Offer retinal assessment at 16–20 weeks to women with pre-existing diabetes who showed signs of diabetic retinopathy at the first antenatal appointment.
20 weeks	Offer four chamber view of the fetal heart and outflow tracts plus scans that would be offered at 18–20 weeks as part of routine antenatal care.
28 weeks	Offer ultrasound monitoring of fetal growth and amniotic fluid volume. Offer retinal assessment to women with pre-existing diabetes who showed no diabetic retinopathy at their first antenatal clinic visit.
32 weeks	Offer ultrasound monitoring of fetal growth and amniotic fluid volume. Offer to nulliparous women all investigations that would be offered at 31 weeks as part of routine antenatal care.
36 weeks	Offer ultrasound monitoring of fetal growth and amniotic fluid volume. Offer information and advice about: • timing, mode and management of birth • analgesia and anaesthesia • changes to hypoglycaemic therapy during and after birth • management of the baby after birth • initiation of breastfeeding and the effect of breastfeeding on glycaemic control • contraception and follow-up.
38 weeks	Offer induction of labour, or caesarean section if indicated, and start regular tests of fetal wellbeing for women with diabetes who are awaiting spontaneous labour.
39 weeks	Offer tests of fetal wellbeing.
40 weeks	Offer tests of fetal wellbeing.
41 weeks	Offer tests of fetal wellbeing.

[a] Women with diabetes should also receive routine care according to the schedule of appointments in 'Antenatal care: routine care for the healthy pregnant woman' (NICE clinical guideline 62), including appointments at 25 weeks (for nulliparous women) and 34 weeks, but with the exception of the appointment for nulliparous women at 31 weeks.

There were no research recommendations relating to the timetable of antenatal appointments for women with diabetes.

5.9 Preterm labour in women with diabetes

Description of the evidence

Incidence of preterm birth

A prospective cohort study[303] examined the importance of glycaemic control and risk of preterm birth in women with type 1 diabetes who have normoalbuminuria and no pre-eclampsia during pregnancy. Seventy-one women with complete data on HbA_{1c}, insulin dose and albumin excretion rate measured at 12 weeks of gestation and every second week thereafter were recruited and followed. The overall rate of preterm birth was 23%; women who experienced preterm birth had higher HbA_{1c} throughout pregnancy. Regression analysis showed that HbA_{1c} was the strongest predictor of preterm birth from 6–32 weeks of gestation and that the risk of preterm birth was more than 40% when HbA_{1c} was above 7.7% at 8 weeks of gestation. [EL = 2+]

Antenatal steroids

Antenatal steroids are administered to women who have a spontaneous or planned preterm birth to accelerate fetal lung development and prevent respiratory distress syndrome. The use of steroids in women with diabetes is associated with a significant worsening of glycaemic control requiring an increase in insulin dose.

Two studies were identified that reported on approaches to increasing insulin in women with diabetes undergoing treatment with antenatal steroids.

The first study reported on a test of an algorithm for improved subcutaneous insulin treatment during steroid treatment (intramuscular administration of betamethasone 12 mg repeated after 24 hours).[304] The algorithm was as follows:

- on day 1 (the day on which the first betamethasone injection is given), the night insulin dose should be increased by 25%
- on day 2, all insulin doses should be increased by 40%
- on day 3, all insulin doses should be increased by 40%
- on day 4, all insulin doses should be increased by 20%
- on day 5, all insulin doses should be increased by 10–20%
- during days 6 and 7, the insulin doses should be gradually reduced to their levels before treatment.

The study involved 16 women, eight of whom were treated before the introduction of the algorithm (cohort 1) and another eight who were treated after its introduction (cohort 2). Women in cohort 1 had insulin doses adjusted individually based on the level of blood glucose obtained. The median blood glucose over the 5 days was 6.7 mmol/litre, 14.3 mmol/litre, 12.3 mmol/litre, 7.7 mmol/litre and 7.7 mmol/litre in cohort 1 and 7.7 mmol/litre, 8.2 mmol/litre, 9.6 mmol/litre, 7.0 mmol/litre and 7.4 mmol/litre in cohort 2 ($P < 0.05$ for days 2 and 3). None of the women developed ketoacidosis or severe hypoglycaemia. [EL = 2+]

The second study reported on the use of a supplementary intravenous sliding scale to indicate the required dosage of supplementary insulin infusion in six women receiving antenatal steroids.[305] The supplementary insulin was in addition to the woman's usual subcutaneous insulin regimen and usual dietary programme. The additional infusion was commenced immediately before the first steroid injection and continued for at least 12 hours after the second injection. If blood glucose levels were too high on the initial regimen (glucose 10.1 mmol/litre or more for 2 consecutive hours) the dosage regimen was moved up to the next level. If the blood glucose level was less than 4 mmol/litre the dosage regimen was reduced by one level. Data were collected on six women receiving dexamethasone. Significant amounts of supplementary intravenous insulin were required (median dose 74 U, range 32–88 U) in order to achieve glucose control following administration of dexamethasone. Seventy-five percent of all glucose measurements were within 4–10 mmol/litre. [EL = 3]

Tocolytic agents

Tocolytic agents are used to inhibit uterine contractions. They may help to delay birth and allow women to complete a course of antenatal steroids. Betamimetics have been widely used for tocolysis, although they are no longer recommended as the first choice for general use.[306] Betamimetics increase blood glucose concentrations[307–309] and several cases of ketoacidosis have been reported in women with diabetes following administration of these drugs (see Section 5.3).[310–314]

Current practice
CEMACH undertook a descriptive study of all pregnancies of women with pre-existing diabetes who gave birth or booked between 1 March 2002 and 28 February 2003.[2] Of the 3474 women in this study with a continuing pregnancy at 24 weeks of 328 gave birth before 34 weeks of gestation. Thirty-five of these pregnancies resulted in a stillbirth. Of the remaining 293 women, 70.3% received a full course of antenatal steroid therapy. The most common reason given for non-administration of antenatal steroids was birth of the baby before the full course could be given. In a small group of women diabetes was considered a contraindication to antenatal steroid use. [EL = 3]

Evidence statement

The use of antenatal steroids for fetal lung maturation in women with diabetes is associated with a significant worsening of glycaemic control.

Two studies that reported on approaches to modifying insulin dose in women undergoing antenatal steroid treatment showed that glycaemic control could be improved by increasing the insulin dose immediately prior to and during administration of antenatal steroids. However, the two protocols evaluated were only moderately successful in keeping blood glucose levels at the desired level (less than 7 mmol/litre).

Evidence shows that administration of betamimetics to suppress labour induces hyperglycaemia and ketoacidosis.

From evidence to recommendations

The evidence supports the use of increased insulin dose immediately before and during antenatal administration of steroids. Since the two protocols that have been evaluated were only moderately successful in achieving glycaemic control, women receiving additional insulin during administration of antenatal steroids should be closely monitored according to an agreed protocol in case the insulin dose requires further adjustment.

When tocolysis is indicated in women with diabetes an alternative to betamimetics should be used to avoid hyperglycaemia and ketoacidosis.

Recommendations for preterm labour in women with diabetes

Diabetes should not be considered a contraindication to antenatal steroids for fetal lung maturation or to tocolysis.

Women with insulin-treated diabetes who are receiving steroids for fetal lung maturation should have additional insulin according to an agreed protocol and should be closely monitored.

Betamimetic drugs should not be used for tocolysis in women with diabetes.

There were no research recommendations relating to preterm labour in women with diabetes.

6   Intrapartum care

6.1   Timing and mode of birth

Description of the evidence

Eight epidemiological studies were identified that examined the effect of diabetes on timing and mode of birth. Nine studies were identified that investigated different methods of intervening in timing and mode of birth in women with diabetes. Five studies were identified in relation to optimal timing of birth in women with diabetes. Three studies were identified that examined vaginal birth after previous caesarean section (VBAC) in women with diabetes.

Effect of diabetes on mode of birth

A retrospective case–control study based on administrative data ($n = 776\,500$) from Canada examined obstetric intervention and complication rates for women with and without pre-existing diabetes.[315] The proportion of women with diabetes in 1996 was 8.42 per 1000 deliveries, but this increased to 11.90 per 1000 deliveries by 2001. The study found that women with pre-existing diabetes were significantly more likely to have caesarean section or induced labour than women without diabetes ($P < 0.0001$). Pregnancies in women with pre-existing diabetes were also more likely to be complicated by obstructed labour ($P = 0.01$), hypertension ($P < 0.0001$), pre-eclampsia ($P < 0.0001$) and shoulder dystocia ($P < 0.0001$). However, the study noted marked increases in all these outcomes between 1996 and 2001 in women without diabetes. The study concluded that women with pre-existing diabetes needed close monitoring during pregnancy. [EL = 2–]

A retrospective cohort study ($n = 12\,303$) from the USA examined the relationship of diabetes and obesity on risk of caesarean section.[316] The study found that diet-controlled gestational diabetes ($P < 0.0001$), insulin-controlled gestational diabetes ($P < 0.0001$) and pre-existing diabetes ($P < 0.0001$) were risk factors for having caesarean section. However, multiple regression analysis showed that only pre-existing diabetes was an independent risk factor for having caesarean section. [EL = 3]

A prospective cohort study ($n = 166$) from the USA examined route of birth of women with gestational diabetes.[317] The study found that 110 women had vaginal births and 56 had caesarean section. Multiple regression analysis showed that maternal nulliparity, fetal position and fetal fat were factors associated with caesarean section. [EL = 3]

A prospective case–control study ($n = 3778$) from Canada examined the relationship between caesarean section rates and gestational glucose intolerance (3 hour 100 g OGGT).[318] The study identified four groups: negative gestational diabetes ($n = 2940$), false-positive gestational diabetes ($n = 580$), untreated borderline gestational diabetes ($n = 115$) and known treated gestational diabetes ($n = 143$). Women with gestational diabetes had higher rates of macrosomia (28.7% versus 13.7%, $P < 0.001$) and caesarean section (29.6% versus 20.2%, $P = 0.02$). Treatment of gestational diabetes reduced rates of macrosomia (more than 4000 g) to 10.5% compared with 28.7% in the untreated group and 13.7% in the women without diabetes, but caesarean section rates were 33.6% compared with 29.6% in the untreated group and 20.2% in the women without diabetes. Multivariate analysis found that being treated for gestational diabetes was the most significant factor in determining caesarean section (OR 2.1, 95% CI 1.3 to 3.6); untreated gestational diabetes was not a significant risk factor (OR 1.6, 95% CI 0.9 to 2.7). [EL = 2+]

A retrospective case–control study ($n = 2924$) undertaken in the USA compared the outcomes of macrosomic babies (4000 g or more) with those of babies weighing 3000–3999 g.[319] The rate of injury to the baby during birth was 1.6% for the macrosomic group (RR 3.1, 95% CI 2.5 to 3.8). The study concluded that more research was needed to determine suitable interventions. [EL = 2+]

A prospective cohort study from the USA (*n* = 53 518) examined the association between perinatal death and presence of gestational diabetes.[320] The study found 33.8 per 1000 perinatal deaths in the group without gestational diabetes and 70.3 per 100) in the group with gestational diabetes. However, the rate in the women without diabetes who had induced labour or caesarean section was 33.2 per 1000 compared with 14.8 per 100 in the women without gestational diabetes who had spontaneous birth. The study also found that babies of women with gestational diabetes who were equal to or greater than the 90 percentile in birthweight were more likely to have retarded lung development (*P* < 0.005). The study also examined biochemical markers in the placenta, umbilical cord and fetal membranes. Maternal risk factors were not examined and the study was undertaken in 1978 since when the neonatal survival rate has improved. [EL = 3]

A population-based cohort from the UK (*n* = 11791) examined antenatal risk factors associated with a woman having a caesarean section.[321] The study found that having gestational diabetes increased the risk of having a caesarean section (OR 2.60, 95% CI 1.38 to 4.92), as did pre-existing diabetes (OR 8.50, 95% CI 4.27 to 16.9). However, a number of other factors were also identified, including obstetric history and medical history. Multiple regression showed that diabetes was a risk factor for caesarean section alongside maternal age, previous caesarean section, outcome of last pregnancy, parity, birthweight, neonatal head circumference, gestational age at birth and fetal presentation. However, the study did not examine any health professional- or healthcare-related factors. [EL = 2+]

A cross-sectional study[322] assessed routes of birth and pregnancy outcomes in 10369 births in the USA. The study showed that diabetes was associated with increased caesarean section, resuscitation of babies with positive pressure ventilation and low Apgar score (less than 3) at 1 minute and 5 minutes. [EL = 3]

Regimens for inducing labour and their impact
An RCT (*n* = 200) from the USA involving women with insulin-requiring diabetes compared the outcomes of active induced labour (accurate measurement of gestational development and induction of labour with intravenous oxytocin, *n* = 100) with expectant management (close monitoring and insulin treatment, *n* = 100).[323] Those enrolled had gestational diabetes (*n* = 187) or pre-existing diabetes (*n* = 13). There were no differences between the groups at baseline. In the active induction group 70 women had induction of labour, eight had caesarean section and 22 had spontaneous labour. In the expectant management group 49 women had induction, seven had caesarean section and 44 had spontaneous labour. There were significantly more LGA babies in the expectant management group compared with the active induction group (23% versus 10%, *P* = 0.02). There were three cases of 'mild' shoulder dystocia in the expectant management group and none in the active induction group. The study concluded that active induction of labour at 38 weeks of gestation should be considered in women with insulin-requiring diabetes. [EL = 1+]

A cohort study from Israel (*n* = 1542) examined the effect of intensive management of diet and three protocols for active elective management of route of birth on outcomes in women with gestational diabetes.[324] The results for the three periods of different protocols were compared (period A, estimated fetal weight for caesarean section more than 4500 g; period B, mean glucose less than 5.8 mmol/litre, estimated fetal weight for caesarean section more than 4000 g, time of elective induction 40 weeks of gestation; period C, mean glucose 5.3 mmol/litre, estimated fetal weight for caesarean section more than 4000 g, time of elective induction 38 weeks of gestation). The results were as follows (period A versus period B versus period C): macrosomia (more than 4000 g) 17.9% versus 14.9% versus 8.8% (*P* < 0.05); LGA 23.6% versus 21.0% versus 11.7% (*P* < 0.05); caesarean section 20.6% versus 18.4% versus 16.2%; shoulder dystocia 1.5% versus 1.2% versus 0.6%; induction of labour 11.0% versus 17.0% versus 35.0%. The study concluded that intensive management of diet and active management of birth were beneficial to women with gestational diabetes and their babies. [EL = 2+]

A case–control study (*n* = 2604) undertaken in the USA examined the outcome of elective caesarean section due to macrosomia in women with diabetes.[325] The study compared two time periods (before and after introduction of a protocol based on ultrasound estimates of fetal weight, with AGA fetuses being managed expectantly, those more than 4250 g being born via caesarean section, and those LGA but less than 4250 g being born vaginally after induction of labour. The rate of shoulder dystocia was lower in macrosomic babies in the induced grouped compared with the non-induced group (7.4% versus 18.8%, OR 2.9). The rate of caesarean section was higher postprotocol compared with pre-protocol (25.1% versus 21.7%, $P < 0.04$). The study recommended the use of ultrasound to estimate fetal weight and using this to determine method of birth. [EL = 2–]

A retrospective cohort study using routinely collected data ($n = 108487$) undertaken in the USA examined whether induction of labour increased caesarean section rates in women with diabetes.[326] Women with diabetes were more likely to have a caesarean section than women without diabetes (OR 2.00, 95% CI 1.83 to 2.19). The caesarean section rate was lower in women who had induction of labour than those who did not have induction of labour (OR 0.77, 95% CI 0.50 to 0.89). [EL = 2+]

An RCT ($n = 273$) undertaken in Israel compared induction of labour with expectant management in the presence of macrosomia (4000–4500 g).[327] At baseline the women in the induction group were significantly older than the expectant management group (30.8 years versus 29.5 years, $P = 0.02$). There were no significant differences in the mode of birth between the groups (induction of labour group, 91 spontaneous vaginal births, 17 instrumental births and 26 caesarean sections; expectant management group, 91 spontaneous vaginal births, 18 instrumental births and 30 caesarean sections), nor in the mean birthweight (4062.8 g versus 4132.8 g, $P = 0.24$). There were five cases of shoulder dystocia in the induction group compared with six in the expectant management group. The study concluded that estimated fetal weight between 4000 g and 4500 g should not be considered an indication for inducing birth. However, the study was not explicitly conducted on women with diabetes. [EL = 1+]

An RCT ($n = 120$) undertaken in the USA compared misoprostol with placebo for inducing birth in women with diabetes.[328] There was no difference between the groups at baseline. The study found no difference between the groups during outpatient observation, time from induction to birth ($P = 0.23$), total oxytocin dose ($P = 0.18$) or neonatal characteristics. The study concluded that misoprostol was not beneficial for induction of labour in women with diabetes. [EL = 1+]

A quasi-randomised study ($n = 84$) undertaken in the USA compared the outcomes of caesarean section ($n = 44$) and vaginal births ($n = 40$, 26 spontaneous and 14 induced) in women with gestational diabetes (3 hour 100 g OGTT).[329] The complications recorded for caesarean section versus vaginal birth were: morbidity (9 versus 0), blood transfusions (2 versus 0), wound separation (2 versus 0), macrosomia more than 4000 g (5 versus 3), prematurity by weight (6 versus 5), neonatal infection (1 versus 1), neonatal hypoglycaemia (1 versus 0) and hyperchloraemic acidosis (1 versus 0). The study concluded that there was no advantage to preterm caesarean section in women with gestational diabetes. [EL = 2+]

A case–control study ($n = 388$) undertaken in the USA examined the risk of wound complication after caesarean section in women with pre-existing diabetes and women without diabetes.[330] At baseline women with pre-existing diabetes were more likely to be obese ($P < 0.01$) and have a positive group B streptococcus status ($P < 0.01$). During caesarean section the women with diabetes were more likely to have estimated blood loss above 1000 ml ($P < 0.01$), postpartum haemorrhage ($P = 0.05$) and to spend longer in the operating theatre ($P = 0.01$), but they were less likely to have meconium present ($P = 0.01$). Women with diabetes were more likely to have wound infection (OR 2.7, 95% CI 1.2 to 6.1), wound separation (OR 6.1, 95% CI 1.8 to 21.2) and wound complications (OR 3.7, 95% CI 1.8 to 7.7). The study concluded that diabetes was a risk factor for wound complications after caesarean section. However, analysis did not take into account baseline and surgical differences between groups. [EL = 2–]

Optimal timing of birth
An RCT ($n = 200$) from the USA compared the outcomes of birth after 38 weeks of gestation in women with insulin-requiring diabetes.[323] Those enrolled had gestational diabetes ($n = 187$) or pre-existing diabetes ($n = 13$). In women with pre-existing diabetes, the expectant management of pregnancy after 38 weeks of gestation did not reduce the incidence of caesarean section, but rather led to an increased prevalence of LGA babies (23% versus 10%) and shoulder dystocia (3% versus 0%). Given the risk associated with birth after 38 weeks of gestation, the study suggested that active induction of labour at 38 weeks of gestation should be considered in women with insulin-requiring diabetes, but if this is not pursued careful monitoring of fetal growth should be performed. [EL = 1+]

A case–control study (n = 260) from Israel compared inducing labour at 38–39 weeks of gestation with allowing pregnancy to continue naturally in women with type 1 diabetes.[331] There were no differences between the two groups at baseline. The rate of shoulder dystocia was 1.4% in the induction of labour group compared with 10.2% in the non-induced group who gave birth beyond 40 weeks of gestation ($P < 0.05$). No differences in caesarean section rates or birthweights of babies were found. The rate of shoulder dystocia was lower in the babies of women who had induction of labour at 38–39 weeks of gestation than in those without induction (1.4% versus 10.2%, $P < 0.05$). The study recommended elective induction of labour for women with insulin-requiring diabetes in order to reduce the rate of shoulder dystocia. [EL = 2–]

A case–control study (n = 3778) from Canada examined the relationship between gestational glucose intolerance (3 hour 100 g OGGT) and fetal outcomes.[318] The study identified four groups: negative gestational diabetes (n = 2940), false-positive gestational diabetes (n = 580), untreated borderline gestational diabetes (n = 115) and known treated gestational diabetes (n = 143). There were no significant differences in gestational age at birth (39.8 ± 1.8 weeks for women without diabetes, 39.8 ± 1.8 for women with borderline diabetes and 39.3 ± 1.6, $P > 0.20$ for women with gestational diabetes). There were no differences among the groups in the rates of fetal distress or shoulder dystocia. [EL = 2+]

A cohort study (n = 317) from Israel conducted between 1993 and 1995 examined the effect of intensive management of gestational diabetes with diet in relation to birth timing and outcomes and compared the effect with that for women without diabetes.[324] The gestational age at birth for women with gestational diabetes was 39 ± 2.5 weeks and that of women without diabetes was 39 ± 1.5 weeks. [EL = 2+]

A case–control study (n = 428) from the USA examined the mean gestational ages at birth of babies of women with gestational diabetes and those in a control group without maternal diabetes.[332] The study found no significant difference between women with diabetes and the controls in gestational age at birth (38. 4 ± 2.8 weeks versus 39 ± 2.9 weeks), shoulder dystocia, Apgar scores, neonatal death or prolonged hospital stay after birth. The study suggests that if pregnancy is not interrupted then the gestational age at birth is similar between women with diabetes and those without diabetes, and neonatal outcomes do not differ between the two groups. [EL = 2–]

Vaginal birth after previous caesarean section

A retrospective case-series (n = 10110) from the USA examined the success of VBAC in women with previous obstetric complications, including gestational diabetes.[333] Sixty-two percent of women who attempted VBAC were successful. The factors associated with unsuccessful VBAC were birthweight more than 4000 g, cephalopelvic disproportion, prolonged labour, dysfunctional labour, pre-existing diabetes and gestational diabetes, hypertension, induced labour, sexually transmitted disease, fetal distress and breech birth. [EL = 3]

A retrospective cohort study (n = 25079) from the USA examined whether women with diet-controlled gestational diabetes were at increased risk of failed VBAC compared with women who did not have diabetes.[334] The study involved 13396 women who attempted VBAC. Data on 423 women with diet-controlled gestational diabetes and 9437 women without diabetes were analysed. After controlling for birthweight, maternal age, race, tobacco use, chronic hypertension, hospital setting, labour management and obstetric history, 49% of the women with gestational diabetes and 67% of the women without diabetes attempted VBAC. The study found that gestational diabetes was not an independent risk factor for VBAC. The success rate for attempted VBAC among women with gestational diabetes was 70% compared to 74% for women without diabetes, and the proportion of babies weighing more than 4000 g was 18% compared with 13% ($P < 0.05$). The VBAC group had more previous pregnancies (3.4 versus 3.1, $P < 0.001$), different ethnic mix ($P < 0.05$), different insurance profile ($P < 0.001$), seen in university hospital (56% versus 42%, $P < 0.001$), previous vaginal birth or VBAC (40% versus 17%, $P < 0.001$) and birthweight more than 4000 g (18% v 33%, $P < 0.001$). Logistic regression analysis showed that age, birthweight, white ethnic origin, induced labour, augmented labour and previous vaginal birth were all predictors of successful VBAC, whilst diet-controlled gestational diabetes and chronic hypertension were not. [EL = 2+]

A retrospective cohort study ($n = 428$) conducted in the USA compared attempted VBAC in women with gestational diabetes to that in women without diabetes.[332] One hundred and fifty-six women with gestational diabetes were matched with 272 controls. The parities were similar for the two groups, but the women with gestational diabetes were significantly older than the control group ($P < 0.001$) and more likely to be white or Hispanic ($P = 0.006$). The study found that those with previous gestational diabetes were more likely to have a future caesarean section (35.9% versus 22.8%, $P < 0.001$), less likely to have a vaginal birth (64.1% versus 77.2%, $P < 0.001$) and more likely to have induction of labour (38.5% versus 22.4%, $P < 0.001$). There was no difference in failure of VBAC in the induced labour group (63.2% versus 68.9%, $P = 0.540$) but significant difference in failure of VBAC in the spontaneous labour group (18.7% versus 9.5%, $P = 0.20$). There were no differences for pre-eclampsia, lacerations or shoulder dystocia. The birthweight in the gestational diabetes group was significantly greater than the control (3437.8 g versus 3191.9 g, $P = 0.001$), but there were no significant differences in outcome Apgar scores or neonatal deaths. [EL = 2+]

No evidence was identified to suggest that the indications for caesarean section in preference to induction of labour are different for women with diabetes compared to women without diabetes.

Current practice
The CEMACH enquiry reported that women with pre-existing diabetes had high rates of obstetric intervention with a 39% induction of labour rate compared with 21% in the general maternity population. The reasons given for induction of labour were that it was routine for women with diabetes (48.4%), general obstetric complications (13.9%), presumed fetal compromise (9.4%), large baby or polyhydramnios (8.5%) and diabetes complications (2.1%), and the remainder were other clinical reasons, preterm rupture of membranes, maternal request, or unknown or inadequately described.[2] [EL = 3–4]

The caesarean section rate was 67%, which is three times higher than the general maternity population (24%). The indications for elective and emergency caesarean section were presumed fetal compromise (28.3%), previous caesarean section (24.9%), general obstetric complication (14.2%), failure to progress in labour (13.9%), large baby (3.7%), diabetes complications (2.5%) and routine for diabetes (1.9%), and the remainder were due to other clinical reasons, maternal request, reason unknown or inadequately described. [EL = 3–4]

The preterm birth rate was 35.8% compared with 7.4% in the general maternity population. Of the total births 26.4% were iatrogenic and 9.4% were spontaneous preterm births (including preterm rupture of the membranes requiring induction) which is higher than in the general maternity population. The majority of iatrogenic preterm births were due to preterm caesarean sections, 21.9% of which were for previous caesarean section, large baby, maternal request or routine for maternal diabetes. [EL = 3–4]

The enquiry case–control study found that 8% (15/178) of women with poor pregnancy outcomes and 2% (4/202) of women with good pregnancy outcome had no details of discussion about timing and mode of birth in their medical records.[33] A lack of discussion was associated with poor pregnancy outcome (OR 4.0, 95% CI 1.2 to 12.7, adjusted for maternal age and deprivation). Additional case–control analysis showed an association with fetal or neonatal death, but not with fetal congenital anomaly, although it is important to note that women who did not have a discussion also gave birth at an earlier gestational age. The majority of women (65% of 382 women) were assessed as having optimal care during labour and birth and there was no association of sub-optimal care and pregnancy outcome. The most frequent issues noted were poor management of maternal risks, inappropriate decisions relating to birth and inadequate fetal surveillance during labour or delay in acting on signs of fetal compromise. [EL = 3–4]

The condition of the baby at birth was reported by the CEMACH enquiry: 2.6% of live births had an Apgar score of less than 7 at 5 minutes. The corresponding figure for the general maternity population is 0.76%. [EL = 3–4]

The enquiry found that 6.9% (261/3808) of pregnancies led to *in utero* losses (there were also two early neonatal deaths, twins born live at 20 weeks of gestation who both died within 1 hour of birth). This is thought to be an underestimate of the actual number of pregnancies that ended before 24 weeks of gestation due to many women not accessing maternity services during the early stages of pregnancy. [EL = 3–4]

Of the pregnancies continuing at 24 weeks of gestation 87/3474 ended in stillbirth and 3449 live births. The stillbirth rate (26.8 per 1000 live births and stillbirths, 95% CI 19.8 to 33.8, adjusted for maternal age) was significantly higher than the national rate of 5.7 per 1000 live births and still births (RR 4.7, 95% CI 3.7 to 6.0). Of the stillbirths 17.2% occurred at 24–27 weeks of gestation, 13.8% at 28–31 weeks of gestation, 41.4% at 32–36 weeks of gestation and 27.6% at 37–41 weeks of gestation. No stillbirths were reported after 42 weeks of gestation. [EL = 3–4]

The perinatal death rate (the number of stillbirths and early neonatal deaths per 1000 live and stillbirths; 31.8, 95% CI 24.2 to 39.4 adjusted for maternal age) was significantly higher than the national rate of 8.5 per 1000 live births and stillbirths (RR 3.8, 95% CI 3.0 to 4.7). [EL = 3–4]

The neonatal death rate (number of neonatal deaths per 1000 live births; 9.3, 95% CI 5.2 to 13.3, adjusted for maternal age) was significantly higher than the national rate of 3.6 per 1000 live births (RR 2.6, 95% CI 1.7 to 3.9). Of the neonatal deaths 38.5% occurred at 24–27 weeks of gestation, 7.7% at 28–31 weeks of gestation, 38.5% at 32–36 weeks of gestation and 15.4% at 37–41 weeks of gestation. No neonatal deaths were reported after 42 weeks of gestation. [EL = 3–4]

The enquiry recommended that women should be involved in the decision–making process regarding timing and mode of birth. [EL = 3–4]

Existing guidance

The NICE induction of labour guideline[12] recommended that women with pregnancies complicated by diabetes should be offered induction of labour before their estimated date for delivery. Although the guideline reported that there were insufficient data clarifying the gestation-specific risk for unexplained stillbirth in pregnancies complicated by diabetes, the GDG that developed the induction of labour guideline considered that it was usual practice in the UK to offer induction of labour to women with type 1 diabetes before 40 weeks of gestation. The induction of labour guideline is currently being updated and induction of labour for women with diabetes is excluded from the scope having been incorporated into the scope for the diabetes in pregnancy guideline.

The NICE intrapartum care guideline[10] contains recommendations in relation to routine intrapartum care, including electronic fetal monitoring.

The NICE caesarean section guideline[13] contains recommendations in relation to caesarean section, including VBAC and provision of information for women.

The NSF for diabetes[20] states: [EL = 4]

> 'Women with pre-existing diabetes: During labour, a midwife experienced in supporting women with diabetes through labour should be present and an appropriately trained obstetrician should be available at all times. The woman's blood glucose level should be maintained within the normal range in order to reduce the risk of neonatal hypoglycaemia. Continuous electronic fetal heart monitoring should be offered to all women with diabetes during labour and fetal blood sampling should be available if indicated. Arrangements should be in place to enable the rapid transfer of women with diabetes who choose not to deliver in a consultant-led obstetric unit, should difficulties arise.

> Women who develop gestational diabetes: In the second and third trimesters of pregnancy, the main risks to the baby are macrosomia (excessive fetal growth), affecting approximately 30% of the offspring of women with type 1 diabetes, and neonatal hypoglycaemia, which occurs in approximately 24% of babies. Jaundice is also more common, but other complications, such as respiratory distress syndrome, hypoglycaemia and polycythaemia, are now rare.

> Macrosomia is associated with an increased risk of fetal injury and damage to the birth canal. The risk of macrosomia can be reduced by the achievement of near normal blood glucose levels during the third trimester. Problems during the neonatal period can be reduced by the achievement of tight blood glucose control during labour.

Improving pregnancy outcomes: The rate of shoulder dystocia can be decreased by the use of ultrasound monitoring and elective delivery of those babies weighing over 4250 g. In one study, ultrasound was found to determine accurately the presence or absence of macrosomia in 87% of women scanned.

Diabetic pregnancy is associated with an increased risk of complications during labour and delivery. Close monitoring and prompt intervention can improve outcomes for both the mother and her baby. For example, tight blood glucose control during labour can reduce the risk of neonatal hypoglycaemia and hence reduce the need for admission to a neonatal intensive care unit. However, it should be remembered that some women's experience of a "medicalised" and high-intervention labour and delivery is a negative and frightening one. This need not be the case if they are helped to feel in control, are involved in decision-making and kept informed, and if they are supported by calm and competent professionals.'

Evidence statement

Eight studies examined the epidemiology of women with diabetes requiring intervention in the timing and mode of birth. The studies showed that stillbirth and shoulder dystocia were the greatest risks involved. Diabetes during pregnancy and macrosomia were the greatest risk factors affecting outcome of birth. However, evidence shows that factors related to the behaviour of healthcare professionals and the organisation of health service impact on outcome. For example, caesarean section rates remain high even when diabetes is controlled and macrosomia is not present.

Nine studies investigated different methods of intervening in the timing and mode of birth. There is evidence that fetal weight and risk of stillbirth are the determining factors in whether women with diabetes undergo caesarean section. Caesarean section rates were lower in women who were actively managed for induction of labour, and caesarean section was associated with higher levels of complications and adverse outcomes than vaginal birth. However, the majority of the studies were conducted in the USA where sociocultural and health service factors are different to the UK.

Five studies were considered in relation to optimal timing of birth in women with diabetes. An RCT involving women with insulin-requiring diabetes and a case–control study involving women with type 1 diabetes compared elective induction of labour at 38–39 weeks of gestation with expectant management. There were more LGA babies and cases of shoulder dystocia in the expectant management groups. Routine induction of labour at 38–39 weeks of gestation did not increase the rate of caesarean section. The remaining studies allowed comparison of gestational ages at birth between babies of women with diabetes and those of women without diabetes, but these none of these studies was specifically designed to address the optimal timing of birth in women with diabetes.

Three studies examined VBAC and showed that birthweight was the main factor in determining success. Women with diabetes were more likely to have unsuccessful VBAC compared to women without diabetes, but diabetes was not a complete contraindication.

From evidence to recommendations

Evidence shows that women with diabetes are more likely to undergo induction of labour and/or caesarean section than women without diabetes. The reasons for intervention in the mode of birth in women with diabetes are to prevent stillbirth and shoulder dystocia, which are associated with fetal macrosomia. Healthcare professionals should, therefore, inform women with fetal macrosomia of the risks and benefits of vaginal birth, induction of labour and caesarean section. No evidence was identified to suggest that induction of labour should be conducted differently in women with diabetes compared to other women (including oxytocin protocols and electronic fetal monitoring). Preparation for surgical birth (caesarean section) is considered in Section 6.2.

Routine induction of labour for women with diabetes at 38–39 weeks of gestation reduces the risk of stillbirth and shoulder dystocia without increasing the risk of caesarean section. However, there was insufficient evidence to determine the precise gestational age at which elective induction of labour should be offered. The GDG's discussions highlighted the need to balance the risk of fetal lung immaturity which may be associated with induction at 36–37 weeks of gestation against the risk of stillbirth associated with later induction. In the absence of evidence to determine whether elective birth through induction of labour, or elective caesarean section if indicated, should be offered before 38 weeks of gestation, the GDG's view was that elective birth should be offered after 38 completed weeks of gestation. No evidence was identified to suggest that the indications for elective caesarean section in preference to induction of labour in women with diabetes would be any different to those in women without diabetes.

Evidence shows that diabetes should not be considered a contraindication to attempting VBAC.

Recommendations for timing and mode of birth

Pregnant women with diabetes who have a normally grown fetus should be offered elective birth through induction of labour, or by elective caesarean section if indicated, after 38 completed weeks.

Diabetes should not in itself be considered a contraindication to attempting vaginal birth after a previous caesarean section.

Pregnant women with diabetes who have an ultrasound-diagnosed macrosomic fetus should be informed of the risks and benefits of vaginal birth, induction of labour and caesarean section.

There were no research recommendations relating to the timing and mode of birth for women with diabetes or for the implications for future pregnancies and births.

6.2   Analgesia and anaesthesia

Description of the evidence

Labour and birth can be stressful for any woman. In women with diabetes these stresses may make diabetes more difficult to control, resulting in otherwise preventable morbidities and even mortality. Any interventions during labour and birth should, therefore, be considered carefully in terms of the effect on the woman and the baby. Relevant factors to consider in terms of women with diabetes are glycaemic control, prevention of metabolic disturbances (abnormal acid–base status leading to ketoacidosis) and haemodynamic control (with an emphasis on prevention of hypotension).[335] Additional factors to consider are comorbidities such as neuropathy and obesity, which may complicate obstetric analgesia and anaesthesia.

Glycaemic control
No clinical studies were identified in relation to the effects of analgesia or anaesthesia on perioperative glycaemic control in women with diabetes. However, an RCT compared epidural anaesthesia plus general anaesthesia with general anaesthesia alone in people undergoing colorectal surgery for non-metastatic carcinoma.[336] Epidural anaesthesia plus general anaesthesia reduced the perioperative increase in blood glucose compared with general anaesthesia alone (intra-operative glucose production, 8.2 ± 1.9 micromol/kg/min versus 10.7 ± 1.4 micromol/kg/min, $P < 0.05$; postoperative glucose production, 8.5 ± 1.8 micromol/kg/min versus 10.5 ± 1.2 micromol/kg/min, $P < 0.05$). Although this was a small study with only eight people without diabetes in each treatment group, it suggests that there may be a benefit in regional anaesthesia for women with diabetes facing caesarean section compared with general anaesthesia. [EL = 1+]

A narrative non-systematic review reported that pain and/or stress following surgery and trauma impairs insulin sensitivity by affecting non-oxidative glucose metabolism.[337] While these observations were not drawn from labouring women with diabetes the suggestion is that glucose regulation can be improved with administration of analgesia (pain relief) in stressful states. [EL = 4]

Acid–base status
One cohort study and one case–control study investigated acid–base status (and neonatal Apgar scores) in women with diabetes undergoing elective caesarean section with epidural or spinal anaesthesia.

The cohort study assessed whether epidural anaesthesia in women with diabetes undergoing elective caesarean section was associated with abnormal acid–base and glucose status in the woman and baby compared with epidural anaesthesia in women without diabetes.[338] At birth there were no significant differences between women with diabetes and those without diabetes in terms of arterial blood acid–base status, nor in terms of neonatal umbilical venous or arterial blood acid–base status or neonatal Apgar scores. However, women with diabetes and their babies had a 25–50% reduction in pyruvate concentrations in maternal venous blood and neonatal umbilical venous and arterial blood compared to women without diabetes and their babies ($P = 0.001$). The study suggests that epidural anaesthesia in women with diabetes is associated with normal acid–base status in the mother and baby. [EL = 2+]

The case–control study, which was undertaken in the 1980s, involved ten women with rigidly controlled type 1 diabetes and ten healthy women without diabetes.[335] All the women were scheduled for elective primary or repeat caesarean section using spinal anaesthesia at term. Dextrose-free intravenous solutions were used for volume expansion before induction of anaesthesia, and hypotension was prevented in all women. There were no significant differences in acid–base values between women with diabetes and those without diabetes, nor between babies of women with diabetes and babies in the control group. Mean maternal artery pH in women with diabetes and women without diabetes were 7.40 (standard error (SE) 0.006) and 7.42 (SE 0.01), respectively. Mean umbilical vein pH in women with diabetes and women without diabetes were 7.33 (SE 0.01) and 7.35 (SE 0.01), respectively. Mean umbilical artery pH in women with diabetes and women without diabetes were 7.27 (SE 0.01) and 7.30 (SE 0.01), respectively. Apgar scores were similar in both groups, with one baby of a woman with diabetes having a score of less than 7 at 1 minute and the remaining 19 babies in both groups having scores of more than 7 at 1 and 5 minutes. The authors of the study suggested that anaesthetics such as nitrous oxide and intravenous agents such as thiopentone are virtually free of metabolic effects and may, therefore, be preferred for women with diabetes. They also suggested that sedatives, narcotic analgesics and muscle relaxants are similarly of benefit to women with diabetes. However, no clinical data were provided to support either of these statements. [EL = 2+]

Haemodynamic control

No clinical studies were identified in relation to the effects of analgesia or anaesthesia on perioperative haemodynamic control in women with diabetes.

Neuropathy

A retrospective cohort study was identified in relation to the effects of coexisting neuropathy on analgesia and anaesthesia in women with diabetes.[339] The study involved 567 people with pre-existing peripheral sensorimotor neuropathy or diabetic polyneuropathy who were investigated for neurological injury after neuraxial blockade. Two people (0.4%, 95% CI 0.1% to 1.3%) experienced new or progressive postoperative neurological deficits and 65 technical complications occurred in 63 people (11.1%). The most common complications were unintentional elicitation of paraesthesia (7.6%), traumatic needle placement (evidence of blood; 1.6%) and unplanned dural puncture (0.9%). There were no infectious or haematological complications. The study concluded that the risk of severe postoperative neurological injury is high in the population of people with pre-existing neuropathy and healthcare professionals should be aware of this when developing and implementing regional anaesthetic care plans. [EL = 2+]

Obesity

No clinical studies were identified in relation to the effects of coexisting obesity on analgesia or anaesthesia in women with diabetes. However, a narrative non-systematic review reported that obesity is a risk factor for obstetric analgesia and anaesthesia.[340] [EL = 4]

No further clinical studies were identified in relation to factors affecting the choice of analgesia or anaesthesia in women with diabetes. However, a narrative non-systematic review suggested that increased risks were associated with general anaesthesia. One risk was that women with diabetes tend to have a higher resting gastric volume (slower gastric emptying) than women without diabetes, increasing the risk of Mendelson syndrome, which results from aspiration of gastric contents into the lungs following vomiting or regurgitation in obstetrical patients.[335] Another risk was that irreversible brain damage could occur if hypoglycaemia was allowed to develop during general anaesthesia and surgery. The review also noted the possibility of women with diabetes inadvertently being given glucose orally rather than intravenously, and that irreversible brain damage could occur if hypoglycaemia was allowed to develop during general anaesthesia and surgery. It was also suggested that a delay in returning to consciousness following general anaesthesia could prolong the time before routine metabolic management with insulin could be reinstituted. [EL = 4]

The review also reported that regional anaesthesia (as used for caesarean section), which includes epidural anaesthesia and spinal anaesthesia, carries risks for women with diabetes. In particular it was reported that regional anaesthesia can accentuate haemodynamic distortions in women with diabetes in the presence of polyhydramnios and increased segmental spread of the nerve blockade.[335] Vomiting is a consequence of hypotension caused by sympathetic nerve blockade and it may exacerbate metabolic disturbances. For labour analgesia, an epidural nerve blockade may reduce metabolic expenditure and avoid the emetic effects of opioids. [EL = 4]

Existing guidance

The NICE guideline for the management of type 1 diabetes recommends that hospitals ensure that protocols for inpatient procedures and surgical operations are in place and used. Such protocols should ensure that near-normoglycaemia is maintained without the risk of acute decompensation, and that this should normally be achieved through adjustment of intravenous insulin delivery in response to regular blood glucose testing.

Evidence statement

No clinical studies were identified in relation to the effects of analgesia or anaesthesia on perioperative glycaemic control in women with diabetes. A small RCT in people undergoing colorectal surgery showed that epidural anaesthesia plus general anaesthesia reduced the perioperative increase in blood glucose compared with general anaesthesia alone. A narrative non-systematic review suggested that glucose regulation could be improved with administration of analgesia in stressful states.

Two observational studies showed that epidural anaesthesia and spinal anaesthesia are associated with normal acid–base status in women with diabetes undergoing elective caesarean section and with normal acid–base status and Apgar scores in their babies.

No clinical studies were identified in relation to the effects of analgesia and anaesthesia on perioperative haemodynamic control in women with diabetes.

A cohort study showed that neuraxial blockade carries an increased risk of severe postoperative neurological injury in people with pre-existing neuropathy.

No clinical studies were identified in relation to the effects of coexisting obesity on analgesia and anaesthesia in women with diabetes. However, a narrative non-systematic review highlighted that obesity is in itself a risk factor for analgesia and anaesthesia.

From evidence to recommendations

Evidence suggests that epidural anaesthesia and spinal anaesthesia are associated with normal acid–base status in women with diabetes. No evidence was identified to suggest that epidural or spinal anaesthesia should be used any differently (in terms of monitoring, dose or provision of fluids) in women with diabetes, and so the GDG has not made any recommendations specific to epidural or spinal anaesthesia. However, the GDG's discussion included consideration of the possibility of prolonged labour with epidural anaesthesia increasing the risk of DKA. The presence of DKA would alter the management of the need for urgent birth. The GDG's view is that diabetes is not in itself a contraindication to restrict the duration of labour, provided that fluids, blood glucose concentrations, etc., are satisfactory.

Long duration of diabetes, hyperglycaemia and any opioid are thought to slow gastric emptying and increase risks for anaesthesia. Evidence shows that the presence of (symptomatic) autonomic neuropathy in women with diabetes is a risk factor for obstetric anaesthesia. Although no clinical evidence was found specifically in relation to coexisting diabetes and obesity as risk factors for obstetric anaesthesia, obesity alone has been reported to increase problems with intubation, risk of thromboembolism, stress response with pre-eclampsia and risk of post-epidural neurological problems. It is, therefore, important that anaesthetists have access to a complete medical history including information about the extent of neuropathy (particularly autonomic neuropathy) and obesity to assess fitness for anaesthesia and that monitoring begins before anaesthesia is initiated.

Very few women are likely to undergo general anaesthesia during labour and birth. However, general anaesthesia carries a risk of hypoglycaemia and women recovering from general anaesthesia will lack hypoglycaemia awareness. The woman's need for insulin will decrease significantly after the birth (see Section 8.1) and this can also lead to hypoglycaemia. Regular blood glucose monitoring during anaesthesia is, therefore, recommended for women with diabetes: monitoring should occur at 30 minute intervals to prevent hypoglycaemia remaining undetected and/or untreated for longer periods, and it should continue after the birth until the woman is fully conscious.

Recommendations for analgesia and anaesthesia

Women with diabetes and comorbidities such as obesity or autonomic neuropathy should be offered an anaesthetic assessment in the third trimester of pregnancy.

If general anaesthesia is used for the birth in women with diabetes, blood glucose should be monitored regularly (every 30 minutes) from induction of general anaesthesia until after the baby is born and the woman is fully conscious.

Research recommendations for analgesia and anaesthesia

What are the risks and benefits associated with analgesia and anaesthesia in women with diabetes?

Why this is important
The increasing number of women with diabetes and the high rate of intervention during birth emphasise the need for clinical studies to determine the most effective methods for analgesia and anaesthesia in this group of women. The research studies should investigate the effect of analgesia during labour, and the cardiovascular effects of spinal anaesthesia and vasopressors on diabetic control.

6.3 Glycaemic control during labour and birth

Description of the evidence

Neonatal hypoglycaemia
Neonatal hypoglycaemia can occur for two reasons, with some overlap in individual cases. Some fetuses develop a pattern of hyperinsulinaemia to cope with the regular excessive glucose transfer across the placenta where the maternal diabetes is poorly controlled[122] (see Section 4.1). As newborns these babies have a persisting autonomous insulin secretion which, in the absence of adequate glucose intake, will lead to severe and prolonged hypoglycaemia. Other babies who have not developed hyperinsulinaemia in fetal life may respond to maternal hyperglycaemia in labour with sufficient insulin production in the 1–2 hours following birth to cause transient hypoglycaemia. In contrast the term baby of a woman without diabetes demonstrates rather sluggish insulin responses to glycaemic stimuli and shows a tendency to a relatively high blood glucose levels after feeding in the newborn period.

Eight observational studies were identified that considered the effect of maternal blood glucose control during labour and birth on neonatal blood glucose levels. Four studies involved only women with type 1 diabetes, one study included women with type 1 and type 2 diabetes and one study involved only women with gestational diabetes. All six studies found maternal hyperglycaemia during labour to be associated with neonatal hypoglycaemia.

A retrospective study of 53 babies born to women with type 1 diabetes[342] measured plasma glucose concentrations at birth and 2 hours later. The maternal blood glucose concentration at birth correlated positively with the neonatal blood glucose concentration at birth ($r = 0.82$, $P < 0.001$) and negatively with the neonatal blood glucose concentration 2 hours after birth ($r = -0.46$, $P < 0.001$). Thirty-seven percent (11/30) of babies born to women whose blood glucose concentration at birth was 7.1 mmol/litre or more developed hypoglycaemia (plasma glucose 1.7 mmol or less). No babies born to women whose blood glucose concentration was less than 7.1 mmol/litre developed hypoglycaemia. Babies with blood glucose concentrations less than 1.7 mmol/litre were treated using intravenous glucose. [EL = 2+]

A prospective study included 122 pregnancies in 100 women with type 1 diabetes.[343] Intravenous glucose and/or insulin was infused during labour to maintain CBG concentrations at 3.9–5.6 mmol/litre. Forty-seven percent (36/76) of babies born to women who had CBG concentrations above 5 mmol/litre before birth developed neonatal hypoglycaemia (less than 1.7 mmol/litre) compared with 14% (6/42) of babies born to women with CBG concentrations less than 5 mmol/litre ($P = 0.0003$). [EL = 2++]

A prospective study included 233 women with insulin-requiring diabetes (77 with type 1 diabetes, 156 with type 2 diabetes).[344] On the day of birth all women received an intravenous infusion of 10% invert sugar (5% fructose, 5% glucose) at a rate of 125 ml/hour. The rate was adjusted if plasma glucose level was less than 2.8 mmol/litre. Intravenous insulin was administered with an infusion pump at a rate of 1–4 U/hour to maintain plasma glucose concentration at 3.3–5 mmol/litre. Boluses of 2–5 units of regular insulin were given additionally if the plasma glucose level exceeded 5.5 mmol/litre. The incidence of neonatal hypoglycaemia (plasma glucose concentration less than 1.7 mmol/litre) was 16.5% (38 babies). Babies with plasma glucose concentration less than 1.7 mmol/litre received enteral feeds or intravenous glucose as dictated by their clinical condition. The degree of hypoglycaemia was mild and rarely required admission to intensive care or intravenous treatment. The mean intrapartum blood glucose level was significantly lower in mothers of babies without hypoglycaemia ($P < 0.05$). The authors reported that the best results were achieved when the desired glucose control was maintained for at least 8 hours before birth. [EL = 2++]

A standardised intravenous protocol for insulin and dextrose therapy in labour and birth was assessed in 25 women with insulin-treated diabetes.[345] Adjustments to insulin infusion rates were determined by trends in blood glucose as well as by absolute concentration. The protocol was as follows:

- nil by mouth until after the birth of the baby
- start intravenous dextrose 10% in 500 ml, 100 ml/hour via IMED® pump
- hourly blood glucose estimation by glucose meter
- insulin infusion by intravenous pump mounted onto the intravenous line, initially at 2 U/ hour when blood glucose more than 7 mmol/litre (50 U human soluble insulin in 50 ml, 0.9% saline, 2 ml/hour)
- adjust insulin infusion rate to maintain blood glucose 4.0–7.0 mmol/litre according to glucose meter:
  - if less than 4.0 mmol/litre and not rising, then decrease by 1 U/hour to a minimum of 0.5 U/hour
  - if more than 7.0 mmol/litre and not falling, then increase by 0.5 U/hour
- after delivery of the placenta:
  - halve the rate of insulin infusion, to a minimum of 0.5 U/hour
  - adjust as before to maintain blood glucose 4.0–7.0 mmol/litre
  - refer to medical record or contact diabetes team for advice about subcutaneous insulin dose before next main meal
  - stop intravenous fluids and insulin 30 minutes after subcutaneous insulin.

Blood glucose was maintained at 6.0 ± 1.8 mmol/litre for a mean of 6 hours (range 1–29 hours) before birth. Blood glucose at birth was 6.3 ± 2.1 mmol/litre. There was only one case of maternal hypoglycaemia. Neonatal hypoglycaemia (plasma glucose less than 2.0 mmol/litre) occurred in 11 babies. Babies with blood glucose less than 2.0 mmol/litre were all treated routinely with intravenous glucose for 3–24 hours with none showing symptoms of hypoglycaemia. Neonatal blood glucose correlated with maternal blood glucose at birth ($r = -0.58$, $P < 0.01$). Introduction of the protocol was associated with a decrease in the incidence of hypoglycaemia in babies born to women with diabetes from 68% to 39% ($P < 0.01$). [EL = 2++]

A study involving women with type 1 diabetes compared CSII (insulin pump therapy) ($n = 28$) with constant intravenous insulin infusion ($n = 37$).[346] Mean blood glucose during labour in women treated using CSII was 4.8 ± 0.6 mmol/litre (range 3.8–5.8). Mean blood glucose in women treated using constant intravenous insulin infusion was 7.2 ± 1.1 mmol/litre (range 5.6–8.3, $P < 0.025$). In the constant intravenous insulin infusion group there were eight cases of neonatal hypoglycaemia (less than 1.7 mmol/litre), whereas in the CSII group there were no cases of neonatal hypoglycaemia ($P < 0.05$). Babies with hypoglycaemia were treated using intravenous glucose. [EL = 2++]

A prospective study of 85 women with gestational diabetes[347] (54 insulin-treated) was undertaken with the aim of assessing a standardised protocol for maintaining glycaemic control during labour and the effect of maternal glycaemic control during labour on neonatal hypoglycaemia (two or more glucose values less than 1.7 mmol/litre). The protocol consisted of: intravenous glucose (8.3 g/hr); intravenous insulin infusion by syringe pump adjusted according to hourly CBG measurements; and urine testing for ketone bodies. The target CBG range for metabolic control was 2.8–6.9 mmol/litre (ideally 3.3–6.1 mmol/litre). Mean CBG during labour was 4.7 ± 1.1 mmol/litre and in 82.3% of women CBG was within the desired range. Five babies developed hypoglycaemia. After logistic regression (HbA_{1c} in third trimester, SGA, preterm birth, insulin treatment) maternal blood glucose in the last 2 hours of labour was associated with neonatal hypoglycaemia ($P < 0.05$). [EL = 2+]

An observational study[348] compared the effect of a policy change following an intensive effort to improve pre-pregnancy care and advice with a relaxation of targets for blood glucose control during labour. There was no relationship between neonatal blood glucose and HbA_{1c} throughout the third trimester ($r = -0.11$), mean HbA_{1c} throughout pregnancy ($r = 0.10$) or HbA_{1c} at booking ($r = 0.28$). In period 1, neonatal hypoglycaemia was recorded in seven babies (less than 2.2 mmol/litre; with intravenous glucose used in four), in period 2, neonatal blood glucose was measured as less than 2.2 mmol/litre in 19 babies; with intravenous glucose used in 14). Mean maternal blood glucose at birth was 7.7 ± 3.8 mmol/litre in the group with neonatal blood glucose levels less than 2.2 mmol/litre, compared with 4.9 ± 2.8 mmol/litre in all other women ($P = 0.05$). When maternal blood glucose was over 10 mmol/litre, the neonatal blood glucose was always low (1.3 ± 0.8 versus 2.5 ± 1.5 for all others; $P < 0.02$). [EL = 2+]

An observational study of 107 consecutive singleton pregnancies in women with type 1 diabetes[349] measured maternal HbA_{1c} throughout pregnancy, maternal blood glucose throughout labour and birth and neonatal blood glucose. There was a significant negative correlation between neonatal blood glucose and mean maternal blood glucose in labour ($r = -0.33$, $P < 0.001$). When maternal blood glucose stayed within the target of 4.0–8.0 mmol/litre there was no relationship with neonatal blood glucose. When maternal blood glucose was greater than 8.0 mmol/litre, neonatal blood glucose was less than 2.5 mmol/litre, in all except two women. If the maternal blood glucose was above 9.0 mmol/litre neonatal blood glucose was always less than 2.5 mmol/litre. [EL = 3]

Fetal distress

Two observational studies were identified that considered the effect of maternal blood glucose control during labour and birth on fetal distress. Both studies found maternal hyperglycaemia during labour to be associated with fetal distress.

A prospective study of 149 babies of women with type 1 diabetes[350] found perinatal asphyxia in 27% (40). Maximum maternal blood glucose during labour was higher in babies with perinatal asphyxia than in those without (9.5 ± 3.7 versus 7.0 ± 3.0, $P < 0.0001$). Perinatal asphyxia was also associated with gestational age and development of vasculopathy during pregnancy but not with vasculopathy before pregnancy, maternal age, duration of diabetes or White's classification of diabetes. [EL = 2++]

A study compared CSII (28 women with type 1 diabetes) with constant intravenous insulin infusion (37 women with type 1 diabetes).[346] Mean blood glucose during labour in women treated using CSII was 4.8 ± 0.6 mmol/litre (range 3.8–5.8). Mean blood glucose in women treated using constant intravenous insulin infusion was 7.2 ± 1.1 mmol/litre (range 5.6–8.3, $P < 0.025$). In the constant intravenous insulin infusion group there was acute fetal distress in 27% of cases and a caesarean section rate of 38%. In the CSII group there was fetal distress in 14.3% of cases ($P < 0.001$) and a caesarean section rate of 25% ($P < 0.05$). [EL = 2++]

Controlling glycaemia during labour and birth

An RCT investigated whether continuous intravenous insulin infusion provided a greater degree of intrapartum maternal glycaemic control in women with gestational diabetes than rotating between glucose-containing and glucose-free intravenous fluids.[351] There was no difference in mean intrapartum maternal CBG levels in the rotating fluids and intravenous insulin groups (5.77 ± 0.48 mmol/litre versus 5.73 ± 0.99 mmol/litre, $P = 0.89$). Neonatal hypoglycaemia (blood glucose less than 0.6 mmol/litre within the first 24 hours was found to be 6.7% in the rotating group and 19% in the continuous intravenous insulin infusion group, but the difference was not statistically significant. Birthweight, Apgar scores at 1 minute and 5 minutes, respiratory distress, shoulder dystocia, admission to the NICU, and hyperbilirubinaemia were also similar between the two treatments. The study suggests that in women with insulin-requiring gestational diabetes, continuous intravenous insulin infusion and a rotation of intravenous fluids between glucose-containing and glucose-free fluids achieve similar intrapartum glycaemic control. [EL = 1+]

A non-randomised study compared CSII (28 women with type 1 diabetes) with constant intravenous insulin infusion (37 women with type 1 diabetes).[346] Mean blood glucose during labour in women treated using CSII was 4.8 ± 0.6 mmol/litre (range 3.8–5.8). Mean blood glucose in women treated using constant intravenous insulin infusion was 7.2 ± 1.1 mmol/litre (range 5.6–8.3, $P < 0.025$). However, the lack of randomisation may have meant that women who used CSII during labour and birth were self-selected as those who had better glycaemic control.

Current practice

The CEMACH enquiry found sub-optimal glycaemic control during labour and/or birth was not associated with poor pregnancy outcome in women with pre-existing diabetes. Among women with poor pregnancy outcome 49% (79/162) were documented as having sub-optimal control in the first trimester compared with 48% (97/202) of the women with good pregnancy outcome. The enquiry panels identified cases of inappropriate intravenous insulin/dextrose regimen, delay in starting intravenous insulin/dextrose regimen, poor management of sliding scale, sub-optimal blood glucose monitoring, hypoglycaemia due to clinical practice, poor management of hypoglycaemia and other clinical practice issues in both groups of women.[33] [EL = 3–4]

The CEMACH enquiry (comparison of women with type 1 and type 2 diabetes) reported that 47% of the women with type 1 diabetes and 41% of the women with type 2 diabetes had sub-optimal glycaemic control during labour and birth ($P = 0.28$). Ten percent of the women with type 1 diabetes and 29% of the women with type 2 diabetes were not given intravenous insulin and dextrose during labour and/or birth ($P < 0.001$).[33] [EL = 3–4]

Existing guidance

The NSF for diabetes recommends tight glucose control during labour to reduce the risk of neonatal hypoglycaemia.[20]

Evidence statement

Eight studies were found that showed that neonatal hypoglycaemia is more likely to occur in babies of women with high blood glucose concentration during labour and birth. Two studies found maternal hyperglycaemia during labour to be associated with fetal distress. Maintaining maternal blood glucose in the range 4–7 mmol/litre during labour and birth reduces the incidence of neonatal hypoglycaemia and reduces fetal distress.

An RCT found continuous intravenous insulin infusion and rotating between glucose-containing and glucose-free intravenous fluids resulted in similar maternal blood glucose levels in women with insulin-requiring gestational diabetes during labour and birth. A non-randomised comparative study found that CSII was associated with better glycaemic control in women with type 1 diabetes during labour and birth than was intravenous insulin infusion. However, the lack of randomisation in the study means that self-selection of CSII by women who were better at controlling their blood glucose cannot be ruled out.

From evidence to recommendations

Evidence shows that maintaining blood glucose in the range 4–7 mmol/litre during labour and birth reduces the incidence of neonatal hypoglycaemia and fetal distress. In formulating their recommendations, the GDG placed a high value on recommending that blood glucose be maintained in this range during labour and birth without being prescriptive about how it is maintained. This leaves the possibility for women who are able to maintain their blood glucose in the range 4–7 mmol/litre using MDI insulin injections or CSII to experience labour and birth without having intravenous insulin regimens. The GDG noted that these options may be associated with greater maternal satisfaction because of the psychological benefits of allowing women to take control of their diabetes during labour and birth, and the practicalities such as permitting greater mobility. However, no clinical studies were identified that evaluated the optimal method of maintaining glycaemic control during labour and birth. In the absence of such evidence the GDG's consensus view was that intravenous dextrose and insulin infusion should be considered for women with type 1 diabetes from the onset of established labour, and that intravenous dextrose and insulin infusion is recommended for women with diabetes whose blood glucose is not maintained between 4–7 mmol/litre.

Recommendations for glycaemic control during labour and birth

During labour and birth, capillary blood glucose should be monitored on an hourly basis in women with diabetes and maintained at between 4 and 7 mmol/litre.

Women with type 1 diabetes should be considered for intravenous dextrose and insulin infusion from the onset of established labour.

Intravenous dextrose and insulin infusion is recommended during labour and birth for women with diabetes whose blood glucose is not maintained at between 4 and 7 mmol/litre.

Research recommendations for glycaemic control during labour and birth

What is the optimal method for controlling glycaemia during labour and birth?

Why this is important
Epidemiological studies have shown that poor glycaemic control during labour and birth is associated with adverse neonatal outcomes (in particular, neonatal hypoglycaemia and respiratory distress). However, no randomised controlled trials have compared the effectiveness of intermittent subcutaneous insulin injections and/or CSII with that of intravenous dextrose plus insulin during labour and birth. The potential benefits of intermittent insulin injections and/or CSII over intravenous dextrose plus insulin during the intrapartum period include patient preference due to the psychological effect of the woman feeling in control of her diabetes and having increased mobility. Randomised controlled trials are therefore needed to evaluate the safety of intermittent insulin injections and/or CSII during labour and birth compared with that of intravenous dextrose plus insulin.

7 Neonatal care

7.1 Initial assessment and criteria for admission to intensive or special care

Description of the evidence

A number of morbidities present in babies born to women with diabetes (including pre-existing type 1 and type 2 diabetes and gestational diabetes). These include fetal macrosomia, infant respiratory distress syndrome, cardiomyopathy, hypoglycaemia, hypocalcaemia, hypomagnesaemia, polycythaemia and hyperviscosity. Hypoxia causes polycythaemia and hyperviscosity.[352] Thrombosis is a rare, but serious, complication necessitating admission to a NICU. Risk factors include maternal diabetes, maternal factors resulting in IUGR, polycythaemia and the use of intravascular catheters in preterm babies.[353] Information on incidence and presentation of thrombosis is very limited and has been gathered mainly from case reports and case series.

While some of the morbidities listed above correct themselves within a period of few hours to a few weeks (e.g. transient tachypnoea normalises within 3 days of birth),[354] it is still important that treatment is provided promptly for those requiring it (e.g. hyaline membrane disease, for which babies may require surfactant, or respiratory and metabolic support).[354]

Incidence of neonatal morbidities
A cohort study[355] assessed the effect of rigorous management of type 1 diabetes during pregnancy on perinatal outcome by comparing 78 pregnant women with type 1 diabetes managed prospectively with 78 matched controls who did not have diabetes. The women with diabetes used insulin by infusion pump or split-dose therapy, with the goal of normalising fasting blood sugars and HbA_{1c}. Women with type 1 diabetes had higher rates of preterm birth (31% versus 10%, $P = 0.003$), pre-eclampsia (15% versus 5%, $P = 0.035$) and caesarean section (55% versus 27%, $P = 0.002$). Complications of babies born to women with diabetes included LGA (41% versus 16%, $P = 0.0002$), hypoglycaemia (14% versus 1%, $P = 0.0025$), hyperbilirubinaemia (46% versus 23%, $P = 0.0002$) and respiratory distress (12% versus 1%, $P = 0.008$). Apgar scores and mortality rates were similar for the two groups. Congenital malformations occurred in 7.7% of babies of women with diabetes and 1.3% of controls ($P = 0.05$).

The incidence of respiratory distress syndrome and mortality was assessed in a cohort study[356] involving 23 babies selected from a total of 30 babies born to women with diabetes who developed hypoglycaemia after birth. These babies were divided into the following three groups: 12 babies treated with intravenous glucose; seven babies treated with long-acting epinephrine plus intravenous glucose; and four babies treated with long-acting epinephrine only. There were no significant differences in incidence of respiratory distress syndrome or mortality rates between the three groups. [EL = 2+]

A case–control study[357] investigated factors that contribute to neonatal hypoglycaemia in babies of women with diabetes. Timing of blood glucose levels, symptoms of hypoglycaemia and interventions provided were assessed. None of the 66 babies investigated developed symptomatic hypoglycaemia or required intravenous glucose. Nearly all the low blood glucose determinations (less than 1.7 mmol/litre) occurred in the first 90 minutes of life, which is the period of greatest risk of low blood glucose occurring in babies born to women with diabetes. [EL = 2+]

A cross-sectional study[322] assessed routes of delivery and pregnancy outcomes in 10 369 births in the USA. Diabetes was associated with increased caesarean section rates, resuscitation of babies with positive pressure ventilation and low Apgar scores (less than 3) at 1 minute and 5 minutes. [EL = 3]

Another cross-sectional study[358] assessed types and frequencies of complications occurring in babies of women with diabetes. Immediately after birth, babies of women with diabetes were admitted to a NICU and detailed maternal history and physical examination were performed to detect any congenital anomalies. The caesarean section rate was high, as was the rate of birth injuries among those who had vaginal birth. The number of babies with asphyxia, congenital anomalies, hypoglycaemia, hypocalcaemia and hyperbilirubinaemia was high. The overall mortality rate of 7.5% was high. The study recommended that women with diabetes should be offered regular antenatal care to maintain good glycaemic control during pregnancy, the birth should be attended by experienced paediatricians to minimise complications and when there is clinical evidence of macrosomia caesarean section should be offered to reduce birth injuries. [EL = 2–]

Neonatal assessment
No clinical studies were identified that addressed the assessments that babies of women with diabetes should undergo. The following evidence is drawn from two narrative non-systematic reviews.[354,359] [EL = 4]

Fetal macrosomia:
The investigation of birth trauma in macrosomic babies of women with gestational diabetes has been described as necessary. Manifestations included fractures of the clavicle and/or humerus. Brachial plexus (Erb palsy), phrenic nerve or cerebral injuries were also reported. In cases where a fracture is suspected, a chest radiograph may be used to confirm the presence of fractures. The startle reflex could also be used to confirm the presence of fractures, as the baby may show an asymmetric reflex or limited use of the arm on the affected side.[359] As most fractures of this nature heal without treatment, admission to a NICU is probably not necessary. [EL = 4]

Respiratory distress:
Use of chest radiographs has been suggested for babies displaying signs of respiratory distress syndrome. An enlarged heart or diffuse, fine granular densities are consistent with respiratory distress syndrome. Together with arterial blood gas results, the need for respiratory support and replacement surfactant therapy could be determined. Where left ventricular outflow obstruction was suspected, an echocardiogram was prescribed in order to prevent congestive heart failure.[359] [EL = 4]

Polycythaemia:
For babies displaying clinical signs of polycythaemia (respiratory distress syndrome, apnoea, hepatomegaly, jitteriness, irritability, seizures, feeding intolerance, hypoglycaemia, decreased urine output), venous haematocrit measurements are indicated.[359][EL = 4]

Hypocalcaemia:
Signs and symptoms of hypocalcaemia include coarse tremors, twitching, irritability and seizures. These should indicate monitoring of serum calcium levels. If levels are 1.75 mmol/litre or more, calcium replacement should be started.[359][EL = 4]

Hyperbilirubinaemia:
Where there has been lethargy, delayed feeding, polycythaemia and birth trauma, bilirubin levels should be monitored.[359] A review addressing medical concerns in the neonatal period described jaundice in the first 24 hours of life as pathological and requiring immediate evaluation and therapy as bilirubin in high concentrations is considered a cellular toxin.[354] [EL = 3]

Severe asphyxia:
If severe asphyxia has occurred at birth, the presence of hypotonia, seizures, poor perfusion and/or absence of respirations in the baby should be assessed to determine whether endotracheal intubation and respiratory support is needed.[359][EL = 4]

Hypoglycaemia:
The prevention and treatment of neonatal hypoglycaemia is addressed separately in Section 7.2.

Criteria for admission to intensive/special care

Amniotic fluid erythropoietin:

A case–control study investigated whether chronic fetal hypoxia, as indicated by amniotic fluid erythropoietin (EPO) levels, was associated with neonatal complications in pregnancies complicated by type 1 diabetes.[360] An amniotic fluid sampled for EPO measurement was taken from 157 women with type 1 diabetes who gave birth by caesarean section before the onset of labour (one vaginal birth), either within 2 days of birth or at birth. EPO measurements were compared with those from 19 healthy, non-smoking women delivered by elective caesarean section with an uneventful singleton pregnancy producing a healthy newborn baby. The median amniotic fluid EPO level was significantly higher in the women with diabetes (14.0 mU/ml, range 2.0 to 1975, $n = 155$) than in control pregnancies (6.3 mU/ml, range 1.7 to 13.7, $n = 19$; $P < 0.0001$). Amniotic fluid EPO levels above 63.0 mU/ml were considered to indicate fetal hypoxia and these elevated values were observed in 14.1% of the women with diabetes who were divided into three groups: low EPO less than 13.8 mU/ml, intermediate EPO 13.8–63.0 mU/ml and high EPO more than 63.0 mU/ml. Newborn babies in the high EPO group were significantly more likely to be macrosomic ($P = 0.0005$) and acidotic ($P < 0.0001$) and had significantly lower pO_2 levels than those in the intermediate and low EPO groups ($P < 0.0001$). Neonatal hypoglycaemia (blood glucose less than 2.0 mmol/litre more than 6 hours after birth; $P < 0.0001$), admission to neonatal intensive care ($P = 0.03$), cardiomyopathy ($P < 0.0001$) and hyperbilirubinaemia ($P = 0.002$) occurred significantly more often in the high EPO group than in the low EPO group. After adjusting for the effects of maternal age, maternal BMI, gestational age at birth, birthweight z-score, last amniotic fluid EPO level and last maternal HbA_{1c} level, amniotic fluid EPO was the only variable to remain independently associated with low umbilical artery pH ($P < 0.0001$) and neonatal hypoglycaemia ($P = 0.002$). Low pO_2 at birth was associated with amniotic fluid EPO ($P < 0.0001$) and birthweight z-score ($P = 0.004$). [EL = 2+]

Neonatal hypoglycaemia:

A prospective cohort study investigated the frequency and risk factors for neonatal hypoglycaemia and long-term outcomes of promptly treated neonatal hypoglycaemia.[361] Of the 4032 babies born in the study hospital, 1023 were admitted to NICU. Ninety-four (9.18%) were evaluated as having hypoglycaemia. Evaluations were performed if symptoms such as hypothermia, apnoea, lethargy, poor feeding or seizures were observed, or if risk factors such as SGA, LGA, preterm birth, sepsis or the mother having diabetes were present. The cohort was followed for 24 months, during which time they were assessed neurologically and developmentally using the Bayley motor and developmental scales. The study found that 51.1% of babies were preterm (37 weeks or less), 34.1% of babies were born to women with pre-existing maternal diabetes or gestational diabetes and 12.8% were SGA. SGA babies required the longest duration of intravenous dextrose infusion (5.16 days compared with 3.74 days for AGA babies). In 26.6% of the babies no known risk factors for hypoglycaemia were observed. Of the 48 babies undergoing Bayley's psychometric evaluations, two showed a motor deficit at 6 months and one showed a language deficit at 24 months. [EL = 2+]

Gestational age, respiratory distress syndrome and higher birthweight:

A retrospective cohort study conducted in the USA over a 3 year period acquired data for 530 babies born to 332 women with gestational diabetes and 177 women with type 1 diabetes. The study found 47% (247) of babies were admitted to a NICU.[362] Seventy-six babies had a gestational age of 33 weeks or less, 22 babies had congenital malformations, ten were described as having miscellaneous conditions (apnoea, cardiac arrhythmias, poor feeding or neonatal depression), 103 babies with a gestational age of 34 weeks or more had respiratory distress syndrome and 32 babies had hypoglycaemia as the only diagnosis. For the 182 babies (34%) presenting with respiratory distress syndrome of varying severity, the highest rates (56%) were seen in women with type 1 diabetes which had been diagnosed before the age of 10 years, had had diabetes for 20 years or longer or had complications of diabetes, decreasing to 25% in babies of women with gestational diabetes requiring no insulin. Similarly, babies of women with gestational diabetes requiring no insulin had the lowest representation of LGA babies (25%), while those born to women with type 1 diabetes which had been diagnosed before the age of 10 years and had a duration of 20 years had the highest rate (62%). The frequency of SGA babies was equal among the classes. Seventy-four (14%) of the 530 babies had macrosomia and 57%

(42/74) of this group were delivered by caesarean section. Among those delivered by caesarean section, there were 21 cases of hypoglycaemia, three of polycythaemia, one of hypocalcaemia and 12 of hyperbilirubinaemia. Thirty percent of macrosomic babies had respiratory distress syndrome. [EL = 2+]

Blood glucose levels were recorded for 514 babies. One or more hypoglycaemic episodes occurred in 27% (137) of these babies. While 90% of the babies responded rapidly to treatment, 10% had two or more episodes lasting several hours. Neonatal hypoglycaemia was similar among babies born to women with gestational diabetes requiring no insulin (23%), those with gestational diabetes requiring insulin (24%) and those with type 1 diabetes with age of onset 20 years or more, or a duration less of than 10 years with no vascular lesions (25%). The prevalence of neonatal hypoglycaemia was lower in these babies ($P < 0.05$) than the babies of women with type 1 diabetes with age of onset 10–19 years or duration 10–19 years with no vascular lesions (35%), the babies of women with type 1 diabetes which had been diagnosed before the age of 10 years, and the babies of women who had had diabetes for 20 years or longer or had complications of diabetes (38%). Thirty of the 137 babies with hypoglycaemia were born before 34 weeks of gestation, 55 were LGA, 50 were AGA and two were SGA. Among the 74 babies who were macrosomic, 21 were also hypoglycaemic. Of the 244 babies (46% of total group) assigned to 'well baby nurseries' for routine care and enteral feeding, 32 had hypoglycaemia.

The study found 5% (13) of the 276 babies who had their haematocrit assessed were polycythaemic (haematocrit 0.65 or more). Of the 530 babies, 25% (125) were treated for hyperbilirubinaemia and, of these, 61 were delivered at 33 weeks of gestation or less. The rate of treatment for non-diabetic, full-term babies delivered during the same 2 year period was 5%.

Of the 244 babies admitted to well baby nurseries for routine care, 18% (43) were then transferred to the NICU (19 with respiratory distress syndrome as the main reason for transfer, 16 for treatment of hypoglycaemia, seven for respiratory distress syndrome plus hypoglycaemia and one for poor feeding). Advanced maternal diabetes and lower gestational age were shown by logistic regression to be the strongest predictors of subsequent NICU care. Logistic regression analysis also showed that after controlling for gestational age and type of diabetes, breastfed babies were more likely to succeed with routine care and enteral feeding. [EL = 2+]

Myocardial hypertrophy and respiratory distress syndrome:
A cross-sectional study looked at the association between poorly controlled maternal diabetes and myocardial hypertrophy.[363] Twelve neonates were admitted to NICU with respiratory distress and cardiomegaly. Ten babies were macrosomic and had myocardial hypertrophy as determined by echocardiograph. Two of these babies died from cardiorespiratory failure within 48 hours of birth. Two babies were AGA and had cardiomegaly resulting from ventricular dilation in association with hypoglycaemia and acidaemia. Of the surviving babies, 80% (8/10) had clinical findings suggesting respiratory distress syndrome. The presence of hyaline membranes at autopsy of the other two babies lends support to an association between respiratory distress syndrome and myocardial hypertrophy. [EL = 3]

Gestational age and mode of birth:
A clinical audit was conducted at the National Women's Hospital in New Zealand[364] which serves a multi-ethnic population with a high background prevalence of type 2 diabetes. In total 136 babies of women with diabetes were admitted to NICU. Tweny-nine percent (112/382) of the babies of women with gestational diabetes were admitted and 40% (24/60) of the babies of women with type 2 diabetes were admitted. Fifty-six percent (58/104) of the gestational diabetes was reclassified as normal, IGT or type 2 diabetes after postpartum 75 g OGTTs. Infant outcomes according to maternal antenatal and postpartum diagnoses were recorded. The study found 46% (63/136) babies were delivered preterm (before 37 weeks). Women with gestational diabetes that was reclassified postpartum as IGT or type 2 diabetes accounted for the highest rates of preterm babies (86% [12/14] and 63% [12/19], respectively). The rate of emergency lower segment caesarean section in women with gestational diabetes or type 2 diabetes was 25%. The rate of emergency lower segment caesarean section of women with gestational diabetes or type 2 diabetes whose babies were admitted to NICU was 38% (52/136). When a similar comparison was made for preterm birth the rates were 19% compared with 46% (63/136). The most common indication for admittance to NICU was hypoglycaemia, which was documented in 51% of the

babies. This was followed by respiratory distress in 40% of babies. Rates of respiratory distress in the preterm babies and term babies were not significantly different (39% [26/67] versus 43% [31/70], $P = 0.34$). A third of women with type 2 diabetes antenatally or postpartum had babies weighing more than 4000 g. These birthweights were significantly higher than for the IGT group ($P < 0.05$) and significantly more common than in the IGT or normal group ($P < 0.05$). [EL = 2+]

Current practice
The CEMACH enquiry covered neonatal care of term babies born to women with pre-existing type 1 or type 2 diabetes.[33] In the 112 babies selected for the neonatal enquiry that had medical records available, 70 were admitted to a postnatal ward, transitional care unit, stayed on the labour ward or in a maternal dependency unit and 42 were admitted to a NICU for special care. The three main indications for admission to a NICU were a hospital policy of routine admission of healthy babies of women with diabetes 29% (12/42), asymptomatic hypoglycaemia in a healthy baby 26% (11/42) and a clinical need for admission such as poor feeding or respiratory problems 43% (18/42). The enquiry panels assessed that 57% (24/42) of the admissions were unavoidable and that subsequent care of 63% (15) of the babies was compromised, especially in the area of feeding (50%, 12/24 babies). There was evidence of a clear written care plan for 73% (51/70) of babies who remained with their mothers and 57% (24/42) of babies admitted to a NICU. The care plan was not fully followed for 35% (18/51) of babies remaining with their mothers; aspects of the care plan that were not followed included blood glucose management, feeding and temperature. The enquiry also discussed the importance of early skin-to-skin contact between babies and their mothers (see Section 7.2) and recommended that all units where women with diabetes give birth should have written policy for management of the baby and that the policy should assume that babies will remain with their mothers in the absence of complications. [EL = 3–4]

A 2002 CEMACH audit of units expected to provide maternity care for women with diabetes in England, Wales and Northern Ireland reported that 30% (64/213) had a policy of routinely admitting babies of women with diabetes to the neonatal or special care unit.[32] [EL = 3]

Existing guidance

The NSF for diabetes[20] recommends that 'Neonatal intensive care is only indicated for babies who display persistent hypoglycaemia after 3 hours of age.'

Evidence statement

Five observational studies have reported on the incidence of neonatal morbidity in babies born to women with diabetes. Complications reported in these studies included asphyxia, birth trauma (e.g. shoulder dystocia), congenital malformations, hyperbilirubinaemia, hypoglycaemia, hypocalcaemia, LGA, respiratory distress syndrome and associated mortality.

No clinical studies were identified in relation to neonatal assessment that babies of women with diabetes should undergo, but two narrative non-systematic reviews described the clinical signs of the most frequently occurring neonatal complications in babies of women with diabetes.

A further four observational studies and a clinical audit investigated neonatal complications (including fetal hypoxia, hypocalcaemia, hypoglycaemia, macrosomia, myocardial hypertrophy (hypertrophic cardiomyopathy), polycythaemia and respiratory distress syndrome) and indications for admission to a NICU for babies of women with pre-existing type 1 or type 2 diabetes and gestational diabetes. None of the studies reported incidence of hypoxic ischaemic encephalopathy or hypomagnesaemia, although babies of women with diabetes are believed to be at increased risk of these complications.

One of the observational studies reported that persistent or recurrent hypoglycaemia in the neonatal stage can lead to neurodevelopmental deficits later in life. The authors of the study recommended that high-risk babies be screened at regular intervals in the first 48 hours of life if not being fed, or before the first three or four feedings, and in the presence of clinical signs of hypoglycaemia.

Other observational studies showed that prematurity and birth by emergency caesarean section were predictors for NICU admission in women with type 2 diabetes and those with gestational diabetes. Several of the studies suggested that babies of women with diabetes should be closely monitored and admitted to intensive care only in unavoidable circumstances where there are clinical signs of hypoglycaemia and/or respiratory distress, thus avoiding unnecessary separation of mothers and babies.

The clinical audit reported that the most frequent indications for admission to NICU were hypoglycaemia and respiratory distress syndrome, and one of the observational studies reported that the prevalence of these complications was higher with increasing duration of diabetes.

Cost-effectiveness

The effectiveness of criteria for admission to neonatal intensive/special care for babies of women with diabetes was identified by the GDG as a priority for health economic analysis. The NSF for diabetes[20] recommends that admission to a NICU should be made only for babies with persistent hypoglycaemia. However, the CEMACH audit reported that 30% of units still routinely admit babies of mothers with diabetes to the neonatal or special care unit and that the most frequent reasons for admission to a NICU were routine policy and asymptomatic hypoglycaemia. Thus no health economic modelling is needed to demonstrate that reinforcing the NSF recommendation, to keep babies with their mothers except when there is a clinical reason to separate them, represents a cost saving to the NHS.

From evidence to recommendations

Evidence shows that birth trauma, congenital malformations (cardiac and central nervous system), hyperbilirubinaemia, hypocalcaemia, hypoglycaemia, hypomagnesaemia, myocardial hypertrophy (hypertrophic cardiomyopathy), neonatal encephalopathy, polycythaemia and hyperviscosity, and respiratory distress (several of which are potentially life-threatening) are more prevalent in babies of women with pre-existing diabetes and gestational diabetes. Healthcare professionals assessing such babies should, therefore, be competent to recognise and manage these conditions and women with diabetes (including gestational diabetes) should be advised to give birth in hospitals where advanced neonatal resuscitation skills are available 24 hours a day.

The GDG's view is that blood glucose testing should be carried out routinely (at 2–4 hours after birth) for babies of women with diabetes because of the risk of complications arising from asymptomatic hypoglycaemia (see Section 7.2). However, blood tests for polycythaemia, hyperbilirubinaemia, hypocalcaemia and hypomagnesaemia, and investigations for congenital heart malformations and cardiomyopathy should be reserved for babies with clinical signs of these complications, thus avoiding unnecessary investigations, which will represent cost savings to the NHS and should provide reassurance for parents.

Babies of women with diabetes should be kept with their mothers unless there is a clinical complication or abnormal clinical signs that warrant admission for intensive or special care, in accordance with the recommendations contained in the NSF for diabetes,[20] thus bringing cost savings to the NHS and maximising the opportunity for early skin-to-skin contact between babies and their mothers and initiation of breastfeeding (see Section 7.2).

Some babies with clinical signs of the conditions listed above may be cared for in a transitional care unit, depending on local guidelines, facilities and care pathways. Where such facilities are unavailable, babies with these conditions should be admitted to a neonatal unit.

Neonatal metabolic adaptation in babies of women with diabetes is generally completed by 72 hours of age. Transfer to community care is not recommended before 24 hours and not before healthcare professionals are satisfied that the baby is maintaining blood glucose levels and has developed good feeding skills because of the risk of recurrent hypoglycaemia in the early neonatal period. Early community midwifery support for these babies should be more intense than average.

Recommendations for initial assessment and criteria for admission to intensive or special care

Women with diabetes should be advised to give birth in hospitals where advanced neonatal resuscitation skills are available 24 hours a day.

Babies of women with diabetes should be kept with their mothers unless there is a clinical complication or there are abnormal clinical signs that warrant admission for intensive or special care.

Blood glucose testing should be carried out routinely in babies of women with diabetes at 2–4 hours after birth. Blood tests for polycythaemia, hyperbilirubinaemia, hypocalcaemia and hypomagnesaemia should be carried out for babies with clinical signs.

Babies of women with diabetes should have an echocardiogram performed if they show clinical signs associated with congenital heart disease or cardiomyopathy, including heart murmur. The timing of the examination will depend on the clinical circumstances.

Babies of women with diabetes should be admitted to the neonatal unit if they have:

- hypoglycaemia associated with abnormal clinical signs
- respiratory distress
- signs of cardiac decompensation due to congenital heart disease or cardiomyopathy
- signs of neonatal encephalopathy
- signs of polycythaemia and are likely to need partial exchange transfusion
- need for intravenous fluids
- need for tube feeding (unless adequate support is available on the postnatal ward)
- jaundice requiring intense phototherapy and frequent monitoring of bilirubinaemia
- been born before 34 weeks (or between 34 and 36 weeks if dictated clinically by the initial assessment of the baby and feeding on the labour ward).

Babies of women with diabetes should not be transferred to community care until they are at least 24 hours old, and not before healthcare professionals are satisfied that the babies are maintaining blood glucose levels and are feeding well.

There were no research recommendations relating to the initial assessment of babies and criteria for admission to intensive/special care.

7.2 Prevention and assessment of neonatal hypoglycaemia

Description of the evidence

The working definition for neonatal hypoglycaemia is blood glucose less than 2.6 mmol/litre.[193,365,366] This threshold is not used to diagnose the condition, but rather to indicate the level at which intervention (additional feeding and, if this does not reverse the hypoglycaemia, intravenous dextrose) should be considered. It is based on a study that found adverse neurodevelopmental outcomes to be associated with repeated values below this level.[367] The study involved 661 preterm babies and used multiple regression to show that reduced developmental scores were associated independently with plasma glucose concentration less than 2.6 mmol/litre. [EL = 2+]

A consensus statement[368] discussed the definition of neonatal hypoglycaemia. The statement considered term babies, babies with abnormal clinical signs, babies with risk factors for compromised metabolic adaptation, preterm babies and babies receiving parenteral nutrition. Close surveillance should be maintained in babies with risk factors for compromised metabolic adaptation if the plasma glucose concentration is less than 2.0 mmol/litre; at very low concentrations (1.1–1.4 mmol/litre) an intravenous glucose infusion is indicated to raise the glucose level above 2.5 mmol/litre. [EL = 4]

The characteristics of neonatal hypoglycaemia in babies of women with diabetes are very early onset (first hour after birth), generally asymptomatic, non-recurrent and good response to intravenous dextrose.[368]

Early feeding
Two studies were found that investigated the effect of timing of first feed on blood glucose levels. The studies were undertaken in the 1960s when delaying the initial feed was common.

The first study compared 27 preterm babies allocated to an 'early fed' group (fed with formula from 6 hours of age) with 41 babies fasted for 72 hours.[369] At 72 hours 24/41 babies in the fasted group had blood glucose levels below 1.4 mmol/litre. In the early fed group no babies had blood glucose values below this level. Statistical significance was not reported. [EL = 2+]

The second study compared 118 preterm babies fed at 3 hours with undiluted breast milk with 121 fed at a later stage, usually at 12 hours. There were no cases of symptomatic hypoglycaemia in the early fed group compared with four cases in the later fed group. Blood sugar estimation was introduced in phase three of the trial. The lowest level was less than 1.1 mmol/litre in 5/44 in the 'immediate fed' group compared with 10/54 in the 'later fed' group.[370] Statistical significance was not reported. [EL = 2+]

Frequent feeding
One study was identified that looked at the effect of frequency of initial feeds on blood glucose levels.

The study was a cross-sectional study of 156 term babies.[371] A multiple regression analysis with method of feed, between-feed interval, volume of feed and postnatal age as independent variables found only between-feed interval (minutes) to be significantly correlated with blood glucose concentration ($B = -0.003$, SE = 0.001, $\beta = -0.32$, $P < 0.05$). [EL = 2+]

Breastfeeding
Ten studies were found that had implications for choice of feeding method.

The first study compared 45 breastfed babies with 34 formula-fed babies.[372] The babies were 6 days old and matched for gestation and birthweight. Breastfed babies had significantly higher levels of ketones. [EL = 2+]

The second study compared 71 breastfed babies with 61 formula-fed babies.[371] All babies were term babies less than 1 week old. Breastfed babies had significantly lower mean blood glucose concentration ($P < 0.05$) and significantly higher ketone body concentrations ($P < 0.001$). Breastfed babies had higher total gluconeogenic substrate concentrations ($P < 0.01$). [EL = 2+]

A cohort study investigated the glucose concentration of breast milk of women with diabetes and its relationship with the quality of metabolic control.[373] The study involved 11 women with type 1 diabetes and 11 age-matched women without diabetes. The women with diabetes had intensified insulin treatment and their average HbA_{1c} values were significantly higher than those in women without diabetes ($8.1 \pm 0.9\%$ versus $6.2 \pm 0.5\%$, $P < 0.01$). The glucose concentration of breast milk taken from women with diabetes did not differ from that of women without diabetes (0.68 ± 0.50 versus 0.66 ± 0.55 mmol/litre). No correlation was found between the maternal blood glucose (HbA_{1c}) and the glucose concentration of breast milk. [EL = 2−]

A prospective cohort study[374] investigated whether children born to women with diabetes were at increased risk of developing obesity and IGT in childhood. A total of 112 children of women with diabetes (type 1 diabetes, $n = 83$ and gestational diabetes, $n = 29$) were evaluated prospectively for impact of ingestion of either breast milk from a woman with diabetes or banked donor breast milk from women without diabetes during the early neonatal period (days 1–7 of life) on relative body weight and glucose tolerance at a mean age of 2 years. There was a positive correlation between the volume of breast milk from women with diabetes ingested and risk of overweight at 2 years of age (OR 2.47, 95% CI 1.25 to 4.87). In contrast, the volume of banked donor breast milk from women without diabetes ingested was inversely correlated to body weight at follow-up ($P = 0.001$). Risk of childhood IGT decreased by increasing amounts of banked donor breast milk ingested neonatally (OR 0.19, 95% CI 0.05 to 0.70). Stepwise regression analysis showed volume of breast milk from women with diabetes to be the only significant predictor of relative body weight at 2 years of age ($P = 0.001$). The results suggest that early neonatal ingestion of breast milk from women with diabetes may increase the risk of becoming overweight and, consequently, developing IGT during childhood. [EL = 2+]

A prospective cohort study[375] investigated whether intake of breast milk of women with diabetes during the late neonatal period and early infancy influenced subsequent risk of overweight (adipogenic) and IGT (diabetogenic) in children born to women with diabetes. One hundred and twelve children born to women with diabetes were evaluated for influence of ingesting their mother's breast milk during the late neonatal period (second to fourth neonatal week) and early infancy on relative body weight and glucose tolerance in early childhood. Exclusive breastfeeding was associated with increased childhood relative body weight ($P = 0.011$). Breastfed children of women with diabetes had an increased risk of overweight (OR 1.98, 95% CI 1.12 to 3.50). Breastfeeding duration was also positively related to childhood relative body weight ($P = 0.004$) and 120 minute blood glucose during an OGTT ($P = 0.022$). However, adjustment for the volume of breast milk from women with diabetes ingested during the early neonatal period (i.e. the first week of life), eliminated all these relationships with late neonatal breastfeeding and its duration. No relationship was observed between maternal blood glucose in the middle of the third trimester and neonatal outcomes. The study suggests that neither late neonatal breast milk intake from women with diabetes nor duration of breastfeeding has an independent influence on childhood risk of overweight or IGT in children born to women with diabetes. The first week of life appears to be the critical window for nutritional programming in children of ingestion of breast milk from women with diabetes. [EL = 2+]

Another cohort study[376] investigated whether late neonatal ingestion of breast milk might independently influence neurodevelopment in 242 children of women with diabetes. There was no impact of ingestion of breast milk of women with diabetes on psychomotor parameters, but it negatively influenced onset of speaking with children of women with diabetes who were fed solely on breast milk taking the longest time to initiate speech. Adjusting for the amount of breast milk ingested during the early neonatal period weakened the hazard ratio towards non-significance. The data suggest that neonatal ingestion of breast milk of women with diabetes, particularly during the first week of life, may delay speech development, an important indicator of cognitive development. [EL = 2++]

Another cohort study investigated the extent to which early breastfeeding or exposure to cow's milk affected psychomotor and cognitive development in children of women with diabetes.[377] Children of women with diabetes with early breast milk ingestion achieved early psychomotor developmental milestones (lifting head while prone, following with eyes; $P = 0.002$). However, children who had ingested larger volumes of milk of women with diabetes had a delayed onset in speaking compared to those with lower milk intake ($P = 0.002$). The data suggest that ingesting larger volumes of milk of women with diabetes may normalise early psychomotor development in babies of these women, but may delay onset of speaking. [EL = 2++]

A systematic review[378] summarised the clinical evidence relating a short duration of breastfeeding or early cow's milk exposure to the development of type 1 diabetes. People with type 1 diabetes were more likely to have been breastfed for less than 3 months during their infancy (pooled OR 1.43, 95% CI 1.15 to 1.77) and to have been exposed to cow's milk before 4 months (pooled OR 1.63, 95% CI 1.22 to 2.17) compared to those without diabetes. The study suggests that early exposure to cow's milk may be an important determinant of subsequent type 1 diabetes and may increase the risk approximately 1.5 times. [EL = 2++]

Another systematic review[379] evaluated the relationship between early infant diet and the risk of developing type 1 diabetes in later life via a meta-analysis of 17 case–control studies involving 21 039 people who were either breastfed or introduced early to cow's milk. The effect of exposure to breast milk substitutes on developing type 1 diabetes was small. [EL = 2++]

A case–control study investigated the association between the type of feeding in infancy and the development of type 1 diabetes.[380] The study involved 100 children with type 1 diabetes and 100 children without diabetes matched for sex and age. Information on feeding patterns during the first year of life was collected using a questionnaire. A larger proportion of children with diabetes had been breastfed. There was no clear difference between children with diabetes and those without diabetes in terms of duration of breastfeeding (children with diabetes, median duration 3 months; children without diabetes, median duration 2 months). The data do not support the existence of a protective effect of breastfeeding on the risk of type 1 diabetes, or that early exposure to cow's milk and dairy products influences the development of type 1 diabetes. [EL = 2+]

Barriers to breastfeeding in women with diabetes in pregnancy
One study was identified that compared breastfeeding initiation and maintenance in 33 women with type 1 diabetes to those of 33 women in a control group and 11 women in a reference sample.[381] The control group consisted of women without diabetes selected using gestational age at delivery, method of delivery, sex of baby and prior lactation experience. The reference group consisted of women without diabetes who were within 90–110% of ideal body weight prior to conception, had uncomplicated pregnancies and delivered vaginally. The study found women with diabetes were more likely to experience difficulties establishing and continuing breastfeeding than control and reference groups. All differences were significant ($P < 0.05$). The difference between groups was attributed to differences in postpartum care. Hospital protocol placed all babies of women with diabetes in the neonatal unit after birth for monitoring for hypoglycaemia. This meant that women with diabetes saw their babies the least amount of time in the first 3 days postpartum, waited the longest to begin breastfeeding their babies and breastfed their babies fewer times. Other possible contributory factors were that 70% of the women with diabetes had undergone caesarean section and that 30% of the babies of women with diabetes were macrosomic. Women with diabetes cited baby sleepiness as the most common baby-feeding problem. A sleepy baby was not identified as a problem by any of the women in the control group and by only one woman in the reference group. [EL = 2+]

A case–control study[382] investigated factors influencing the initiation and maintenance of breastfeeding in 22 women with type 1 diabetes and 22 women without diabetes. Diabetes was not a principal factor in the decision to breastfeed or bottle-feed for the majority of the women. Women who considered diabetes in their decision to breastfeed had on average 2 years more of education than those who did not (14.82 years versus 12.94 years). Although the women did not perceive diabetes as influencing their breastfeeding experiences, they found that maintaining good control of diabetes required greater effort and flexibility during breastfeeding. [EL = 2+]

Banking colostrum before birth
Two publications were identified in relation to production of colostrum from women with diabetes and banking colostrum before birth for use in the neonatal period.

A cohort study compared the composition of macro- and micronutrients in milk from six women with tightly controlled type 1 diabetes (median glycosylated haemoglobin concentrations at parturition of 5.2% (range 4.9–5.3%) and 6 weeks later of 6.1% (range 5.0–6.3%), reference range 5.0–6.4%) with that from five women without diabetes.[383] Milk samples were collected halfway through a single breastfeed at days: 3–5 (colostrum); 7, 9 and 10 (transitional milk); and 12, 15, 17, 21, 25, 29 and 35 (mature milk). There were no differences between the two groups in terms of concentrations of macronutrients (triglycerides, lactose and protein), cholesterol, glucose or myoinositol, nor in fatty acid composition. The duration of colostrum lactation was the same for women with diabetes and those without diabetes (3–5 days in both groups). [EL = 2–]

A narrative non-systematic review considered expressing and banking colostrum antenatally for use in the neonatal period.[384] The review suggested that women with conditions that may delay breastfeeding and those who wish to lessen known familial health problems for their expected babies (including women with type 1 diabetes or gestational diabetes) would benefit from antenatal expression of colostrum. The risk of nipple stimulation initiating oxytocin release and, therefore, preterm contractions, labour and preterm birth was discussed and a protocol for expressing and storing colostrum was suggested. The review concluded that expressing and storing colostrum is advantageous to babies and confidence building for women and should, therefore, be supported for any condition which healthcare professionals consider to be relevant. [EL = 4]

Testing for neonatal hypoglycaemia
A systematic review by the WHO[366] found that screening for hypoglycaemia using glucose oxidase-based reagent strips had poor sensitivity and specificity. The report recommended that 'less frequent but more accurate laboratory or ward-based glucose electrode measurements among babies at risk are preferable'.

Intravenous dextrose for neonatal hypoglycaemia
There is a consensus that intravenous dextrose should be administered for symptomatic hypoglycaemia and for asymptomatic hypoglycaemia that fails to respond to feeding.[366,386,387] However, no clinical studies were identified in relation to evaluation of protocols for the treatment of neonatal hypoglycaemia using intravenous dextrose.

Current practice
The CEMACH enquiry[33] reported that the opportunity for early skin-to-skin contact after birth was achieved in 29% (30) of the 102 babies whose medical records were available. In eight cases, skin-to-skin contact was not possible due to the condition of the woman and/or the baby. Ninety-five percent of babies remaining with their mothers received their first feed on the labour ward compared with 50% of those admitted to a neonatal unit ($P < 0.001$). Twenty-six percent (29/112) of women received help with breastfeeding within 1 hour of birth (34% of women on labour wards and 12% of women in the neonatal unit). Thirty-one percent of women whose babies were admitted to the neonatal unit had documented evidence in their medical records that they were shown how to breastfeed and maintain lactation. Infant formula was given at the first feed for 63% (67/106 babies) and this was the first choice for women in 46% (32/70) of cases. Breast milk was the first feed for 50% (34/68) of babies that remained with their mothers and 21% (8/38%) of babies in the neonatal unit ($P = 0.001$). The first feed given was not the mother's intended type of feed for 28% (27/96) of babies (16% of women who stayed with their babies and 50% of those admitted to the neonatal unit, $P < 0.001$). [EL = 3–4]

CEMACH undertook a descriptive study of all pregnancies of women with pre-existing diabetes who gave birth or booked between 1 March 2002 and 28 February 2003.[2] The study found that 40.1% of all babies (1382/3451) were fed within 1 hour and 78.8% (2717/3451) by 4 hours. Among term babies 46.5% (1031/2216) were fed within 1 hour and 87.7% (1837/2216) within 4 hours. Exclusive breastfeeding was the choice at birth for 53% (1762/3342) of women with pre-existing diabetes compared with 69% in the general population. At 28 days after birth the proportion of exclusively breastfed babies was 23.8%, half the proportion who had intended to breastfeed at birth. A history of low blood glucose alone was the main reason (36.7%) for giving term babies of women with diabetes supplementary milk or glucose. In 9% of cases babies were given supplementary milk or glucose routinely according to local practice, possibly compromising establishment of breastfeeding. Of the 3451 babies in the study, 83.2% were tested within 6 hours and 47.3% were tested within 1 hour. Testing this early may, however, simply detect the normal drop in blood glucose that can be expected after birth. One-third of term babies were admitted to a neonatal unit for special care. Examining the reasons for admission suggested that many (67%) were avoidable. [EL = 3]

The CEMACH enquiry[33] reported that neonatal blood glucose testing was mainly carried out using reagent strips. It supported the WHO's recommendation that reagent strip testing is unreliable and recommended that when considering the diagnosis of hypoglycaemia at least one laboratory value should be obtained. The enquiry also recommended that women with diabetes should be informed antenatally of the beneficial effects of breastfeeding on metabolic control for them and their babies and that blood glucose testing performed too early should be avoided in well babies without signs of hypoglycaemia. [EL = 3–4]

A standard textbook of neonatology[388] supports this evidence.

Existing guidance

The NSF for diabetes advises that babies born to women with diabetes should be fed as soon as possible after birth.[20] It also recommends breastfeeding for babies of women with diabetes, but that women should be supported in the feeding method of their choice. [EL = 4]

The NICE guideline for routine postnatal care recommends that women should be encouraged to have skin-to-skin contact with their babies as soon as possible after birth and that initiation of breastfeeding should be encouraged as soon as possible after birth and ideally within 1 hour.[11]

Evidence statement

The blood glucose concentration used to guide intervention for neonatal hypoglycaemia (i.e. additional feeding and, if this does not reverse hypoglycaemia, intravenous administration of dextrose) is 2.6 mmol/litre. Close surveillance should be maintained in babies with risk factors for compromised metabolic adaptation if the plasma glucose concentration is less than 2.0 mmol/litre; at very low concentrations (1.1–1.4 mmol/litre) an intravenous glucose infusion is indicated to raise the glucose level above 2.5 mmol/litre.

Two studies showed that early feeding of babies was associated with lower incidence of hypoglycaemia than late feeding (more than 12 hours after birth). However, these studies involved preterm babies who may demonstrate different metabolic adaptation to term babies.

Another study showed between-feeding interval to be correlated with blood glucose levels, suggesting that frequent feeding should be encouraged to prevent neonatal hypoglycaemia.

Three studies relating to choice of infant-feeding method for women with diabetes suggested that: breastfeeding may enhance ketogenesis and that ketones may be an important alternative to glucose for brain metabolism in the neonatal period; breastfeeding babies of women with diabetes was not associated with increased exposure of the babies to high glucose levels; and, where possible, separation of mother and baby should be avoided to enable early feeds, frequent feeds and breastfeeding, with the possibility that supplementary feeding with infant formula may be required for women with diabetes who breastfeed. However, the first of these studies involved 6-day-old babies and therefore has limited relevance to hypoglycaemia in babies of women with diabetes, who are at greatest risk of hypoglycaemia in the first 12 hours.

A further seven observational studies, including two systematic reviews of observational studies, examined associations between feeding method and long-term outcomes. Three of the studies showed that obesity, IGT and impaired cognitive development were associated with ingestion of breast milk from women with diabetes. However, the two systematic reviews, which showed an association between breastfeeding and subsequent development of diabetes, were not specific to children of women with diabetes.

Two studies reported that initiation and maintenance of breastfeeding was more difficult for women with diabetes because of routine separation of babies from their mothers at birth or clinical reasons for separation such as the woman having undergone caesarean section or the baby having macrosomia. Although diabetes was not a major factor in deciding whether to breastfeed, women with diabetes found that maintaining good control of diabetes required greater effort and flexibility during breastfeeding. These findings suggest that, where possible, separation of the mother and baby should be avoided to facilitate early, frequent feeds and breastfeeding. Supplementary feeding with infant formula may be required for women with diabetes who breastfeed.

No clinical studies were identified in relation to the potential benefits of expressing and storing colostrum antenatally for the purposes of supporting early feeding to prevent hypoglycaemia in babies of women with diabetes.

A systematic review by the WHO noted low sensitivity and specificity of reagent strip blood glucose testing to identify neonatal hypoglycaemia and recommended laboratory or ward-based glucose electrode measurements for babies at risk of neonatal hypoglycaemia.

No clinical studies were identified in relation to the evaluation of protocols for treatment of neonatal hypoglycaemia using intravenous dextrose.

From evidence to recommendations

In the absence of high-quality evidence, the GDG's recommendations for the prevention and treatment of neonatal hypoglycaemia are based on group consensus. The GDG's view is that all maternity units should have a local written protocol for the prevention, detection and management of hypoglycaemia in babies of women with diabetes. Breastfeeding is recommended to prevent neonatal hypoglycaemia (by promoting successful metabolic adaptation) alongside other known benefits. Early commencement of breastfeeding is more important in babies of women with diabetes because of the risk of neonatal hypoglycaemia and is encouraged by skin-to-skin contact. Babies of women with diabetes should, therefore, feed as soon as possible after birth and at frequent intervals thereafter. While the target level for blood glucose is 2.6 mmol/litre, the GDG has set the threshold for initiating intravenous administration of dextrose at 2.0 mmol/litre on two consecutive readings, despite maximal support for feeding. Babies of women with diabetes should not be treated with invasive procedures (such as tube feeding or intravenous dextrose) unless they have clinical signs of hypoglycaemia or unless their blood glucose values persist below the threshold for initiating intravenous dextrose.

Blood glucose measurements should be obtained using ward-based glucose electrode or laboratory analysis because these have greater sensitivity and specificity than reagent strip testing. In making this recommendation the GDG noted the findings of the CEMACH enquiry, which reported that reagent strip testing is still commonplace. The GDG's view is that blood glucose should be tested before feeding the baby.

Recommendations for prevention and assessment of neonatal hypoglycaemia

All maternity units should have a written policy for the prevention, detection and management of hypoglycaemia in babies of women with diabetes.

Babies of women with diabetes should have their blood glucose tested using a quality-assured method validated for neonatal use (ward-based glucose electrode or laboratory analysis).

Babies of women with diabetes should feed as soon as possible after birth (within 30 minutes) and then at frequent intervals (every 2–3 hours) until feeding maintains pre-feed blood glucose levels at a minimum of 2.0 mmol/litre.

If blood glucose values are below 2.0 mmol/litre on two consecutive readings despite maximal support for feeding, if there are abnormal clinical signs or if the baby will not feed orally effectively, additional measures such as tube feeding or intravenous dextrose should be given. Additional measures should only be implemented if one or more of these criteria are met.

Babies of women with diabetes who present with clinical signs of hypoglycaemia should have their blood glucose tested and be treated with intravenous dextrose as soon as possible.

Research recommendations for prevention and assessment of neonatal hypoglycaemia

Is systematic banking of colostrum antenatally of any benefit in pregnancies complicated by diabetes?

Why this is important
Babies of women with diabetes are at increased risk of neonatal hypoglycaemia and may need frequent early feeding to establish and maintain normoglycaemia. Additionally, the opportunity for early skin-to-skin contact and initiation of breastfeeding is not always achieved in pregnancies complicated by diabetes because of the increased risk of neonatal complications requiring admission to intensive/special care. Antenatal expression and storage of colostrum may, therefore, be of benefit to babies of women with diabetes. There have been no clinical studies to evaluate the effectiveness of antenatal banking of colostrum in women with diabetes. Randomised controlled trials are needed to determine whether this practice is clinically and cost-effective. Encouraging women with diabetes to express and store colostrum before birth might be viewed as an additional barrier to breastfeeding in this group of women who already have lower breastfeeding rates than the general maternity population. There is also a putative risk of precipitating uterine contractions through antenatal expression of colostrum and an accompanying release of oxytocin. These factors should be explored in the randomised controlled trials.

8 Postnatal care

8.1 Breastfeeding and effects on glycaemic control

Description of the evidence

Two small cohort studies and a case series were identified that considered the effect of breastfeeding on glycaemic control in women with diabetes. Two cohort studies were identified that considered the effects of oral hypoglycaemic agents on breast milk and infant hypoglycaemia. Factors affecting the choice between breastfeeding and bottle-feeding for babies of women with diabetes are considered in Section 7.2.

Insulin

The first cohort study involved 36 women with type 1 diabetes.[389] Breastfeeding was initiated by 15 women in the first 24 hours. At 7 days and 1 month postpartum 28 women were breastfeeding and at 2 months postpartum 24 women were breastfeeding. On discharge from hospital women were prescribed an insulin regimen two-thirds of the third-trimester requirements and advised to adjust pre-meal insulin doses to glycaemic response. Women were advised to keep to regular meal times and eat before the baby's feeding times. If this was not possible, women were advised to have a glass of juice (during the day) or milk (at night). The study compared glycaemic control and insulin requirements of breastfeeding and bottle-feeding women over four periods: preconception, the first 7 days postpartum, the first month postpartum and the second month postpartum. In all women mean blood glucose values were significantly lower during the first week postpartum (6.7 ± 1.1 mmol/litre) than at preconception (7.7 ± 0.9 mmol/litre) or during the second month postpartum (7.6 ± 1.3 mmol/litre). The percentage of blood glucose readings below 3 mmol/litre did not differ during the four periods. In all women insulin requirements were significantly lower during the first week postpartum (0.56 ± 0.15 U/kg/day) than at preconception (0.68 ± 0.16 U/kg/day) and they remained significantly lower over the first and second months postpartum (0.56 ± 0.15 U/kg/day and 0.56 ± 0.11 U/kg/day, respectively). There was no difference in glycaemic control or insulin requirements between breastfeeding and bottle-feeding women, with the exception of mean blood glucose values during the first week postpartum which reached borderline significance (6.6 ± 0.6 versus 7.0 ± 0.9 mmol/litre, $P = 0.050$). Fewer hypoglycaemic episodes in breastfeeding women were associated with breastfeeding sessions (4.0 ± 3.5) than at other times (12.2 ± 7.1, $P = 0.002$). [EL = 2+]

The second cohort study followed 30 women with type 1 diabetes from birth to 6 weeks postpartum.[390] Six women breastfed exclusively, nine women stopped breastfeeding before 6 weeks and 14 women bottle-fed. Insulin dosages did not differ between the three groups. Six week postpartum FBG levels were significantly lower in women who breastfed exclusively (4.6 ± 2.2 mmol/litre) compared with those in women who stopped breastfeeding before 6 weeks (8.1 ± 2.1 mmol/litre) and women who bottle-fed (6.7 ± 1.7 mmol/litre). [EL = 2+]

The case series involved 24 women with type 1 diabetes.[391] Of these, 18 established breastfeeding and 16 continued until the 6 week postnatal clinic. Insulin doses were reduced below the pre-pregnancy dose immediately after birth and then adjusted according to blood glucose concentrations. After birth women who breastfed ($n = 18$) reduced their insulin dose by a mean of 11.6 units (26%) from their pre-pregnancy dose (95% CI 8.9 to 14.3 units, $P < 0.001$). Women who bottle-fed ($n = 6$) reduced their insulin dose by a mean of 5.2 units (11.3%) from their pre-pregnancy dose (95% CI 1.1 to 9.3 units, not significant). [EL = 3]

Oral hypoglycaemic agents

A cohort study[392] investigated excretion of metformin into breast milk and the effect on nursing babies. Five women with type 2 diabetes and two women without diabetes were started on metformin on the first day after caesarean section. Four women dropped out, leaving only three for analysis. The results are not meaningful and the study is not considered further. [EL = 2−]

Another cohort study[393] investigated whether glibenclamide and glipizide may be excreted into breast milk and whether breastfeeding from women taking these drugs causes infant hypoglycaemia. Eight women who received a single oral dose of 5 mg or 10 mg glibenclamide were studied by measuring drug concentrations in maternal blood and breast milk for 8 hours after the dosing schedule. Another five women treated with 5 mg/day of glibenclamide or glipizide starting on the first day postpartum were assessed by measuring the concentration of the drugs in maternal blood and milk. Infant blood glucose was measured 5–16 days after birth. Neither glibenclamide nor glipizide were detected in breast milk and blood glucose was normal in the three babies (one glibenclamide and two glipizide) who were wholly breastfed. The results suggest that glibenclamide and glipizide are safe and compatible with breastfeeding at the doses investigated. [EL = 2+]

A reference guide to drugs in pregnancy and lactation reports that women taking metformin can breastfeed.[77] The review included evidence from two small observational studies in breastfeeding women which found that metformin is excreted in milk. The average metformin concentration was under 0.3% of the maternal weight-adjusted dose. Both studies concluded that metformin was safe to use during breastfeeding. [EL = 3]

The reference guide reported that acarbose, nateglinide, pioglitazone, rosiglitazone, glibenclamide, glimepiride and glipizide are probably compatible with breastfeeding.[77] Although no studies have investigated their use in women who are breastfeeding, the reference guide suggested nateglinide, pioglitazone and rosiglitazone-related material may be present in low levels in breast milk. The reference guide also suggested that the amount of acarbose available for transfer to breast milk is very small because less than 2% of the acarbose dose is absorbed systemically, and that data on safety during breastfeeding are needed. The reference guide suggested that glimepiride and glipizide are likely to be present in breast milk. [EL = 3]

The reference guide reported that repaglinide, chlorpropamide and tolbutamide are potentially toxic to babies if they are taken by breastfeeding women. Chlorpropamide and tolbutamide are excreted into breast milk. No studies have investigated the use of repaglinide in breastfeeding women, but the reference guide suggested that it may produce skeletal deformities.[77] [EL = 3]

There was no information about gliclazide or gliquidone in the reference guide.

The British National Formulary reports that metformin is present in breast milk and the manufacturer advises women who are breastfeeding to avoid it.[78] The manufacturers of nateglinide, repaglinide, pioglitazone and rosiglitazone advise women who are breastfeeding to avoid them. The manufacturer of acarbose advises women who are breastfeeding to avoid it. Sulphonylureas have a theoretical possibility of causing hypoglycaemia in the baby.

Angiotensin-converting enzyme inhibitors
A reference guide to drugs in pregnancy and lactation reported that there are limited data for the use of the ACE inhibitors enalapril and trandolapril, and suggested that they are probably compatible with breastfeeding. There were no data for the use of lisinopril, moexipril hydrochloride, perindopril or quinapril in women who are breastfeeding, but the reference guide suggested that they are probably compatible with breastfeeding. There was no information about captopril, cilazapril, fosinopril sodium, imidapril hydrochloride or ramipril.[77] [EL = 3]

The British National Formulary reports that quinapril, captopril, fosinopril and lisinopril have been found to be present in breast milk and they should be avoided by women who are breastfeeding. The manufacturers of trandolapril advise pregnant women to avoid it. Cilazapril, imidapril, moexipril, perindopril and ramipril have no information available and so the manufacturer advises women who are breastfeeding to avoid them. The manufacturers state that enalapril is probably present in breast milk in an amount too small to be harmful.[78]

Angiotensin-II receptor blockers
A reference guide to drugs in pregnancy and lactation reported that there were no data for the use of ARBs in women who are breastfeeding, but it suggests that they are probably compatible with breastfeeding.[77] [EL = 3]

The British National Formulary states that olmesartan has been found to be present in breast milk and recommends that it should be avoided by women who are breastfeeding. Candesartan, eprosartan, irbesartan, losartan, telmisartan and valsartan have no information available so the manufacturers advise women who are breastfeeding to avoid them.[78]

Statins

A reference guide to drugs in pregnancy and lactation reported that statins are contraindicated in women who are breastfeeding.[77] Studies have shown that fluvastatin and pravastatin appear in breast milk. No data were available for simvastatin, atorvastatin or rosuvastatin. [EL = 3]

The British National Formulary notes that pravastatin has been found to be present in a small amount in breast milk and should be avoided by women who are breastfeeding. There is no information available for the use of atorvastatin, fluvastatin, rosuvastatin and simvastatin during breastfeeding and women who are breastfeeding are advised to avoid them.[78]

Calcium-channel blockers

A reference guide to drugs in pregnancy and lactation reported that there are no data for the use of the calcium-channel blockers amlodipine, felodipine, isradipine, nicardipine or nisoldipine in women who are breastfeeding, but suggested that they are probably compatible with breastfeeding. The reference guide reported that there are limited data for the use of diltiazem, nifedipine, nimodipine and verapamil in women who are breastfeeding and it suggested that they are probably compatible with breastfeeding. No data were available for lacidipine or lercanidipine hydrochloride.[77] [EL = 3]

The British National Formulary states that verapamil has been found to be present in breast milk in an amount too small to be harmful.[78] Diltiazem has been found to be present in a significant amount in milk and although there is no evidence of harm the manufacturer advises pregnant women to avoid it unless there is no safer alternative. Felodipine is present in milk. Isradipine may be present in breast milk and the manufacturer advises women who are breastfeeding to avoid it. Nifedipine is found in breast milk, but in an amount too small to be harmful; however, the manufacturer advises breastfeeding women to avoid it. There is no information available for amlodipine, lacidipine, lercanidipine, nicardipine or nisoldipine and the manufacturers advise breastfeeding women to avoid them. There is no information available for nimodipine.

Obesity drugs

A reference guide to drugs in pregnancy and lactation reported that there were no data for the use of the obesity drug orlistat in women who are breastfeeding, but that it is probably compatible with breastfeeding. The reference guide reported that there were no data for the use of sibutramine in women who are breastfeeding and it suggests there may be toxicity to the baby. There was no review for rimonabant.[77] [EL = 3]

The British National Formulary recommends that rimonabant be avoided by women who are breastfeeding. The manufacturers of orlistat and sibutramine recommend that they be avoided in women who are breastfeeding, but no further information is given.[78]

Evidence statement

There are no high quality studies that show that breastfeeding affects glycaemic control. A small cohort study showed that insulin requirements and blood glucose levels fell in all women with diabetes following birth. Blood glucose levels fell only for the first week postpartum. There was no difference between groups in hypoglycaemic episodes, however breastfeeding women were advised to eat a meal or snack before feeds and the small numbers in the study limits comparison between groups.

A small cohort study found lower FBG levels 6 weeks after birth in women who breastfed than in women who bottle-fed or discontinued breastfeeding before 6 weeks.

A case series found a significant reduction in insulin requirements in breastfeeding women following birth, but the study was underpowered to detect a difference in insulin requirements between breastfeeding and bottle-feeding women.

There is limited evidence from two cohort studies and a reference guide in relation to the safety of oral hypoglycaemic agents, ACE inhibitors, ARBs, statins, calcium-channel blockers and obesity drugs in women who are breastfeeding. The reference guide and the manufacturers of the drugs recommend that these preparations are avoided by women who are breastfeeding.

From evidence to recommendations

Given the lack of clinical evidence in relation to the effect of breastfeeding on glycaemic control the GDG's recommendations are based on consensus within the group on best current practice. Women with insulin-treated pre-existing diabetes should, therefore, be advised to reduce their insulin dose immediately after birth and to monitor their blood glucose levels to establish the appropriate dose. Women with insulin-treated pre-existing diabetes who are breastfeeding should be informed that they are at increased risk of hypoglycaemia when breastfeeding and to have a meal or snack available before or during feeds. Women who have been diagnosed with gestational diabetes should discontinue hypoglycaemic treatment immediately after birth.

The safety of oral hypoglycaemic agents, ACE inhibitors, ARBs, statins, calcium-channel blockers and obesity drugs in women who are breastfeeding has not been established. However, it is the GDG's view that women with pre-existing type 2 diabetes who are breastfeeding can resume or continue to take metformin and glibenclamide immediately following birth. Women with diabetes who are breastfeeding should, therefore, continue to avoid any drugs for the treatment of diabetes and its complications that were discontinued for safety reasons in the preconception period.

Recommendations for breastfeeding and effects on glycaemic control

Women with insulin-treated pre-existing diabetes should reduce their insulin immediately after birth and monitor their blood glucose levels carefully to establish the appropriate dose.

Women with insulin-treated pre-existing diabetes should be informed that they are at increased risk of hypoglycaemia in the postnatal period, especially when breastfeeding, and they should be advised to have a meal or snack available before or during feeds.

Women who have been diagnosed with gestational diabetes should discontinue hypoglycaemic treatment immediately after birth.

Women with pre-existing type 2 diabetes who are breastfeeding can resume or continue to take metformin* and glibenclamide* immediately following birth but other oral hypoglycaemic agents should be avoided while breastfeeding.

Women with diabetes who are breastfeeding should continue to avoid any drugs for the treatment of diabetes complications that were discontinued for safety reasons in the preconception period.

There were no research recommendations relating to breastfeeding and effects on glycaemic control in women with diabetes.

8.2   Information and follow-up after birth

Description of the evidence

Gestational diabetes
In the postnatal period, glucose metabolism in women who have been diagnosed with gestational diabetes may return to normal, or there may be ongoing impaired glucose regulation (IGT or impaired fasting glycaemia) or frank diabetes (including pre-existing type 1 or type 2 diabetes that was unrecognised before pregnancy).[31]

One systematic review and nine additional or subsequent studies examining the likelihood of women who have been diagnosed with gestational diabetes later developing type 1 or type 2

---

* This drug does not have UK marketing authorisation specifically for pregnant and breastfeeding women at the time of publication (March 2008). Informed consent should be obtained and documented.

diabetes were identified. Two RCTs and a cross-sectional study on the effect of lifestyle/educational interventions on the development of type 2 diabetes were identified. A further systematic review on the effectiveness of pharmacological and lifestyle interventions to prevent or delay type 2 diabetes in people with IGT was identified. Two studies on alternatives to a 6 week OGTT for women who have been diagnosed with gestational diabetes were identified.

Epidemiology:
Women who have been diagnosed with gestational diabetes are likely to have gestational diabetes in future pregnancies. Recurrence rates for gestational diabetes vary between 30% and 84% after the index pregnancy, and the recurrence rate is about 75% in women with a history of insulin-treated gestational diabetes (see Section 4.1).

A systematic review (28 studies) examined risk factors associated with developing type 2 diabetes in women who had been diagnosed with gestational diabetes.[394] The studies included in the review reported rates of conversion to type 2 diabetes from 2.6% to 70% over periods from 6 weeks to 28 years. The epidemiological data showed that the incidence of type 2 diabetes increased most rapidly in the first 5 years after pregnancy. Fasting glucose levels from OGTTs administered during pregnancy were predictive of developing type 2 diabetes after pregnancy. There was no clear pattern for risk factors such as BMI, maternal age, previous history of gestational diabetes, family history of diabetes or parity. The review highlighted that the included studies varied in ethnicity, length of follow-up and criteria for diagnosis of gestational diabetes and type 2 diabetes and that this made comparison and generalisation of results difficult. The review concluded that women with higher fasting glucose levels during pregnancy may need to be tested for type 2 diabetes more often than current guidelines recommend. [EL = 2+]

A cohort study ($n = 753$) from Denmark compared the incidence of diabetes after gestational diabetes in a cohort of women with gestational diabetes recruited between 1978 to 1985 (old cohort, $n = 151$) with a cohort recruited between 1987 and 1996 (new cohort, $n = 330$).[395] Until 1986, a 3 hour 50 g OGTT was used, whereas afterwards a 75 g OGTT was used. The 1999 WHO criteria were used for classification. Both cohorts were followed up in 2002 ($n = 481$) with a median follow-up of 9.8 years. The study found that overall 40% (192) of women had type 1 or type 2 diabetes and 27% (130) had impaired glucose regulation (IGT or impaired fasting glycaemia). Comparing the cohorts, 40.9% in the new cohort had type 1 or type 2 diabetes compared with 18.3% in the old cohort. Multiple regression analysis showed that membership of the new cohort, being overweight before pregnancy (BMI 25 kg/m² or more) and IGT postpartum were statistically significant risk factors for developing diabetes ($P < 0.05$). The study concluded that the incidence of diabetes in the cohort was very high and increasing, and that the increase in BMI in the population seemed to be the main risk factor accounting for this. [EL = 2−]

A cohort study ($n = 302$) undertaken in Germany examined the risk factors associated with developing diabetes after being diagnosed with gestational diabetes.[396] The study used a 75 g OGTT and the American Diabetes Association criteria for classification. The study found that insulin use during pregnancy, BMI more than 30 kg/m² and serum C-reactive protein at 9 months in 2nd to 4th quartiles were statistically significant predictors of developing diabetes. The study found that having a first-degree relative with diabetes, age, duration of pregnancy, birthweight of child and number of previous pregnancies were not predictive of subsequent diabetes. The study recommended that prospective diabetes assessment and intervention should be considered in women with gestational diabetes who are autoantibody positive, require insulin treatment during pregnancy or who are obese. [EL = 3]

A cohort study using routinely collected data ($n = 2956$) from Australia examined risk factors for developing diabetes after being diagnosed with gestational diabetes.[397] The study used a 50 g OGTT and the WHO criteria for classification. The study found that 2.0% (58/2956) of women developed diabetes within the first 6 months postpartum. Multivariate analysis found that severity of gestational diabetes, Asian origin and 1 hour plasma glucose were predictive of developing diabetes, but that insulin treatment during pregnancy, BMI, fetal macrosomia, maternal age and booking status (private or not) were not. The study concluded that these risk factors should be taken into account when deciding follow-up care for women with gestational diabetes. Whilst this study included a large number of women the follow-up period was, at most, 6 months. [EL = 3]

A cohort study (n = 278) from Hong Kong compared women with abnormal glucose tolerance test results with those with normal glucose tolerance test results.[398] The study used a 75 g OGTT and the WHO criteria for classification. The study found that 29.0% (56/193) of women who had been diagnosed with gestational diabetes had IGT (n = 38) or diabetes (n = 18) by 6 years follow-up compared with 13.8% (5/58 and 3/58, respectively) of women without gestational diabetes. The study found that age, BMI, abnormal OGTT at 6 weeks postpartum, diabetes in a first-degree relative, macrosomia, recurrent gestational diabetes and use of oral contraceptives were not predictive of later developing diabetes. [EL = 3]

A case–control study (n = 70) from Sweden compared the incidence of type 2 diabetes at 15 years follow-up between women who had gestational diabetes and those who did not. The study used the 2 hour 75 g OGTT.[399] The study found that 35% (10/28) of women with gestational diabetes had developed type 2 diabetes, whereas none of 52 controls had developed diabetes (P < 0.001). Weight, BMI, fasting blood sugar and HbA$_{1c}$ were all significant predictors of women with gestational diabetes developing diabetes compared to women with gestational diabetes that did not develop diabetes (P < 0.05). The study concluded that better postpartum strategies for control of weight and lifestyle are needed for women who have been diagnosed with gestational diabetes. [EL = 2–]

A case–control study (n = 468, 315 cases and 153 controls) from Sweden compared women with and without gestational diabetes for later development of diabetes.[400] The study used a 2 hour 75 g OGTT and the European Association for the Study of Diabetes criteria for classification. At 1 year follow-up 22% (50/229) of cases and 1.6% (1/60) of controls had developed type 2 diabetes (P < 0.001). Twenty-seven percent (24/90) of women with insulin-treated gestational diabetes and 17% (23/132) women with non-insulin-treated gestational diabetes had 2 hour OGTT values of 7.8–11.0 ml, whereas 20% (18/90) of women with insulin-treated gestational diabetes and 2% (3/132) of women with non-insulin-treated gestational diabetes had 2 hour OGTT values of more than 11.0 mmol/litre, respectively. The study found 2 hour OGTT value and HbA$_{1c}$ at diagnosis were associated with diabetes at 1 year, but BMI, weight increase, estimated fetal weight and birthweight were not associated with developing diabetes. Multiple regression analysis found that the results of OGTT test during pregnancy was predictive for developing diabetes later. [EL = 2+]

A case–control study (n = 870) from Finland compared the incidence of type 1 or type 2 diabetes postpartum in women who had been diagnosed with gestational diabetes (n = 435) with those who had not (n = 435).[401] The study used the Finnish Diabetes Association classification and a 75 g OGTT. Ten percent (43/435) of women in the case group had developed type 1 or type 2 diabetes, whereas none of the women in the control group had developed diabetes. Women treated with insulin during pregnancy were more likely to develop diabetes than those who did not use insulin (P < 0.0001). The women in the control group were significantly younger (27.2 years versus 34.0 years, P < 0.001). Regression analysis showed that age, insulin treatment, positive islet cell antibodies, positive glutamic acid decarboxylase antibodies and being positive for more than one antibody were all predictive of developing diabetes. [EL = 2+]

A cohort study (n = 317) from the USA compared the incidence of type 2 diabetes in Pima Indians who had IGT (75 g) and who were either pregnant or not when the test was undertaken.[402] The study used the WHO criteria for classification and a 75 g OGTT. The study found that 46% (114/244) of non-pregnant women and 23% (17/73) of pregnant women had developed diabetes within the 10 year follow-up period. Using multiple regression analysis the study found that 2 hour plasma glucose, parity and not being pregnant were all statistically significant risk factors in developing diabetes. The authors concluded that IGT outside pregnancy was a stronger predictor of developing diabetes than IGT during pregnancy. This highlights the often transient nature of gestational diabetes. [EL = 2–]

A retrospective case-series (n = 121) from Denmark examined lifestyle changes after pregnancy in women who had been diagnosed with gestational diabetes.[403] The average follow-up period was 24 months. The study found that 19 women had developed diabetes and 22 had IGT. On average the women had gained weight after pregnancy (36 gained weight compared with 18 who lost weight) and they were not exercising as much after pregnancy as before (36 not exercising before pregnancy versus 47 not exercising after pregnancy). However, women had reduced the fat intake in their diets (58 compared with 90 before pregnancy). [EL = 3]

Lifestyle interventions:
An RCT (*n* = 3234) undertaken in the USA of people (women and men) with elevated fasting and post-load plasma glucose concentrations compared placebo plus standard advice (*n* = 1082), metformin plus standard advice (*n* = 1073) and an intensive lifestyle change programme (*n* = 1079) in the prevention of development of type 2 diabetes.[404] The intensive lifestyle change programme involved one-to-one meetings over 24 weeks focusing on changing diet, exercise and behaviour plus group sessions to reinforce behaviour. The groups were comparable at baseline. At 2.8 year follow-up the incidence of diabetes in the placebo group was 11 cases per 100 person-years, whereas for metformin it was 7.8 cases per 100 person-years, and for the lifestyle change programme it was 4.8 cases per 100 person-years. The reduction in incidence between the lifestyle change programme group and metformin group was 39% (95% CI 24 to 51), and for women only (*n* = 2191) the figure was 36% (95% CI 16 to 51). The study shows that intensive lifestyle education reduced the incidence of type 2 diabetes. However, the reduction in development of diabetes for the general population is likely to be greater than those shown in the placebo group because the fact that these people were made aware of the problem is likely to have had some impact. The study involved women and men with an average age of 50.6 years, and it focused on prevention of diabetes rather than management of existing diabetes. The trial was stopped early by the data monitoring committee due to the divergence in the placebo group. Finally no cost data were available to determine the cost-effectiveness of the interventions. [EL = 1+]

An RCT undertaken in Finland (*n* = 522) in people at high risk of developing type 2 diabetes (relatives with type 2 diabetes, BMI more than 25 kg/m², age 40–65 years and IGT) compared the effect of individualised counselling (*n* = 265) with standard information provision (*n* = 257) on the prevention of diabetes, with a mean follow-up of 3.2 years. At 4 year follow-up the cumulative incidence was 11% in the individualised counselling group (95% CI 6% to 15%) and 23% in the standard information group (95% CI 17% to 29%).[405] Cumulative incidence of diabetes in the individualised counselling group was 58% lower than in the standard information group. The study involved women and men with an average age of 55 years with high-risk factors for developing type 2 diabetes, but not specifically women and pregnancy. Therefore, the results may not be applicable to pregnant women. [EL = 1+]

A cross-sectional study[406] examined postpartum patterns of physical activity and related psychosocial factors in women who had been diagnosed with gestational diabetes. The study showed low prevalence of physical activity that was strongly related to social support and self-efficacy. [EL 3]

A systematic review and meta-analysis[407] of 17 RCTs attempted to quantify the effectiveness of pharmacological and lifestyle interventions to prevent or delay type 2 diabetes in people (women and men) with IGT. The study showed that lifestyle and pharmacological interventions reduced the rate of progression to type 2 diabetes. Lifestyle interventions seemed to be at least as effective as pharmacological treatment. No separate analyses for women and men were reported. [EL = 1+]

Follow-up screening:
A retrospective diagnostic study (*n* = 152) from the UK examined whether an FPG test at 6 weeks postpartum could be used to determine which women needed an OGTT.[408] The study compared FPG with OGTT (as the gold standard). A total of 122 women had results available for analysis. Using a cut-off for FPG of 6.0 mmol/litre, the sensitivity was 100% and the specificity was 94% for identifying those who had diabetes compared to OGTT. The study concluded that FPG could be used to determine who should undergo an OGTT. [EL = 2]

A retrospective diagnostic study (*n* = 298) from Singapore examined whether the results of an antenatal OGTT could be used to predict which of those women who had been diagnosed with gestational diabetes would go on to develop diabetes, the aim being to avoid the need for a 6 week follow-up OGTT.[409] The study compared the antenatal OGTT results with the postnatal OGTT results. At a cut-off of 4.5 mmol/litre the sensitivity was 73.9% and specificity was 70.3%. For a 2 hour OGTT the cut-off was 10.5 mmol/litre with a sensitivity of 55.1% and a specificity of 84.7%. The authors concluded that antenatal OGTT results could not be used reliably to predict postnatal OGTT results. [EL = 3]

Type 1 and type 2 diabetes

No clinical studies were identified in relation to the information and follow-up that should be provided for women with type 1 diabetes and type 2 diabetes in the postnatal period.

The CEMACH enquiry described the postnatal care of women with pre-existing type 1 and type 2 diabetes, emphasising the importance of good communication between maternity and diabetes teams and that maternity staff should have good access to expert advice about glycaemic control.[33] It also commented on: the need for a clear written plan for diabetes management in the woman's medical records; offering information and advice about contraception and the importance of planned pregnancy before the woman is discharged from hospital; and offering women a follow-up diabetes appointment after discharge from hospital to discuss ongoing management of diabetes. The enquiry reported that 17% (31/184) of women who had poor pregnancy outcome and 13% (25/188) of women with good pregnancy outcome had no documented plan for postnatal diabetes management and 73% (280/383) had a follow-up diabetes appointment planned. Women who had a poor pregnancy outcome were more likely not to receive contraceptive advice before being discharged from hospital (44%) than those with a good pregnancy outcome (16%; OR 4.2, 95% CI 2.4 to 7.4, adjusted for maternal age and deprivation). Sixty-six percent (133/203) of the women who had a poor pregnancy outcome and 50% (106/211) of the women who had a good pregnancy outcome were classified as having had sub-optimal postnatal diabetes care and advice (OR 1.8, 95% CI 1.2 to 2.7, adjusted for maternal age and deprivation). The enquiry panels expressed concern specifically about the management of glycaemic control, inadequate plans for care after discharge, lack of contact with the diabetes team and lack of contraceptive advice for women with pre-existing type 1 and type 2 diabetes postnatally. [EL = 3–4]

The CEMACH enquiry (comparison of women with type 1 and type 2 diabetes) reported that women with type 1 diabetes were as likely to have a written plan for postnatal diabetes management as women with type 2 diabetes (87% versus 87%, $P = 0.95$) and to receive sub-optimal postnatal diabetes care (53% versus 46%, $P = 0.3$). Women with type 1 diabetes were more likely to have postnatal contraceptive advice compared to women with type 2 diabetes (85% versus 70%, $P = 0.008$).[33] [EL = 3–4]

Existing guidance

The NSF for diabetes[20] recommends that services should be in place for women with pre-existing diabetes and those who have been diagnosed with gestational diabetes.

> 'Pregestational diabetes: Following delivery, all women should be offered the opportunity to be reviewed by the multidisciplinary team and to discuss the future self-management of their diabetes and the implications of breastfeeding. They should all be offered contraceptive advice and should all receive a six-week postpartum check.
>
> Gestational diabetes: Six weeks after delivery, a 75 g oral glucose tolerance test should be undertaken to determine whether the woman:
>
> * still has diabetes; or
> * now has impaired glucose tolerance; or
> * has returned to normal.
>
> Women who are found still to have diabetes should be managed accordingly.
>
> Those who are found still to have impaired glucose regulation and those who have returned to normal should be advised that they have an increased risk of developing:
>
> * gestational diabetes in subsequent pregnancies; and
> * type 2 diabetes later in life, a risk that can be reduced by eating a balanced diet, maintaining a healthy weight and increasing their physical activity levels. They should also be given advice about the symptoms and signs of diabetes.
>
> Those who are found still to have impaired glucose regulation should also be offered a full assessment of their cardiovascular risk and appropriate follow-up.'

The NICE postnatal care guideline[11] recommends that resumption of contraception should be discussed within the first week of birth.

Evidence statement

Evidence shows that women who have been diagnosed with gestational diabetes are likely to have gestational diabetes in future pregnancies. Recurrence rates of gestational diabetes are between 30% and 84%, with recurrence rates in women with a history of insulin-treated gestational diabetes being about 75%.

Results from a systematic review of epidemiological studies and eight additional or subsequent studies show increasing cumulative incidence of type 2 diabetes in the postnatal period in women who have been diagnosed with gestational diabetes. However, the studies are limited by the variation in data recorded, length of follow-up, high attrition rates at follow-up and differing ethnic and cultural populations. The studies highlight various risk factors or identifiers for developing diabetes after having had gestational diabetes, the main ones being obesity, use of insulin during pregnancy, and results of OGTTs during pregnancy.

A systematic review and two RCTs of lifestyle/education interventions showed that the risk of developing type 2 diabetes could be reduced by either lifestyle or pharmacological interventions. However, these studies were undertaken on a general population at risk of developing diabetes rather than women who had been diagnosed with gestational diabetes. In addition, long-term follow-up would be needed to determine the effectiveness of the programmes.

Two diagnostic studies showed that follow-up of women with gestational diabetes was required to accurately identify ongoing disruption of glucose metabolism, suggesting a clinical need for postnatal testing of women who have been diagnosed with gestational diabetes.

No clinical studies that evaluated the information and follow-up that should be provided for women with type 1 diabetes and type 2 diabetes in the postnatal period were identified.

From evidence to recommendations

In the postnatal period, glucose metabolism in women who have been diagnosed with gestational diabetes may return to normal, or there may be ongoing impaired glucose regulation (IGT or impaired fasting glycaemia) or frank diabetes (including pre-existing type 1 or type 2 diabetes that was unrecognised before pregnancy). Women who have been diagnosed with gestational diabetes should, therefore, be offered blood glucose testing before they are discharged from hospital to exclude persisting hyperglycaemia.

Women who have been diagnosed with gestational diabetes are likely to develop type 2 diabetes postnatally and so they should be informed of the symptoms of hyperglycaemia. There is evidence that lifestyle/education interventions are effective for people with IGT to prevent progression to type 2 diabetes and, therefore, women who have been diagnosed with gestational diabetes should be offered lifestyle advice and follow-up to have their blood glucose tested at the 6 week postnatal check and annually thereafter.

There is evidence from a diagnostic study that FPG measurements have high sensitivity and specificity compared with OGTTs (the gold standard). They are also less costly than OGTTs and it is the GDG's view that using OGTTs instead of FPG measurements would not affect outcomes. Women who have been diagnosed with gestational diabetes should, therefore, be offered blood glucose testing using FPG, rather than an OGTT. This represents a change in clinical practice that will bring a cost saving to the NHS.

There is evidence that women who have been diagnosed with gestational diabetes are likely to have gestational diabetes in future pregnancies. In recommending that women who have been diagnosed with gestational diabetes are informed that they are likely to have gestational diabetes in future pregnancies, the GDG is reinforcing the recommendations contained in the NSF for diabetes. There is no clinical evidence to support early self-monitoring of blood glucose (for 1 week) over OGTT in future pregnancies, or *vice versa*, and the costs are probably the same. Women who have had gestational diabetes in a previous pregnancy should, therefore, be offered early self-monitoring of blood glucose or OGTT, and a further OGTT if the results are normal (see Section 4.3).

Given that no clinical studies that evaluated the information and follow-up that should be provided for women with type 1 or type 2 diabetes in the postnatal period were identified, the GDG's recommendation is based on the consensus view of the group. Women with pre-existing type 1 or type 2 diabetes should, therefore, be referred back to their routine follow-up arrangements with the diabetes care team. This care should include consideration of the issues identified in relation to preconception care, including the importance of contraception and planning future pregnancies (see Chapter 3).

The phrase 'women who have been diagnosed with gestational diabetes' is used in the recommendations contained in this section to highlight the fact that the gestational diabetes may have resolved immediately postpartum.

Recommendations for information and follow-up after birth

Women with pre-existing diabetes should be referred back to their routine diabetes care arrangements.

Women who were diagnosed with gestational diabetes should have their blood glucose tested to exclude persisting hyperglycaemia before they are transferred to community care.

Women who were diagnosed with gestational diabetes should be reminded of the symptoms of hyperglycaemia.

Women who were diagnosed with gestational diabetes should be offered lifestyle advice (including weight control, diet and exercise) and offered a fasting plasma glucose measurement (but not an OGTT) at the 6 week postnatal check and annually thereafter.

Women who were diagnosed with gestational diabetes (including those with ongoing impaired glucose regulation) should be informed about the risks of gestational diabetes in future pregnancies and they should be offered screening (OGTT or fasting plasma glucose) for diabetes when planning future pregnancies.

Women who were diagnosed with gestational diabetes (including those with ongoing impaired glucose regulation) should be offered early self-monitoring of blood glucose or an OGTT in future pregnancies. A subsequent OGTT should be offered if the test results in early pregnancy are normal.

Women with diabetes should be reminded of the importance of contraception and the need for preconception care when planning future pregnancies.

Research recommendations for information and follow-up after birth

Are there suitable long-term pharmacological interventions to be recommended postnatally for women who have been diagnosed with gestational diabetes to prevent the onset of type 2 diabetes?

Why this is important
Oral hypoglycaemic agents such rosiglitazone and metformin offer the possibility of pharmacological treatment for prevention of progression to type 2 diabetes in women who have been diagnosed with gestational diabetes. As yet there have been no clinical studies to investigate the effectiveness of oral hypoglycaemic agents in this context. Randomised controlled trials are needed to determine the clinical and cost-effectiveness of such treatments compared to diet and exercise.

Appendix A

Declarations of interest

This appendix includes all interests declared on or before 28 February 2008.

A.1   Guideline development group members

Dominique Acolet

No interests declared

Lynne Carney

Personal non-pecuniary interests: Speaker at Welsh CEMACH conference

Non-current interests – planned: Teacher on specialist antenatal course for women with diabetes

Anne Dornhorst

Personal pecuniary interests – specific: Consultancy for GlaxoSmithKline, Novo Nordisk and Takeda; UK principal investigator for PREDICTIVE post-marketing surveillance study for treatment of type 1 and type 2 diabetes using insulin detemir and insulin aspart funded by Novo Nordisk; conference expenses and/or lecture fees from Aventis, GlaxoSmithKline, Merck Sharp & Dohme Limited, Novo Nordisk and Servier

Personal non-pecuniary interests: Officer of the Royal College of Physicians; Member of the Working Lives intercollegiate committee

Non-personal pecuniary interests – specific: Hospital department receives funding from Novo Nordisk in connection with the PREDICTIVE study and insulin detemir in pregnancy study

Robert Fraser

No interests declared

Roger Gadsby

Personal pecuniary interests – specific: Adviser to Bristol-Myers Squibb, Colgate-Palmolive, Merck Pharma, Merck Sharp & Dohme Limited, Novo Nordisk, Osaki, Pfizer, Sanofi Aventis and Takeda

Personal non-pecuniary interests: Medical adviser to Warwick Diabetes Care, University of Warwick; Chairman of Trustees of Pregnancy Sickness Support, Nuneaton, Warwickshire; Honorary Treasurer of the Primary Care Diabetes Society

Non-personal pecuniary interests – specific: Warwick Diabetes Care receives sponsorship for educational programmes from the British In Vitro Diagnostics Association (BIVDA), Eli Lilly, GlaxoSmithKline, Lifescan, Novo Nordisk, Pfizer, Sanofi Aventis and Servier; the Primary Care Diabetes Society receives sponsorship for educational programmes from Eli Lilly, GlaxoSmithKline, Merck Pharma, Novo Nordisk, Roche Diagnostics, Sanofi Aventis, Servier and Takeda

Non-current interests – previous: Consultancy, conference expenses and/or lecture fees from Bristol-Myers Squibb, GlaxoSmithKline, Merck, Novartis, Novo Nordisk, Roche, Roche Diagnostics, Sanofi Aventis, Servier and Takeda; Warwick Diabetes Care received start-up sponsorship from Aventis, Bristol-Myers Squibb, Eli Lilly, GlaxoSmithKline, Lifescan, Novo Nordisk, Owen Mumford, Pfizer and Takeda

Jane Hawdon

Personal non-pecuniary interests: Chair of neonatal working group for the CEMACH Diabetes in Pregnancy Enquiry; adviser and speaker for Baby Friendly Initiative, BLISS and CEMACH

Richard Holt

Personal pecuniary interests – specific: Investigator for insulin aspart and insulin detemir in pregnancy studies funded by Novo Nordisk; conference expenses and/or lecture fees from Eli Lilly and GlaxoSmithKline

Personal pecuniary interests – non-specific: Consultancy, lecture fees and educational grants from Astra-Zeneca, Eli Lilly, GlaxoSmithKline, Merck Sharp & Dohme Limited, Novo Nordisk, Roche and Takeda

Non-personal pecuniary interests – specific: Investigator for Softsense blood glucose meter in pregnancy study funded by Abbott Laboratories and insulin aspart and insulin detemir in pregnancy studies funded by Novo Nordisk; research funding from GlaxoSmithKline to examine the role of insulin resistance in gestational diabetes

Personal non-pecuniary interests: Chair of the Professional Advisory Council of Diabetes UK

Ann Parker

No interests declared

Nickey Tomkins

No interests declared

Stephen Walkinshaw

No interests declared

Jackie Webb

Personal pecuniary interests – specific: Conference/meeting expenses and/or lecture fees from Abbot Diabetes Care, Bayer, Becton and Dickenson, Eli Lilly, GlaxoSmithKline, Lifescan, Menarini, Novartis, Novo Nordisk, Roche Diagnostics, Sanofi Aventis and the Centre for Pharmacy Postgraduate Education, University of Manchester; funded by Novo Nordisk to work on an out-of-hours helpline and to attend related update meetings

Personal non-pecuniary interests: Member of Diabetes UK and Royal College of Nursing; participation in CEMACH meetings; attended a meeting of the Management of Diabetes for Excellence (MODEL) group

Non-personal pecuniary interests – specific: Adviser on patient education literature for Eli Lilly; adviser on GlucoGel for British BioCell; Department Trust fund receives funding to support attendance at conferences, courses, study days, meetings and patient-support events and meetings from Abbot Diabetes Care, Bayer, Becton and Dickenson, Diabetes UK, Eli Lilly, GlaxoSmithKline, Lifescan, Menarini, Novo Nordisk, Roche Diagnostics and Sanofi Aventis; insulin detemir study funded by Novo Nordisk

Saiyyidah Zaidi

No interests declared

A.2 NCC-WCH staff and contractors

Paula Broughton-Palmer
No interests declared

Michael Corkett
No interests declared

Anthony Danso-Appiah
No interests declared

Paul Jacklin
Non-current interests – planned: Commissioned by Continence-UK to write an article on the health economics of continence care

Lorelei Jones
No interests declared

Moira Mugglestone
No interests declared

Jeffrey Round
No interests declared

Anuradha Sekhri
No interests declared

A.3 External advisers

Anita Holdcroft
Personal pecuniary interests – non-specific: Consultancy for special opioid advisory group, Napp pharmaceuticals

Non-personal pecuniary interests – non-specific: Research funding from Cephalon; sponsorship from various pharmaceutical companies for organising meetings of the Royal Society of Medicine's Section of Anaesthesia

Jo Modder
No interests declared

Peter Scanlon
No interests declared

Roy Taylor
Personal pecuniary interests – non-specific: Adviser to Eli Lilly (protein kinase C (PKC) inhibitor), Merck Sharp & Dohme Limited (cardiovascular preparations), Novartis (dipeptidyl peptidase 4 (DPP-4) inhibitor); conference expenses from Eli Lilly and Merck Sharp & Dohme Limited

Non-personal pecuniary interests – non-specific: Funding from Servier to support production of educational tools (book and website) on retinal screening in diabetes

Appendix B

Clinical questions

Preconception care

1. What information should be offered in relation to outcomes and risks for the mother and the baby?
2. What information should be offered in relation to the importance of planning a pregnancy and the role of contraception?
3. What information should be offered in relation to diet, dietary supplements, body weight and exercise?
4. What are the target ranges for blood glucose in the preconception period?
5. How should blood glucose and ketones be monitored in the preconception period?
6. How cost-effective are self-management programmes for women with diabetes who are planning a pregnancy?
7. Which medications for diabetes are suitable for use during pregnancy and which should be discontinued?
8. Which medications for diabetic complications are suitable for use during pregnancy and which should be discontinued?
9. What are the barriers to uptake of preconception care?
10. When should information be offered to: (i) women of reproductive age with diabetes; and (ii) women with diabetes who are planning a pregnancy?

Gestational diabetes

11. Which women are at high risk of gestational diabetes?
12. How should gestational diabetes be diagnosed?
13. Does diagnosis, monitoring and intervention for gestational diabetes improve outcomes in mothers and babies?
14. What is cost-effective treatment for gestational diabetes?

Antenatal care

15. What are the target ranges for blood glucose during pregnancy?
16. How should blood glucose and ketones be monitored during pregnancy?
17. What special considerations apply to the management of diabetes during pregnancy?
18. When and how often should women be offered retinal assessment?
19. When and by what method should women be offered renal assessment?
20. When and by what method should women be offered screening for congenital malformations and counselling?
21. When and by what methods should fetal growth and wellbeing be monitored?
22. What timetable of antenatal appointments should be offered to women with diabetes?
23. What special considerations in relation to spontaneous or planned preterm birth are appropriate for women with diabetes?

Intrapartum care

24. Does intervening in the timing and mode of birth improve outcomes for women with diabetes and their babies?
25. Does intervening have any implications for future pregnancies and births?
26. What special considerations in relation to analgesia and anaesthesia are appropriate for women with diabetes?
27. How should glycaemic control be monitored and maintained during labour and birth?

Neonatal care

28. What are the criteria for admission to intensive/special care?
29. How should neonatal hypoglycaemia be prevented and treated?
30. What initial assessment should babies undergo?

Postnatal period

31. How does breastfeeding affect glycaemic control?
32. What information and follow-up should be offered to women with gestational diabetes after birth?
33. What information and follow-up should be offered to women with type 1 and type 2 diabetes after birth?

Appendix C

Cost-effectiveness of self-management programmes for women with diabetes who are planning a pregnancy

C.1   Introduction

A review of the health economics literature identified a single study from the USA addressing the cost-effectiveness of preconception care and advice for women with pre-existing diabetes.[410] Although not explicitly described as such, the study used a decision-analytic approach to determine whether, as a result of averted complications, the additional costs of preconception care and advice yielded net savings compared with no preconception care and advice. The study reported that a mixture of literature review, expert opinion and surveys of medical care were used to estimate the costs and clinical consequences of preconception care and advice compared with 'doing nothing'. Doing nothing in this case meant no preconception care and advice, although antenatal care would, of course, be provided in the event of a pregnancy. The study concluded that preconception care and advice would yield cost savings, with each $1 spent on preconception care and advice realising a saving of $1.86 as a result of fewer births, lower antenatal care costs arising from better glycaemic control, and fewer adverse maternal and neonatal outcomes. The authors reported a number of sensitivity analyses, none of which fundamentally altered the results. Furthermore, the study reported that conservative estimates had been used when there was uncertainty with regard to parameter values and that their assumptions were, therefore, generally biased against preconception care and advice. However, the study also noted that the assumption of full adherence to the preconception care and advice programme may have been a limitation of the analysis.

The study is quite dated and therefore the usual caveats about the generalisability of costs from one healthcare setting to another are even more important than normal. Furthermore, changes to parameter values undertaken as part of the sensitivity analysis may not have been quite as conservative as suggested by the authors of the study. Finally, additional clinical studies and a meta-analysis which included more recent data[121] have been published since the cost-effectiveness study. Therefore, a *de novo* health economic model was developed for this guideline.

An economic evaluation has suggested that structured education programmes for people with pre-existing diabetes are cost-effective in the UK setting.[411] This is consistent with existing NICE guidance on self-management of diabetes.[18] Examples of structured education programmes available in the UK are DAFNE[69] for people with type 1 diabetes and DESMOND and X-PERT for people with type 2 diabetes. The evidence suggests that such programmes lead to improved glycaemic control. For women with diabetes who are planning a pregnancy and those who are already pregnant, good glycaemic control has benefits over and above those associated with good glycaemic control outside pregnancy because of the adverse maternal and neonatal outcomes associated with poor glycaemic control in the periconceptional period and pregnancy (see Sections 3.4 and 5.1).

Improvement in glycaemic control is also an important putative benefit of preconception care and advice. However, it is unlikely that studies of preconception care and advice have disentangled whether there are any additional improvements in relation to glycaemic control over and above those which would be achieved with a structured education programme alone. To the extent that there is further improvement in glycaemic control with preconception care and advice, it cannot be assumed that the effect size would be the same as preconception care and advice in the absence of a structured education programme. Indeed, it seems likely that there would be diminishing returns, with further improvement possible, but at a lower rate.

However, there are other benefits of preconception care and advice which are specific to diabetes in pregnancy which by themselves may make its provision clinically effective and possibly cost-effective. For example, advice on preconception folic acid is particularly important given the elevated risk of neural tube defects in babies of women with diabetes (see Sections 3.3 and 5.6). Furthermore, advice on contraception may also improve outcomes by increasing the number of pregnancies in women with diabetes that are associated with good glycaemic control.

A decision tree was developed for the guideline in Microsoft Excel® and also, for validation purposes, in TreeAge Pro 2006® (see Figure C.1).

As shown in the decision tree, it is assumed that a proportion of women are infertile and therefore do not benefit from preconception care and advice even if they accept an offer of such advice and adhere to it. It is assumed that women who are offered and adhere to preconception care and advice have a lower major congenital malformation rate than pregnant women in the no preconception care and advice arm. It is additionally assumed that those women in the preconception care and advice arm who either decline preconception care and advice or do not adhere to advice will have a congenital malformation rate equivalent to women with diabetes in the no preconception care and advice arm. The effectiveness of preconception care and advice is measured in terms of the number of major congenital malformations averted. In addition to the costs of the advice itself, the model also takes into account 'downstream savings' from averted congenital malformations. Considerable uncertainty surrounds the inputs of this model (see below for details) and therefore the results and sensitivity analysis are both undertaken to address the 'what if' in terms of thresholds for cost-effectiveness.

C.2   Model parameters

The parameter values used in the baseline model are shown in Tables C.1, C.2 and C.3. The model assumes that there are administration costs in just offering a preconception care and advice

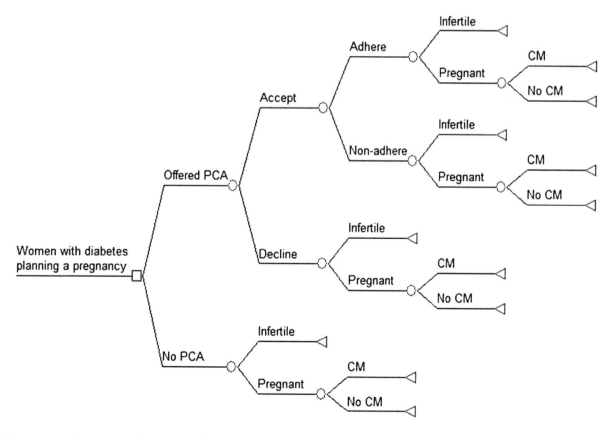

Figure C.1   Preconception care and advice (PCA) versus no preconception care and advice decision tree showing major congenital malformation (CM) rates resulting from pregnancies in women with diabetes

service to women with diabetes who are planning a pregnancy and therefore this is included as a cost parameter. However, it is assumed that this cost can be limited to the population of concern (women with diabetes who are planning a pregnancy). It does not assume that the offer is made to all women with diabetes who are of childbearing age regardless of whether they are actively planning a pregnancy. However, this could be addressed in sensitivity analysis by assuming higher offer costs. The published cost-effectiveness study described above[410] suggested that preconception care and advice would result in lower antenatal costs due to improved glycaemic control during pregnancy. The model structure allows this consideration to be factored in, but at baseline it conservatively assumes that preconception care and advice does not yield any cost saving in this respect compared with the no preconception care and advice alternative. In a similar conservative vein, no QALY gain is attached to averted major congenital malformations at baseline although the results are presented to show a minimum number of QALYs per congenital malformation averted that would be needed for cost-effectiveness given a particular incremental cost of preconception care and advice.

Table C.1   Costs (using 2006 prices)

Resource item	Value	Source	Notes
Offer preconception care and advice	£10	GDG estimate	Administration cost in offering a preconception care and advice service
Preconception care and advice	£615	NICE Technology Appraisal 60, Diabetes (types 1 and 2) – patient education models (2003)[18]	2003 cost of £545 but updated for inflation using the Hospital and Community Health Services (HCHS)[a] Index
Additional costs of antenatal care with poor glycaemic control	£0		At baseline it is conservatively assumed that preconception care and advice does not result in lower antenatal costs
Cost of a major congenital malformation[b]	£81,000	Elixhauser et al. (1993)[410]	Weighted cost of major congenital malformations using an exchange rate of £1 to $2 and the HCHS index to update for inflation[c]

[a]   A price inflation index based on changes to the price of goods and services supplied to the healthcare sector.

[b]   Anencephaly, spina bifida, hydrocephalus, transposition of the great arteries, tetralogy of Fallot, coarctation of aorta, renal agenesis, anal/rectal atresia, caudal regression.

[c]   Clearly there are limitations using these dated US data. As far as we are aware, equivalent UK costings do not exist. The costing of such a wide range of congenital malformations is methodologically complex and time consuming. Therefore, with the resources available for this guideline it was not possible to generate our own cost estimates based on UK NHS data. The known limitations of these data are addressed by sensitivity analysis.

Table C.2   Probabilities

Variable	Value	Source
Decline preconception care and advice	0.5	GDG estimate
Adhere to preconception care and advice	0.8	GDG estimate
Fertile	0.9	Elixhauser et al. (1993)[410]
Major congenital malformation rate (preconception care and advice)	0.021	Ray et al. (2001)[121]
Major congenital malformation rate (no preconception care and advice)	0.065	Ray et al. (2001)[121]

Table C.3   Quality-adjusted life years

Resource item	Value	Source	Notes
Willingness to pay for a QALY	£20,000	NICE guidelines manual (2007)[23]	
QALY gain from averted major congenital malformation	0		A conservative baseline assumption

C.3   Results

The baseline results suggest that preconception care and advice is cost-effective (see Table C.4). In a population of 1000 women with diabetes who are planning pregnancy, the model shows a cost saving of almost £1 million and 16 averted major congenital malformations. There is no necessity to estimate a QALY gain to establish cost-effectiveness as preconception care and advice dominates, being cheaper and more effective than no preconception care and advice.

Table C.4   Baseline results in a population of 1000 women with diabetes who are planning pregnancy

Item	Value
Net costs of preconception care and advice	−£965,540
Major congenital malformations averted	15.84
QALY gain needed per major congenital malformation averted	N/A
Incremental cost-effectiveness ratio (ICER)	Preconception care and advice dominates

C.4   Sensitivity analysis

Considerable uncertainty surrounds the data inputs of the model and therefore sensitivity analysis was used to assess how robust the baseline conclusions would be given different assumptions. This sensitivity analysis was primarily undertaken on a one-way basis, where one parameter value was varied while holding all other parameter values constant. This gives an indication as to whether uncertainty surrounding the exact value of the parameter is likely to have an important bearing on the model's conclusions. Additionally, thresholds for cost-effectiveness were calculated for scenarios where sensitivity analysis indicated that preconception care and advice may not be the dominant strategy. This involved calculating the QALY gain which would be needed to satisfy a cost-effectiveness threshold of £20,000 per QALY where preconception care and advice involved incremental costs relative to no preconception care and advice.

There are potentially many different models of preconception care and advice. At one end of the spectrum there could be a group session with a diabetes specialist nurse, but a more resource-intensive model might involve a one-to-one consultation with a multidisciplinary team. Figure C.2 shows the effect of varying the cost of preconception care and advice between £50

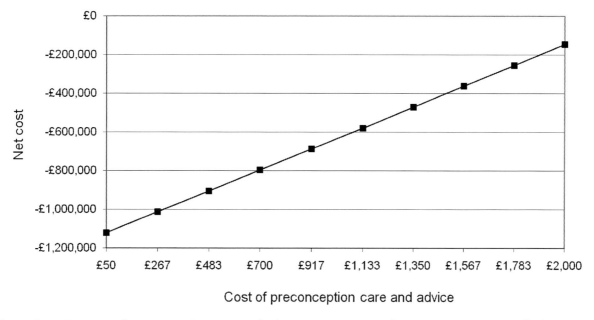

Figure C.2   Net cost of preconception care and advice, varying costs of preconception care and advice

and £2,000. The results suggest that preconception care and advice would be cost saving and hence dominant even at a cost of £2,000 per woman.

Another important source of uncertainty concerns the cost of a major congenital malformation. The baseline estimate was derived from a study conducted in the healthcare setting in the USA. There are a number of reasons why this may not accurately reflect costs to the NHS:

- the healthcare system in the USA differs markedly from that in the UK
- even in the context of the USA, the figures are presented as fairly 'broad brush' estimates
- the original study is quite dated and treatments may have changed.

Figure C.3 shows the impact of varying the cost of a major congenital malformation between £5,000 and £200,000 as part of a one-way sensitivity analysis. This shows that preconception care and advice would be cost saving as long as a major congenital malformation cost more than £20,044. If a major congenital malformation cost £5,000, then a QALY gain of 0.75 per major congenital malformation averted would be required for cost-effectiveness. Given the usually large impact of a major congenital malformation on lifetime health, it can be reasonably assumed that the QALY gain would be sufficient for cost-effectiveness in such a scenario.

The effect of varying the assumption about the effectiveness of preconception care and advice is shown in Figure C.4. The clinical effectiveness of the intervention is given by the absolute difference in the major congenital malformation rate between preconception care and advice and the no preconception care and advice alternative. Figure C.4 shows the situation where the major congenital malformation rate for no preconception care and advice is held constant at 0.065 whilst the major congenital malformation rate for preconception care and advice is varied between the baseline 0.021 (absolute difference 0.044) and 0.064 (absolute difference 0.001). Preconception care and advice is dominant as long as the major congenital malformation rate with preconception care and advice is no more than 0.054 (absolute difference of at least 0.011), which is considerably less than that estimated by a recent meta-analysis.[121] As long as the absolute difference is at least 0.005 then it seems likely that preconception care and advice will be cost-effective. If the absolute difference is less than 0.005 then at least five more QALYs would be needed per averted major congenital malformation and it cannot necessarily be assumed *a priori* that this would be the case.

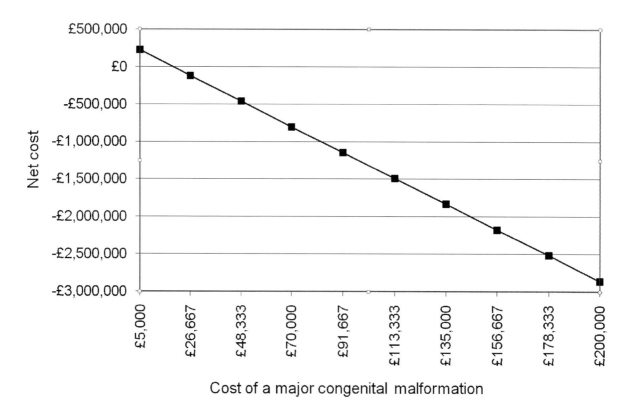

Figure C.3 Net cost of preconception care and advice, varying costs of a major congenital malformation

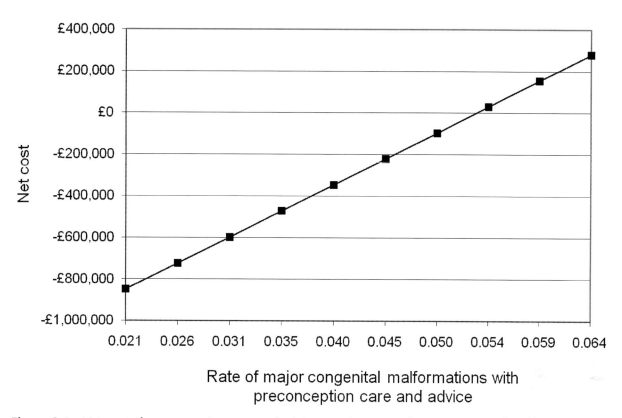

Figure C.4   Net cost of preconception care and advice, varying rates of major congenital malformations with preconception care and advice

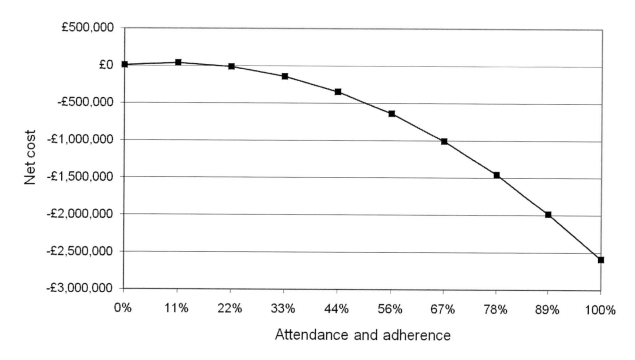

Figure C.5   Net cost of preconception care and advice, varying rates of attendance and adherence with preconception care and advice

Finally, the impact of changing the assumptions about attendance and adherence was assessed by comparing the worst-case scenario (no attendance with zero adherence) with the best-case scenario (full attendance and adherence with the programme). Figure C.5 shows the impact of increasing attendance and adherence in equal proportions between the worst-case and best-case scenarios. Initially, as attendance and adherence increase the net cost of preconception care and advice increases slightly. This is because the costs of providing preconception care and advice are not fully offset by reduced costs of congenital malformations at low adherence rates. However, when attendance and adherence reach a level of 21%, then preconception care and advice is dominant, producing a net cost saving in addition to the reduction in major congenital malformations.

C.5   Discussion

The baseline effectiveness of preconception care and advice in terms of major congenital malformations averted was based on results presented in a recent meta-analysis.[121] The results of the meta-analysis need to be treated with a degree of caution because of the heterogeneous nature of the individual studies included and because of systematic differences reported between women with diabetes who attended preconception care and advice and those who did not. For example, smokers were more prevalent in the no preconception care and advice group (30.2% versus 19.6%) and confounding could plausibly be responsible for at least some of the observed effect. It has been suggested that the availability of a preconception clinic separates women with diabetes into two groups, one containing highly motivated women with well-controlled diabetes who attend and have a low rate of congenital abnormalities and the other containing women who, for various reasons, book late, have worse glycaemic control, and have a congenital abnormality rate of 7.5–10.9%.[412] Furthermore, the effectiveness of preconception care and advice may be diluted when it is offered additionally to structured education programmes rather than as a stand-alone intervention. If a woman's glycaemic control has improved as a result of structured education then the scope for preconception care and advice to achieve further improvement may be limited.

The threshold sensitivity analysis undertaken using the model suggests that only a relatively small reduction in the major congenital malformation rate (as little as 0.005) is necessary for preconception care and advice to be considered cost-effective. This threshold for cost-effectiveness is much less than the absolute difference of 0.044 suggested in the published meta-analysis, and also less than 0.13 (the absolute difference between the upper 95% confidence limit reported in the meta-analysis for the major congenital malformation rate with preconception care and advice (worst case) and the lower 95% confidence limit for the major congenital malformation rate with no preconception care and advice (best case).[121] Preconception care and advice of some sort does, therefore, seem to be justified on economic grounds. The published meta-analysis suggested that the preconception care and advice interventions included were heterogeneous and this raises important questions from an economic perspective in terms of what is the 'best' or most cost-effective form of preconception care and advice. This is particularly important as there is likely to be considerable variation in cost between different models of preconception care and advice and it is important to know what incremental benefits are achieved by more resource-intensive forms of the intervention. If less resource-intensive preconception care and advice is almost as effective then the incremental cost-effectiveness ratio for some preconception care and advice interventions is likely to be unacceptably high.

Appendix D

Cost-effectiveness of screening, diagnosis and treatment for gestational diabetes

D.1 Systematic review of screening

A systematic search of the literature identified 337 studies potentially related to the clinical question. After reviewing the abstracts, 33 articles were retrieved for further appraisal and eight have been included in this section of the review. Six papers were identified that examined the cost-effectiveness of screening for gestational diabetes. Two additional papers were identified that considered the cost-effectiveness of screening for and treatment of gestational diabetes.

D.1.1 Screening and treatment of gestational diabetes

A study conducted in France[441] examined three strategies for screening for gestational diabetes using a decision analysis model. Under strategy one, women deemed to be at higher risk of gestational diabetes based on a series of risk factors (family history of diabetes in a first-degree relative, age over 35 years, BMI greater than 27 kg/m², previous history of gestational diabetes, pre-eclampsia, fetal death after 3 months of gestation or previous macrosomia) were given a non-fasting 50 g OGTT. In strategy two all women were given the 50 g OGTT and in strategy three all women were given a 75 g OGTT. Data on costs were collected through a prospective study of 120 pregnancies and clinical data were taken from a review of published literature. Incremental analysis was reported in terms of cost per additional case prevented of macrosomia, prematurity, perinatal mortality or hypertensive disorder. All strategies were compared with a baseline of no screening for each outcome. The authors recommend strategy one, screening the population of high-risk pregnant women using the 50 g OGTT, based on its favourable ICER for preventing perinatal mortality (€7870*, compared with €8660 and €29,400 for strategies two and three, respectively).

A retrospective study conducted in Italy[442] examined the costs and outcomes for two groups of women. The first group had universal screening using a 50 g GCT while the second were screened based on the presence of given risk factors (history of gestational diabetes, previous macrosomia, family history of diabetes mellitus, age over 30 years and body mass). All women that tested positive in either screening group underwent a 100 g OGTT. Universal screening was found to be more costly than the selective screening approach per case of gestational diabetes diagnosed (€424 and €406, respectively) and that treatment cost €366. No incremental analysis was reported. The authors concluded that, based on the savings from downstream interventions associated with untreated gestational diabetes, such as caesarean section, screening in some form was justified.

D.1.2 Screening for gestational diabetes

A cost–utility analysis[443] examined four screening strategies for gestational diabetes. The strategies were no screening, a 75 g OGTT, a 100 g OGTT and a sequential test (50 g GCT followed by a 100 g OGTT). The authors concluded that the sequential testing strategy was cost-effective, although in a high-prevalence population the 100 g OGTT may be an alternative cost-effective screening strategy. The study was conducted from a societal perspective, which could limit its applicability for decision making in an NHS setting, as this may overestimate costs. References were given for clinical and cost parameters but no specific details of these were reported. No detail was provided on what components comprised the total cost of each strategy and no unit

---

* Exchange rate of £1 = €1.31, from markets.ft.com/ft/markets/currencies.asp on 28 February 2008.

costs were reported. Incremental analysis was undertaken and outcomes reported in quality-adjusted life years (QALYs), with maternal and infant outcomes reported separately. Sources for utility estimates were not provided. Given these drawbacks, the results of this study cannot be generalised to an NHS setting.

One study from the UK[124] examined the cost per case of gestational diabetes detected. Six screening strategies were considered: universal fasting plasma glucose (FPG), universal GCT with 7.8 mmol/litre cut-off, universal GCT with 8.2 mmol/litre cut-off, GCT with 8.2 mmol/litre cut-off in women aged over 25 years, GCT with 8.2 mmol/litre cut-off in women aged over 25 years and risk factors, and universal OGTT. The authors recommended the use of a universal FPG or giving a GCT to those over age 25 years and with risk factors. The FPG detected an additional 6009 cases at a cost of £489 per additional case detected when compared with GCT. A strategy of universal OGTT was predicted to detect an additional 1493 cases compared with the universal FPG, at a cost per additional case detected of £4,665.

Four studies reported in US dollars estimated the cost per case detected of gestational diabetes.[444–447] One study[444] examined the cost per case diagnosed of six different strategies. Incremental analysis was not reported. The authors recommended screening women aged over 25 years using a 50 g 1 hour glucose screening test. In a second study[445] the authors examined the cost per case diagnosed using different thresholds for the diagnosis of gestational diabetes in a high-risk population. The cost per case of gestational diabetes identified by a 50 g oral glucose screening test was $114* at a cut-off of 7.2 mmol/litre and $106 at a cut-off of 8.3 mmol/litre. The authors made no conclusion on the cost-effectiveness of either approach. A third study[446] examined the cost per case diagnosed of gestational diabetes in two groups of women. Group 1 had historical or clinical risk factors for gestational diabetes and Group 2 were offered routine screening. Screening was with a 50 g GCT followed by a OGTT for women with greater than 150 mg/100 ml. The number of cases of gestational diabetes diagnosed did not differ between groups. The cost per case diagnosed of the testing programme was $329. A fourth study[447] was conducted in Iran and reported in US dollars. Women were stratified into high-, intermediate- and low-risk groups based on American Diabetes Association (ADA) criteria. The authors recommended universal screening in a high-prevalence population such as theirs, with a cost per case diagnosed of $80.56. No incremental analysis was reported.

D.2   Introduction to the model

The recently published ACHOIS trial demonstrated potential benefit of treatment for mild gestational diabetes.[153] However, while clinical effectiveness is a necessary condition for cost-effectiveness it is not sufficient. Resources have competing uses and showing that resources yield a benefit does not demonstrate that an even greater benefit could not be produced if those resources were deployed in an alternative use. Furthermore, treatment requires identification of those affected by gestational diabetes using some screening/diagnostic strategy which further reduces scarce resources available to other NHS patients. Therefore, the cost-effectiveness of treatment will partly be determined by the ability to identify patients for treatment via screening in a cost-effective fashion. Similarly, the cost-effectiveness of screening is predicated on an efficacious treatment which gives an acceptable cost per effect given the finite resources available.

Therefore, the cost-effectiveness of screening, diagnosis and treatment for gestational diabetes are highly interdependent. As a result, a single cost-effectiveness model addressing screening, diagnosis and treatment for gestational diabetes was developed jointly by the diabetes in pregnancy and antenatal care GDGs to enable them to make recommendations on this area of care for pregnant women.

However, in addition to this single model incorporating both screening and treatment, a separate cost-minimisation analysis of the various treatment options is also presented. This better illustrates the cost-effectiveness of different treatment alternatives, under the assumption of equivalent effectiveness, where the decision to screen for cases and treat has been accepted on economic grounds.

---

* Exchange rate of £1 = $1.98, from markets.ft.com/ft/markets/currencies.asp on 28 February 28.

D.2.1 The decision tree

The model utilises a decision-analytic approach. In this approach, competing alternatives represent the decisions. Then, by considering the probabilities of different scenarios under each decision, drawing on best available evidence, the expected costs and effects of each decision can be computed and compared.

At its most basic, this cost-effectiveness model can be represented as the decision to screen and treat patients identified with gestational diabetes versus no screening, which was the recommendation of the previous antenatal care guideline (Figure D.1).

Data from the ACHOIS intervention group were used to estimate the outcomes and associated costs of treating true positives. As ACHOIS was limited to those with 'mild' gestational diabetes, the costs and effects may be an underestimate of the true costs and effects in the population under consideration. The outcomes and associated costs of false negatives were estimated from the routine care group in ACHOIS. It is also necessary to consider the cost of providing treatment to women falsely diagnosed with gestational diabetes (false positives). The outcomes for women without gestational diabetes (true negatives and false positives) in the screening arms were not considered as the perinatal outcomes for these pregnancies do not differ from those in the population of otherwise healthy pregnant women.

In Figure D.1 the decision, for diagrammatic simplicity, is depicted as screen versus no screen. However, given an initial decision to screen there is then the decision of how to screen. The various screening options that have been considered in this model are described in the next section.

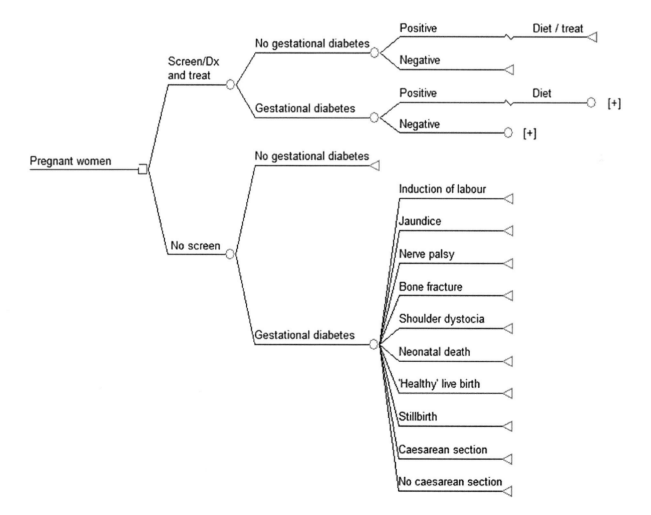

Figure D.1   The basic decision tree structure; [+] denotes that the tree is truncated – see Figure D.3 for the treatment sub-tree; the sub-tree for those with gestational diabetes who are undetected on screening is the same as the sub-tree for women with gestational diabetes who are not screened; Dx = diagnose

The key outputs of each screening strategy are the costs of screening and treating women and the number of women accurately diagnosed with gestational diabetes. There are four possible outcomes when applying a diagnostic test:

- true positive – the patient is diagnosed as positive and has the condition/disease
- false positive – the patient is diagnosed as positive but does not have the condition/disease
- true negative – the patient is not diagnosed with the condition/disease and does not have it
- false negative – the patient is not diagnosed with the condition/disease but does in fact have it.

The number of individuals diagnosed correctly is determined by the accuracy of the diagnostic test applied (sensitivity and specificity) and by the prevalence of the condition in the population being tested. The treatment and outcome sub-trees are identical for each screening strategy in this model but the costs and effects will vary according to the numbers diagnosed as having gestational diabetes or not.

D.3 Screening strategies

Table D.1 contains a list of the various strategies that have been considered as screening strategies for gestational diabetes. All screening methods, including risk factor screening, screening blood tests and universal diagnostic tests, have been considered in isolation. Combinations of these tests have then been considered.

Not all possible strategies have been considered – particularly where they are clinically inappropriate, for example treating patients based on the presence of a risk factor alone. Some strategies have been excluded from further analysis after preliminary analysis showed them to be dominated by alternative strategies. Limitations in the data are discussed in greater detail later in this appendix.

Risk factors that have been considered:

- age ≥ 30 years
- age ≥ 25 years
- high-risk ethnic background (ethnicity; see Table D.5)
- BMI ≥ 27 kg/m² (high BMI)
- family history of diabetes.

Screening blood tests considered:

- FPG
- random blood glucose (RBG)
- 1 hour 50 g GCT.

Diagnostic blood test considered:

- 2 hour 75 g OGTT.

D.3.1 Screening strategy assumptions

Decision analysis is used to help us make decisions about the best treatment or intervention to use, based on grounds of cost and clinical effectiveness. When developing a decision analysis model it is necessary to make simplifying assumptions to highlight what the important elements of the model might be and to reduce the complexity of the model. It is not possible to consider every possible potential outcome in a model and it is important to focus on those with the greatest relevance in answering the question at hand. The assumptions used in the model of screening strategies are given below:

- A 2 hour 75 g OGTT is used as the gold standard diagnostic test (refer to Section 4.2 for details) and is assumed to be 100% sensitive and specific.
- It has not been possible to establish an accurate fertility rate in some population subgroups. It is therefore assumed that the fertility rate among women with a high BMI is the same as the rate among women with a BMI in the normal range. This may overestimate the number of pregnancies in this group, as high BMI is associated with fertility problems.[448]

- The available data on BMI are not consistent. Population level data on BMI from the Office of National Statistics or the Health Survey for England is presented as overweight and obese with a BMI greater than or equal to 25 kg/m², whereas the data presented in the literature[129] used a BMI greater than or equal to 27 kg/m² to define some at risk of gestational diabetes based on BMI. It was assumed initially that the risk of those with a BMI greater than 25 kg/m² is equal to that of those with a BMI greater than 27 kg/m², though this assumption could be relaxed in sensitivity analysis. If there is a genuine difference in the subpopulation (BMI 25–27 kg/m²), this assumption may overestimate the number of cases of gestational diabetes in the at-risk population and lead to a greater number of false positive diagnoses of gestational diabetes.

D.3.2 Screening strategy input parameters

The parameters used to populate the model have been chosen based on the best available evidence, and those relating to screening are listed in Tables D.2 to D.5.

After some initial modelling, the GDG expressed concern that test acceptability might be an additional important consideration. Some women may find the tests inconvenient and unpleasant, especially where they are required to fast for a period beforehand. Table D.6 lists the input parameters relating to test acceptability.

The model assumes that women are more likely to accept a test if they have already been identified as being at higher risk, either by risk factor or a previous screening test. The baseline values reflected the views of the GDG, but clearly considerable uncertainty surrounds the actual test acceptance, and thus sensitivity analysis was undertaken to determine to what extent test acceptance determines the cost-effectiveness conclusions of the model.

Table D.1 List of screening strategies

Strategy number	Risk factor	Screening blood test	Screening diagnostic test
1	–	–	OGTT
2	ADA criteria[a]	FPG	OGTT
3	ADA criteria	RBG	OGTT
4	ADA criteria	GCT	OGTT
5	ADA criteria	FPG	–
6	ADA criteria	–	OGTT
7	ADA criteria	GCT	–
8	–	FPG	–
9	–	RBG	–
10	–	GCT	–
11	–	FPG	OGTT
12	–	GCT	OGTT
13	Age ≥ 30 years	FPG	OGTT
14	Age ≥ 30 years	GCT	OGTT
15	Age ≥ 25 years	FPG	OGTT
16	Age ≥ 25 years	GCT	OGTT
17	Age ≥ 30 years	–	OGTT
18	Age ≥ 25 years	–	OGTT
19	High-risk ethnicity	FPG	OGTT
20	High-risk ethnicity	GCT	OGTT
21	High-risk ethnicity	–	OGTT

[a] Having one or more of the following risk factors: age > 25 years; BMI> 27 kg/m²; family history of diabetes; high-risk ethnic group.

Table D.2 Accuracy of screening and diagnostic blood tests

Test	Sensitivity	Specificity	Source
FPG	0.88	0.78	Reichelt et al. (1998)[449]
RBG	0.48	0.97	Ostlund and Hanson (2004)[450]
1 hour 50 g GCT	0.80	0.43	Seshiah et al. (2004)[451]
2 hour 75 g OGTT	1.0	1.0	Gold standard

Table D.3 Cost of screening and diagnostic blood tests

Variable	Cost	Source
Risk factor screening	£2	GDG estimate
FPG	£5.39	Updated from Scott et al. (2002)[124]
RBG	£5.39	Updated from Scott et al. (2002)[124]
1 hour 50 g GCT	£10.61	Updated from Scott et al. (2002)[124]
2 hour 75 g OGTT	£28.58	Updated from Scott et al. (2002)[124]

Table D.4 Risk factors for gestational diabetes – age

Risk factor	% of population (Source)	% of women with gestational diabetes (source)	PPV (%)
Age ≥ 30 years	48.7 (ONS, 2005)	0.65 (Coustan, 1993)[452]	4.7
Age ≥ 25 years	74.2 (ONS, 2005)	0.85 (Coustan, 1993)[452]	4.0

Table D.5 Risk factors for gestational diabetes other than age

Risk factor	% of population (Source)	% of women with gestational diabetes (source)	PPV (%)
Gestational diabetes in a previous pregnancy	3.5 (HES, 2005)	30 (Weeks et al., 1994)[453]	10.5
Family history of diabetes	10.0 (Davey and Hamblin, 2001)[129]	39.9 (Davey and Hamblin, 2001)[129]	14.0
High-risk ethnic group	8.5 (ONS, 2001)	68.7 (Davey and Hamblin, 2001)[129]	28.1
BMI ≥ 27 kg/m²	35.8 (ONS, 2001)	36.2 (Davey and Hamblin, 2001)[129]	3.5

Table D.6 Test acceptance

Test	Initial test acceptance	Test acceptance if identified as 'at risk'	Source
FPG	0.50	0.90	GDG estimate
RBG	0.90	1.00	GDG estimate
1 hour 50 g GCT	0.70	1.00	GDG estimate
2 hour 75 g OGTT	0.40	0.90	GDG estimate

D.3.3 Incorporating risk factors within the model

General overview

In terms of the decision tree for the gestational diabetes screening/treatment model, risk factors can be thought of analogously to diagnostic tests (Figure D.2).

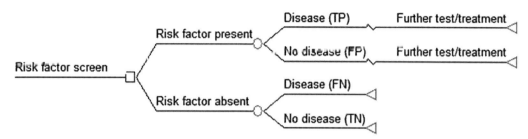

Figure D.2 Decision tree for risk factors; TP = true positive; FP = false positive; FN = false negative; TN = true negative

Positives from a risk factor screen or screen/diagnostic test progress to the next stage of testing or treatment. Negatives do not progress.

The detection rate of a risk factor screen is given by the true positive rate[*]. This detection rate is an important component of the model, as treatment costs and effects are predicated on it. Its flip-side (false negatives) is also important because there may be 'downstream' costs associated with missed cases.

In the economic model of screening we are also concerned with the unnecessary costs of screening which are caused by false negatives. The screening does not lead to improved outcomes in women with gestational diabetes and the scarce resources used in screening have an opportunity cost in terms of the benefit they could have achieved if used elsewhere in the healthcare system[†].

Therefore, the screening strategy with the highest detection rate is not necessarily the most cost-effective. There may be some desirable trade-off between detection and unnecessary testing and treatment.

The methodological problem

The data requirements for the model for any risk factor screening strategy are conceptually straightforward:

- what is the disease prevalence?
- what proportion of the population meets the risk criteria[‡]?
- what proportion of cases is detected in the population who meet the criteria?

With answers to these questions the true positive, false positive, true negative and false negative branches of the decision tree can be completed.

The literature tends to focus on the detection rates of a particular risk factor (or more rarely combination of risk factors). Using Office for National Statistics (ONS) data in combination with the literature it is possible to estimate the true positive, false positive, true negative and false negative rates for a single risk factor screen at baseline prevalence. However, given data limitations, it is much more difficult to derive these estimates for screening strategies based on combinations of risk factors.

Prevalence varies across the country and this is potentially important in the cost-effectiveness of screening as it influences the trade-off between detection and false positives. Therefore, the model has been developed to explore how the conclusion may vary at different disease prevalence. To

---

[*] In our gestational diabetes model, this is complicated by assumptions made about test acceptance.

[†] It is not explicitly addressed in the model, but an undesirable consequence of screening may be the unnecessary inconvenience and worry associated with false positives.

[‡] This information obviously also gives the proportion who do not meet the criteria.

do this required that we model a relationship between changes in disease prevalence and the proportion classed at 'high risk'. This poses further methodological difficulties because of the complex and interdependent relationship between risk factors.

With sufficient individual level data, it is possible to envisage a multiple regression equation which would predict the change in prevalence arising from a change in the proportions with different risk factor (RF) combinations.

$$\text{Prevalence} = a + b_1 RF_1 + b_2 RF_2 + b_3 RF_3 + \ldots + b_n RF_n$$

Such a model could be used to predict individual risk of disease.

However, in this model, risk factor proportion would be the dependent variable. As a result any model change in gestational diabetes prevalence would lead to a change in risk factor proportion. However, in reality , it is likely that different combinations of risk factors are consistent with the same overall disease prevalence. So, for example, a relatively young pregnant population may have the same gestational diabetes prevalence as an older pregnant population, if the younger population has a higher proportion in high-risk ethnic groups. This means that the most cost-effective screening strategy may be determined by the demographic characteristics of a particular population rather than prevalence *per se* (although the latter is a function of the former).

Our approach to modelling risk factor screening
Owing to data limitations and methodological complexity, our approach involved certain simplifying assumptions and the accuracy of the model may ultimately depend on whether these give a sufficiently good approximation to the real world.

Each risk factor screening strategy involves dividing the population in two – those at 'high' risk and those at 'low' risk[*]. Logically, the disease prevalence is the weighted average of the respective prevalence in these two groups. The weights are the proportions in each of the groups.

$$\text{Prevalence} = (\text{proportion high risk} \times \text{high-risk prevalence}) + (\text{proportion low risk} \times \text{low-risk prevalence})$$

The first step is to estimate a PPV for each risk factor screen, i.e. what proportion of the high-risk group had gestational diabetes? This gives the prevalence of gestational diabetes for the high-risk group. Next, an NPV is calculated, i.e. what proportion of the low-risk group did not have gestational diabetes. The prevalence in the low-risk group is given by 1 – NPV. These estimates use a combination of the literature and ONS data and they are probably reasonably good at baseline because they are not based on a simplified model extrapolation[†].

We then assume that the PPV and NPV are independent of prevalence. In a hypothetical scenario where there was just one risk factor for a disease, this would be correct. However, this linear relationship between risk factor proportion and prevalence is clearly a simplifying assumption in this case.

The model does not capture the impact and interdependence of multiple risk factors. As the proportion with a risk factor (e.g. age) increases, there would be concomitant increases in the proportion with multiple risk factors, which would change the PPV in those of 'at risk' age. This would exert an upward pressure on prevalence over and above that arising from the change in a single risk factor. In practice, changes in gestational diabetes prevalence are likely to lead to a smaller change in risk factor proportion than that implied by the model. This is even true for the ADA strategy, as clearly there is no reason why the proportion with multiple risk factors should be constant with respect to prevalence. Similarly, if the low-risk group have some risk factors then their disease prevalence (1 – NPV) is also likely to change with the demographic differences associated with changing disease prevalence.

Recognising these simplifying assumptions as a limitation, it should also be noted that the software developed for modelling included an option to override the relationship between prevalence and risk factors. If this option were chosen, the user of the software would themselves select the 'at risk' proportion and the proportion of cases that would exist in this population. This can be used to reflect better local data, if known, or to conduct sensitivity analysis. Such sensitivity analysis may indicate to what extent the simplifying assumptions drive the cost-effectiveness conclusions.

---

[*] 'High' and 'low' risk should be interpreted as a comparison of two groups, where one has a higher level of risk than the other.

[†] ADA may be a slight exception because the paper used to derive PPV and NPV values was based on a US population with a lower prevalence than our baseline model.

Below we outline in more detail the assumptions that were made for each risk factor screening strategy used in the model.

ADA:
ADA selective screening criteria exclude women who are:

- age < 25 years
- BMI < 27 kg/m²
- low-prevalence ethnic group
- no first-degree relative with history of diabetes.

The PPV and NPV for the ADA criteria were calculated as follows, using a retrospective study by Danilenko-Dixon et al.[454] which compared selective screening (using ADA criteria) with universal screening. The authors estimated that only 10% would be exempt from screening in their population (of which 17.8% were under 25 years), i.e. having none of the ADA risk factors. They found that 3% (17/564) of gestational diabetes cases were missed using ADA criteria*. The prevalence of gestational diabetes in their population was 3% (564/18 504) (see Table D.7).

Table D.7 Calculating PPV and NPV using ADA criteria as a risk factor screen

Parameter	Value
n	18 504
Prevalence = 564 / 18 504	3.05%
High risk = 0.9 × 18 504	16 654
Gestational diabetes cases in high risk = 564 − 17	547
PPV = 547/ 16 654	3.28%
Low risk = 0.1 × 18 504	1,850
Gestational diabetes cases in low risk	17
NPV = 1833/1850	99.1%

In this case, we needed to model the relationship between ADA parameters and prevalence even for our baseline analysis, because the calculations are taken from a population having different disease prevalence.

The key assumption in modelling this was to assume that the PPV and NPV were independent of disease prevalence. The PPV is essentially the disease prevalence in the high-risk group. The gestational diabetes prevalence in the low-risk group is given by 1 − NPV (0.92%).

The overall prevalence can then be seen as a weighted average of the high-risk and low-risk groups. For a given population gestational diabetes prevalence, it is therefore possible to estimate the proportions in the high-risk and low-risk categories. The PPV in conjunction with the high-risk proportion gives the detection rate.

What this modelled relationship implies is that for prevalence of 3.28% or more, all the population would be high risk as defined by ADA and therefore this is what our model assumes for the baseline prevalence (3.5%). This would not be the case in reality for reasons outlined in the preceding section[†].

Ethnicity:
Here 'high risk' is defined as women in a 'high' prevalence ethnic group and 'low risk' is defined as women in a 'low' prevalence ethnic group.

---

* Another study by Williams et al.[462] suggested 4% of gestational diabetes cases would be missed by ADA criteria.

† However, given the study on which our calculations were based, > 90% proportion 'high risk' and > 97% gestational diabetes detection might be considered 'realistic' .

The approach we used was similar to that used for the ADA criteria and is described in Table D.8.

Table D.8 Calculating PPV and NPV in using high-risk ethnicity as a risk factor screen

Parameter	Value	Source
Proportion of high risk	8.5%	ONS
Proportion of gestational diabetes high-risk ethnic group	68.7%	Weeks *et al.* (1994)[453]
Births	645 835	ONS
Births high-risk ethnic groups	54 896	Calculated
Gestational diabetes prevalence	3.5%	GDG estimate
Gestational diabetes births	22 604	Calculated
Gestational diabetes births high-risk ethnic groups	15 529	Calculated
PPV (15 529/54 896)	28.1%	Calculated
NPV (583 864/590 939)	98.8%	Calculated

Again it was assumed that PPV and NPV were independent of disease prevalence. As with the ADA creiteria, these provide prevalence in the high-risk and low-risk group with the overall population prevalence being a weighted average of the two*. Therefore, it is possible to estimate the high-risk ethnic group proportion from any given population gestational diabetes prevalence.

The model suggests that at a population prevalence of 2%, the high-risk ethnic proportion would be 2.98%. At a gestational diabetes prevalence of 10% it predicts 32.6%. On the face of it, these seem fairly plausible estimates but with the caveat that they are derived from a high-risk prevalence which is much higher than the literature would suggest.

BMI of 27 kg/m² or more:
This strategy identifies high-risk women as having a BMI of 27 kg/m² or more and low-risk women has having a BMI of less than 27 kg/m². The proportion of high-risk women in this strategy at baseline was calculated as shown in Table D.9.

Table D.9 Calculating PPV and NPV using a BMI of 27 kg/m² or more as a risk factor screen

Parameter	Value	Source
High-risk BMI proportion	0.358	ONS[a]
Proportion of gestational diabetes high-risk BMI	0.362	Davey and Hamblin (2001)[129]
Births	645 835	ONS
High-risk BMI births	231 209	Calculated
Low-risk BMI births	414 624	Calculated
Gestational diabetes prevalence	0.035	GDG estimate
Gestational diabetes births	22 604	Calculated
High-risk BMI gestational diabetes births	8183	Calculated
Low-risk BMI gestational diabetes births	14 421	Calculated
PPV (8183/231 209)	3.5%	Calculated
NPV (400 203/414 624)	96.5%	Calculated

[a] ONS data are based on proportions with BMI > 25 kg/m² (see earlier discussion).

* A prevalence of 28.1% for 'high-risk' ethnic groups seems considerably higher than values quoted in the literature.

Family history of diabetes:
This strategy identifies high-risk women as having a first-degree relative with a history of diabetes and low-risk women has having no first-degree relative with a history of diabetes. The proportion of high-risk women in this strategy at baseline was calculated as shown in Table D.10.

Table D.10 Calculating PPV and NPV using a first-degree relative with a history of diabetes as a risk factor screen

Parameter	Value	Source
High-risk family history proportion	0.10	Davey and Hamblin (2001)[129]
Proportion of gestational diabetes high-risk history	0.399	Davey and Hamblin (2001)[129]
Births	645 835	ONS
Low-risk family history births	581 252	Calculated
High-risk family history births	64 584	Calculated
Gestational diabetes prevalence	0.035	GDG estimate
Gestational diabetes births	22 604.	Calculated
High-risk family history gestational diabetes births	9,018	Calculated
Low-risk family history gestational diabetes births	13 586	Calculated
PPV (9018/64 584)	14.0%	Calculated
NPV (567 666/581 252)	97.6%	Calculated

Age ≥ 25 years:
This strategy identifies high-risk women as 25 years of age or older and low-risk women being 24 years of age or less. At baseline this gives a high-risk proportion of 74.2% and low-risk proportion of 25.8% (source: ONS).

The detection rate is then derived using a PPV, which is again assumed not to change with disease prevalence. The proportion of high-risk women in this strategy at baseline was calculated as shown in Table D.11.

Table D.11 Calculating PPV and NPV using age 25 years or older as a risk factor screen

Parameter	Value	Source
Total births	645 835	ONS
Total births ≥ 25 years	478 860	ONS
Gestational diabetes prevalence	3.5%	GDG estimate
Gestational diabetes births (0.035 × 645 835)	22 604	Calculated
Proportion detected ≥ 25 years	85%	Coustan (1993)[452]
Gestational diabetes detected (0.85 × 22 604)	19 214	Calculated
PPV (19 214/478 860)	4.01%	Calculated
NPV (163 585/166 975)	98.0%	Calculated

It should be noted that the model assumes that all the population is in the high-risk category for prevalence values of 4.01% and above.

Age ≥ 30 years:
The method is the same as for age ≥ 25 years, but using an older age threshold to define the high-risk and low-risk proportion. At baseline this gives a high-risk proportion of 48.7% and low-risk proportion of 51.3% (source: ONS).

The detection rate is then derived using a PPV, which is again assumed not to change with disease prevalence (Table D.12).

Table D.12   Calculating PPV and NPV using aged 30 years or older as a risk factor screen

Parameter	Value	Source
Total births	645 835	ONS
Total births ≥ 30 years	314 512	ONS
Gestational diabetes prevalence	3.5%	GDG estimate
Gestational diabetes births (0.035 × 645 835)	22 604	Calculated
Proportion detected ≥ 30 years	65%	Coustan (1993)[452]
Gestational diabetes detected (0.65 × 22 604)	14 693	Calculated
PPV (14 693/314 512)	4.7%	Calculated
NPV (323 412/331 323)	97.6%	Calculated

It should be noted that the model assumes that all the population is in the high-risk category for prevalence values of 4.7% and above.

D.4   Treatment

D.4.1   Treatment decision tree

The basic decision tree for treatment is depicted in Figure D.3.

The screening part of the model produces an output of true positives, false negatives, false positives and true negatives and these numbers then inform the probabilities attached to given patient treatment pathways following a positive or negative diagnosis of gestational diabetes.

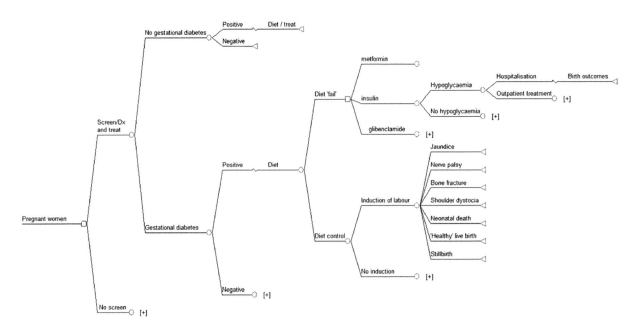

Figure D.3   The basic treatment sub-tree

As far as possible, treatment was modelled according to the ACHOIS protocol, as this is what the effectiveness data were based upon. It is assumed that women with gestational diabetes would start treatment at a gestational age of 27 weeks and that this would continue for 90 days.

The treatment protocol used in the model is outlined below.

Diet
Initial treatment aims to control blood glucose using diet. This part of treatment consists of:

- 30 minutes of individualised dietary advice from a qualified dietitian
- 30 minutes of instruction on self-monitoring of blood glucose provided by a specialist nurse (band 5/6)
- self-monitoring of blood glucose, four times daily (costing of self-monitoring of blood glucose includes one monitor, and assumes one lancet and one test strip per reading)
- 5 minutes of assessment of control after 10 days on diet by a specialist nurse.

At this 10 day assessment, women with gestational diabetes are judged to have achieved adequate control with diet or not. If they have achieved adequate control, they remain on dietary control until the end of their pregnancy, with self-monitoring of blood glucose reduced to twice daily.

If women are deemed not to have achieved adequate control with diet, medical treatment (insulin analogue, glibenclamide, metformin) is then initiated.

Insulin analogue
- 45 minutes of instruction from a diabetes specialist nurse
- daily insulin dose: 20 units
- pre-filled disposable injection device
- twice-daily injections (two needles per day of treatment)
- a proportion of women will experience hypoglycaemia and a small proportion of these will be severe cases requiring an inpatient admission
- self-monitoring of blood glucose, two times daily.

Glibenclamide and metformin, two alternative oral hypoglycaemic treatments to analogue insulin, were also included in the model. An RCT of glyburide (glibenclamide) versus insulin for gestational diabetes showed no statistically significant differences in outcomes. The effectiveness of metformin is currently being investigated as part of the ongoing MIG trial and is therefore a potential treatment option. The basic tree structure for an oral hypoglycaemic treatment, such as glibenclamide, would be as illustrated in Figure D.4.

Glibenclamide
- daily dose: 15 mg.

Metformin
- daily dose: 1.5 g.

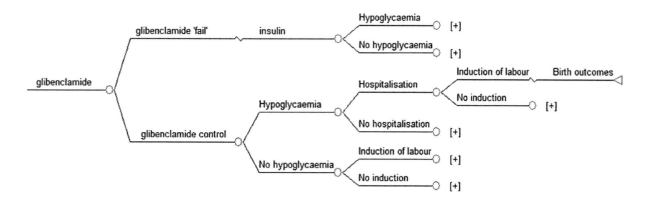

Figure D.4   Glibenclamide treatment sub-tree

D.4.2   Outcomes and downstream costs

The model uses the following outcomes presented in the ACHOIS study to estimate the incremental QALY gain associated with screening, diagnosis and treatment of gestational diabetes:

- stillbirth
- neonatal death
- maternal health state utility.

Furthermore, the following outcomes from ACHOIS are assumed to have downstream cost implications. Costs are assigned to these outcomes and included in the evaluation of incremental costs:

- neonatal death
- shoulder dystocia
- bone fracture
- admission to neonatal unit
- jaundice requiring phototherapy
- induction of labour
- caesarean section.

We used the outcome data of ACHOIS for 'serious perinatal complications' as the measure of the effectiveness in the model. The trial data allow this to be easily done for deterministic sensitivity analysis, with the different event rates giving well-defined relative risks. In order to reflect the individual components of the composite measure, a weighted cost and QALY was calculated for a serious perinatal complication based on the QALY and costs associated with each of the individual components. In order to calculate the weights, it was assumed, based on the lack of statistical significance for any difference, that the proportion of serious perinatal complications accounted for by individual components did not differ according to whether the women were treated for gestational diabetes or not. Therefore, the data on individual events were pooled across both arms of the trial in order to estimate the weighting for individual components (Table D.13).

Table D.13   ACHOIS trial outcome data for serious perinatal complications combined across control and intervention groups

Outcome	Total	Weight
All serious perinatal complications	32	1.00
Stillbirth	3	0.09
Neonatal death	2	0.06
Shoulder dystocia	23	0.72
Bone fracture	1	0.03
Nerve palsy	3	0.09

D.4.3   Treatment model parameters

The baseline parameter values for all model treatment inputs are shown in Tables D.14 to D.20.

Table D.14   Treatment timeframe

Variable	Value (days)	Source	Notes
Treatment duration	90	Diabetes in pregnancy GDG	The diabetes in pregnancy GDG consensus was that treatment would usually commence between 26 and 28 weeks of gestation. Taking the midpoint of 27 weeks, 90 days is a reasonable approximation of the typical time to term.
Exclusive diet	10	Diabetes in pregnancy GDG	The diabetes in pregnancy GDG suggested that diet alone would be given 7–14 days to achieve adequate control.
4 × daily SMBG	10	ACHOIS[153]	The ACHOIS protocol suggested that SMBG be done 4 × daily until glucose levels had been in the recommended range for 2 weeks.

SMBG = self-monitoring of blood glucose.

Table D.15   Cost of healthcare professionals' time

Variable	Time (minutes)	Cost per hour	Source	Notes
Dietary advice	30	£28	Curtis and Netten (2006)[456]	Unit costs of a dietitian for an hour of client contact
SMBG instruction	30	£63	Curtis and Netten (2006)[456] GDG estimate	Unit cost of a nurse specialist (community) for an hour of client contact
Control with diet; assessment/review	5	£63	Curtis and Netten (2006)[456] GDG estimate	Unit cost of a nurse specialist (community) for an hour of client contact
Insulin instruction	15	£63	Curtis and Netten (2006)[456] GDG estimate	Unit cost of a nurse specialist (community) for an hour of client contact
Risk factor screening questions	2	£63	Curtis and Netten (2006)[456] GDG estimate	Unit cost of a nurse specialist (community) for an hour of client contact

SMBG = self-monitoring of blood glucose.

Table D.16   Self-monitoring of blood glucose and treatment costs

Variable	Cost	Source	Notes
Blood glucose monitor	£7.79	BNF 52 (2006)[457]	
Test strips	£0.31 each	BNF 52 (2006)[457]	Many makes, all similarly priced. £15.55 for a pack of 50 was the cheapest found from a small sample.
Lancets	£0.03 each	BNF 52 (2006)[457]	
Needles	£0.09 each	BNF 52 (2006)[457]	£8.57 for a pack of 100 needles
Insulin analogue (Humalog®)	£0.39 per day	BNF 52 (2006)[457]	This is based on a dose of 20 units per day. A pre-filled disposable pen has 1500 units and costs £29.46.
Glibenclamide	£0.16	BNF 52 (2006)[457]	Based on 15 mg daily. A 5 mg 28 tablet pack costs £1.50.
Metformin	£0.10	BNF 52 (2006)[457]	Based on 1.5 g daily. A 500 mg 84 tablet pack costs £2.85.
Treatment of severe hypoglycaemia	£403	Curtis and Netten (2006)[456] NHS Reference Costs 2005–06	Average cost per patient journey for paramedic ambulance: £323. Accident and emergency department admission with low-cost investigation: £80.

Table D.17   Downstream outcome costs

Variable	Cost	Source	Notes
Admission to neonatal unit	£1,676	NHS Reference Costs 2004	Assume 2 days of neonatal intensive care at £838 per day.
Induction of labour	£20	Davies and Drummond (1991)[458] and (1993)[459]	Updated to 2006 prices using Retail Price Index published by ONS.
Neonatal death	£2,568	NHS Tariff 2006 NHS Reference Costs 2004	From NHS Reference Costs 2004 finished consultant episode (FCE) data assume that 25% of neonatal deaths are < 2 days (n = 974). NHS Reference Costs for this is £527. For remaining 75% assume 2 days of neonatal intensive care (£838 × 2) and neonate with one major diagnosis which has an NHS Tariff of £1,572. £1,676 + £1,572 = £3,248
Shoulder dystocia	£629	NHS Tariff 2006	Cost for neonate with one minor diagnosis (HRG N03)
Bone fracture	£629	NHS Tariff 2006	Cost for neonate with one minor diagnosis (HRG N03)
Nerve palsy	£629	NHS Tariff 2006	Cost for neonate with one minor diagnosis (HRG N03)
Phototherapy	£629	NHS Tariff 2006	Cost for neonate with one minor diagnosis (HRG N03)
Emergency caesarean section	£1,205	NHS Reference Costs 2004	Incremental cost over and above that of a normal vaginal birth
Elective caesarean section	£822	NHS Reference costs 2004	Incremental cost over and above that of a normal vaginal birth

HRG = Health Resource Group.

Table D.18   Treatment pathway probabilities

Variable	Value	Source	Notes
Control with diet	0.86	Persson et al. (1985)[172]	–
Control with glibenclamide	0.96	Langer et al. (2000)[74]	GDG member suggested that data from Southampton (their local practice) indicate a higher failure rate (23%).
Control with metformin	0.96	–	Assumed the same as for glibenclamide.
Hypoglycaemia on insulin therapy	0.20	Langer et al. (2000)[74]	–
Hypoglycaemia on insulin analogue	0.20	–	Assumed the same as for insulin.
Hypoglycaemia on glibenclamide	0.02	Langer et al. (2000)[74]	–
Hypoglycaemia on metformin	0.02	–	Assumed the same as for glibenclamide.
Severe hypoglycaemia requiring hospitalisation	0.05	GDG estimate	–

Table D.19   ACHOIS outcome probabilities

Variable	Treatment value	No treatment value	Source
Serious perinatal complications	0.014	0.044	ACHOIS[153]
Admission to neonatal unit	0.706	0.613	ACHOIS[153]
Induction of labour	0.374	0.286	ACHOIS[153]
Elective caesarean section	0.142	0.116	ACHOIS[153]
Emergency caesarean section	0.158	0.197	ACHOIS[153]
Jaundice (phototherapy)	0.087	0.092	ACHOIS[153]

Table D.20   QALYs

Variable	QALY	Source	Notes
Averted death (stillbirth/neonatal)	25		This is the approximate lifetime QALYs from 75 years lived in perfect health with QALYS discounted at 3.5% per annum.
Maternal QALY – treatment (during pregnancy)	0.72	ACHOIS[153]	It is assumed that this QALY gain persists throughout treatment.
Maternal QALY – no treatment (during pregnancy)	0.70	ACHOIS[153]	It is assumed that this QALY gain persists throughout treatment.
Maternal QALY – treatment (3 months postpartum)	0.79	ACHOIS[153]	It is assumed that this QALY gain covers the entire 3 months postpartum period.
Maternal QALY – no treatment (3 months postpartum)	0.78	ACHOIS[153]	It is assumed that this QALY gain covers the entire 3 months postpartum period.

D.5   Baseline results

The baseline results from the modelling exercise are given based on a population of 10 000 pregnant women and assume a baseline prevalence of gestational diabetes of 3.5%. The total cost and QALYs generated for each strategy under the baseline assumptions are presented in Table D.21 and are plotted on a cost-effectiveness plane in Figure D.5. The origin represents the no screening/no treatment option and all costs and QALYs are measured relative to this.

Table D.21 Total QALYs and cost for each screening strategy

Screening strategy[a]	QALYs	Cost
11	16.63	£146,188
1	17.48	£212,816
8	18.48	£304,753
9	18.70	£145,419
3	18.70	£126,929
13	19.46	£119,940
14	20.39	£191,529
19	20.56	£77,465
20	21.55	£89,758
12	21.96	£259,791
10	24.40	£838,561
15	25.45	£160,670
17	25.56	£203,902
16	26.66	£269,731
21	27.01	£99,341
2	29.94	£198,769
4	31.37	£345,932
5	33.26	£489,580
18	33.43	£286,763
7	34.85	£1,172,747
6	39.33	£367,009

[a] Ranked in order of effectiveness (from fewest to most QALYs).

As can be seen from Figure D.5, a number of strategies are more expensive than the two circled and yet offer a lower QALY gain. Such strategies can unambiguously be excluded (they are said to be (strictly) dominated). Once these strategies are excluded the remainder are again ranked in order of effectiveness. Moving down the list, it is possible to calculate the incremental costs and incremental QALYs of selecting a given strategy relative to the next best strategy. From this, the

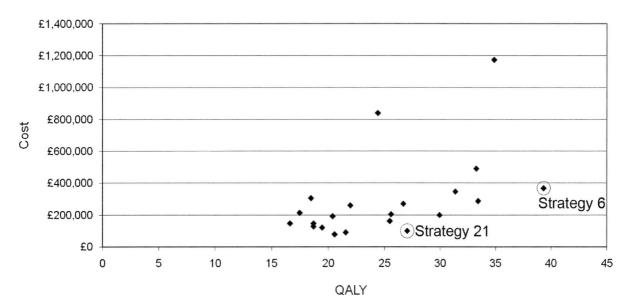

Figure D.5 The cost-effectiveness plane for the baseline analysis

ICER is derived which effectively shows the cost of 'buying' QALYs. It is then possible to exclude certain further strategies on the grounds of 'extended dominance'. Extended dominance occurs when a strategy has a higher ICER than a more effective strategy. If the decision maker was willing to buy QALYs at the cost implied by the ICER of the less effective strategy, they would logically be willing to buy (and prefer) strategies where additional QALYs could be obtained at a lower cost.

In Table D.22 all but two of the strategies are excluded on these dominance grounds. The ICER for strategy 21 is calculated relative to no screening/treatment and the ICER for strategy 6 is calculated relative to strategy 21. The cost-effective option is the most effective strategy which falls within the willingness to pay threshold set by the decision maker.

Table D.22   ICER for non-dominated strategies

Strategy	QALYs	Cost	Incremental QALYs	Incremental cost	ICER
21	27.01	£99,341	27.01	£99,341	£3,677
6	39.33	£367,009	12.31	£267,668	£21,738

The baseline analysis suggests that a strategy of offering women from a high-risk ethnic background a diagnostic test (strategy 21) would be cost-effective when compared with not offering a screening, with an ICER of £3,677. The strategy of offering a diagnostic test to those women who are deemed to be at increased risk according to the ADA criteria (strategy 6) has an ICER of £21,738 when compared with strategy 21. Although it is higher than the £20,000 per QALY threshold suggested by NICE, it is comfortably under the maximum willingness to pay per QALY of £30,000 and may be considered cost-effective under certain circumstances, for example if it is believed some salient piece of information falls outside the model such as the identification of women at higher risk of developing type 2 diabetes in the future. Thus it is possible that strategy 6 could reasonably be argued to be cost-effective.

D.6   Sensitivity analysis

All decision analysis models are subject to uncertainty[460] and there are two common approaches to dealing with this uncertainty – making use of a reference case (that is, a standard of good practice) and sensitivity analysis. This model takes as its reference case the standards for conducting economic evaluations included in the 2007 version of the NICE guidelines manual.[23] The methods and assumptions used in the model are highlighted above in detail and were tested using a second method of examining uncertainty, sensitivity analysis. In the analyses presented below we primarily used a series of one-way and multi-way sensitivity analyses to explore what happened when the value of one or more parameters is changed. This allows us to see what happens to the model results when these values are changed, and thus the implications for our baseline results. The analyses that follow explore the uncertainty in a number of key areas, including:

- the reliability of the trial data on which the likelihood of an event occurring was based
- the prevalence of gestational diabetes in the population
- the proportion of women that would undergo a screening or diagnostic blood test if it were offered as a first-line test or based on identification of a potentially high-risk population
- treatment options
- the efficacy of using risk factors to define high- and low-risk populations, based on the presence of one or more of the risk factors highlighted in the ADA criteria (age over 25 years, BMI greater than 27 kg/m², family history of diabetes or from a high-risk ethnic background).

Tables D.23 to D.27 give the sensitivity analysis ICER for strategies which have not been excluded on the grounds of strict or extended dominance.

Table D.23 Effect on ICER of varying the number of perinatal deaths attributable to gestational diabetes

Strategy	QALYs	Cost	Incremental QALYs	Incremental cost	ICER
Four deaths					
21	21.26	£99,490	21.26	£99,490	£4,680
6	30.95	£367,227	9.69	£267,737	£27,633
Three deaths					
21	15.80	£100,136	15.80	£100,136	£6,336
6	23.01	£368,167	7.20	£268,031	£37,209
Two deaths					
21	10.69	£100,287	10.69	£100,287	£9,385
6	15.56	£368,386	4.87	£268,100	£55,042
One death					
21	5.94	£100,473	5.94	£100,473	£16,913
6	8.65	£368,657	2.71	£268,184	£99,045
No deaths					
21	1.61	£101,069	1.61	£101,069	£62,854
6	2.34	£369,525	0.73	£268,456	£366,272

Table D.24 Gestational diabetes prevalence of 2%

Strategy	QALYs	Cost	Incremental QALYs	Incremental cost	ICER
21	9.41	£48,856	9.41	£48,856	£5,192
2	12.84	£100,583	3.43	£51,727	£15,085
6	16.87	£177,118	4.03	£76,536	£19,005

Table D.25 Gestational diabetes prevalence of 5%

Strategy	QALYs	Cost	Incremental QALYs	Incremental cost	ICER
19	33.97	£113,694	33.97	£113,694	£3,347
21	44.62	£149,825	10.65	£36,131	£3,392
6	56.18	£401,205	11.56	£251,379	£21,738
18	56.18	£401,205	11.56	£251,379	£21,738

Table D.26 Gestational diabetes prevalence of 2% and 100% test acceptance

Strategy	QALY	Cost	Incremental QALY	Incremental cost	ICER
21	10.46	£51,385	10.46	£51,385	£4,915
11	21.12	£163,434	10.66	£112,049	£10,507
1	24.97	£336,113	3.85	£172,679	£44,852

Table D.27 Gestational diabetes prevalence of 5% and 100% test acceptance

Strategy	QALY	Cost	Incremental QALY	Incremental cost	ICER
19	41.93	£130,634	41.93	£130,634	£3,115
21	49.58	£161,816	7.64	£31,183	£4,079
1	62.43	£411,583	12.85	£249,766	£19,439

D.6.1 Outcomes

The outcome that had the greatest influence on the model results was the number of perinatal deaths (stillbirths and neonatal deaths). This is because of the non-negligible weight given to this outcome as a proportion of all serious perinatal complications and the significant gain in QALYs to be made by preventing a perinatal death. In the ACHOIS trial there were five perinatal deaths recorded in those who received no treatment ($n = 524$) while in the treatment arm there were none ($n = 506$). This difference was not statistically significant. The number of deaths in the control group was similar to the number of perinatal deaths that would be expected in the general population according to ONS data on perinatal mortality (in 2005 there were 5.4 stillbirths, 2.6 early neonatal deaths and 3.4 late neonatal deaths per 1000 total births in England and Wales). The authors of the ACHOIS study highlight that at least one death in the control group was unrelated to gestational diabetes.

Table D.23 shows the results of the models when the number of perinatal deaths in each group was assumed to be different to that reported in the ACHOIS trial. As the number of perinatal deaths decreases, the cost-effectiveness of the various strategies changes. When only four deaths in the trial group are attributed to gestational diabetes, the ICERs of both strategies 21 and 6 become less favourable and this continues until only one perinatal death is attributed to gestational diabetes. Even when there is only a single death assumed, there is still a screening, diagnosis and treatment strategy that would be considered cost-effective – in this case strategy 21. However, if no perinatal deaths are attributed to gestational diabetes, then there is no strategy for screening , diagnosis and treatment that could be considered cost-effective.

This result demonstrates that the model is highly sensitive to the potential QALYs gained by preventing even a single perinatal death. The model also potentially underestimates the QALYs to be gained by preventing other adverse outcomes, such as shoulder dystocia or nerve palsy, and may therefore underestimate the cost-effectiveness of screening. However, the ICERs when no deaths are assumed are sufficiently large to suggest that the potential QALY gain from preventing some of these events would not be adequate for these strategies to be cost-effective.

What is clear from this analysis is that the potential benefits to the NHS with respect to QALYs gained from intervention are likely to be felt in the form of preventing perinatal deaths, and the cost-effectiveness of screening, diagnosis and treatment strategies are highly influenced in the model by this one particular adverse outcome.

D.6.2 Gestational diabetes prevalence

The prevalence of a disease can often be a very important determinant of the cost-effectiveness of screening. Tables D.24 and D.25 show how the results of the model varied for different prevalences of gestational diabetes. The results suggest that varying the prevalence over a range of 3 percentage points has little impact on the cost-effectiveness conclusions of the model, but it should be remembered that the simplified model relationship between risk factor proportions and gestational diabetes prevalence has a bearing on these results.

D.6.3 Test acceptance

As noted earlier, test acceptance rates are potentially an important source of uncertainty within the model, especially as with default assumptions there is an inverse relationship between test accuracy and test acceptance. Tables D.26 and D.27 show how the results varied when it was assumed that all women were tested in populations with a relatively low and relatively high disease prevalence, respectively.

The results show that a universal screening strategy using the gold standard diagnostic test becomes more cost-effective as disease prevalence increases. This is because of its advantages over other test options in terms of its detection rate. However, its advantages in terms of detection rate are negated if it is assumed that the test has a low level of acceptance.

A threshold analysis, with all other model parameters at their baseline values, showed that, even if test acceptance for FPG/OGTT in women identified as 'at risk' fell from 90% at baseline to 52%, strategy 6 would remain the preferred option up to a willingness to pay threshold of £20,000 per QALY.

D.6.4   Treatment option

The model also allowed the ICERs for different strategies to be calculated for different treatment options (analogue insulin, glibenclamide and metformin). Table D.28 shows that the choice of treatment option in the model made little difference to the ICERs for the screening strategies. This is because treatment represents a relatively small proportion of the total costs, and because all the incremental analysis is undertaken with treatment cost as a given. For example, a lower treatment cost will reduce the cost of each strategy but may have relatively little impact on the incremental costs.

Table D.28   ICER for strategy 6 for different treatment options in the baseline model

Treatment	ICER
Analogue insulin	£21,738
Glibenclamide	£21,647
Metformin	£21,642

D.6.5   Single risk factors

The baseline analysis suggested that strategy 6 was a borderline cost-effective strategy using a willingness to pay threshold of £20,000 per QALY. However, the GDG expressed concerns over the number of women that would have to undergo a OGTT if strategy 6 were adopted. A large proportion of women tested would be tested based on age criteria alone – under the baseline assumptions as many as 90% might be offered the diagnostic test. This would be a considerable inconvenience to a large number of women, only a small minority of whom would ultimately benefit from the testing process, as well as putting a strain on local services. As a result it was decided that the use of screening based on risk factors other than age should be considered.

The PPVs and NPVs of different risk factor combinations are not accurately known which means that the relative cost-effectiveness of different combinations of any of the single risk factors can not be calculated. However, it may be the case that where single risk factors are cost-effective on their own, then any combination of these is also likely to be cost-effective. Therefore an analysis of the cost-effectiveness of each single risk factor, followed by an OGTT, has been performed, with each risk factor plus OGTT combination compared with a strategy of no screening or treatment. The results are presented in Table D.29.

Table D.29   ICER for single risk factor strategies followed by a diagnostic test when compared with a strategy of no screening or treatment

Strategy	QALY	Cost	ICER
Ethnicity	9.55	£66,226	£6,935
BMI	6.29	£80,109	£12,736
Family history	15.73	£81,915	£5,208

Any strategy where a single risk factor from the ADA criteria other than age is applied alone, followed by a diagnostic test, has an ICER that is below the threshold of £20,000 and could in each case be considered cost-effective on its own.

The above analysis established that screening, diagnosis and treatment of gestational diabetes is generally cost-effective in some populations. Below we consider the cost-effectiveness of the various treatment options for gestational diabetes.

D.7 Cost analysis of different treatment options for gestational diabetes

A systematic review of the literature, targeted at the guideline question on what is cost-effective treatment for gestational diabetes, identified a single paper for inclusion.[461] This paper described a cost model to compare the costs of an oral hypoglycaemic, glyburide (glibenclamide), with those of insulin for the treatment of gestational diabetes. The paper justifies what is essentially a cost minimisation approach on the basis that glyburide and insulin confer similar glycaemic control.[74] Their model, based in a US setting, excluded resource items that were identical in both treatments. Included in the costs for insulin were drug costs, costs of the consumables needed to administer the insulin and the cost of instructing women with diabetes on how to draw up the insulin and inject themselves. The cost of glyburide was based on the average wholesale cost of a milligram of drug multiplied by the weekly dose expected to be necessary for glycaemic control. In addition, it was assumed that 4% of patients would not achieve control with glyburide and would have to switch to insulin. Therefore, the model also incorporated a cost for glyburide treatment failure. Women switching to insulin also incurred the educational costs associated with insulin treatment. Finally, the model also included the downstream costs of hypoglycaemia, which was assumed to be more common in insulin-treated gestational diabetes. In the baseline analysis, glyburide produced an average cost saving of $166 per woman. The authors reported that most sensitivity analyses did not alter the direction of this finding. A threshold analysis suggested that insulin was only less costly than glyburide at the highest wholesale cost of $18.24 per week in conjunction with a daily dose of 18.9 g, which is considerably higher than what is believed to be necessary to achieve good glycaemic control. A similar cost model was developed to compare the cost of insulin analogue (lispro) with that of two oral hypoglycaemics (glibenclamide and metformin) in a UK context.

D.7.1 Introduction

A cost minimisation analysis can be considered to be a special case of cost-effectiveness analysis when the interventions being compared are equally efficacious. In such a scenario, the cheapest option is unambiguously cost-effective as it dominates the alternatives, being cheaper and equally effective. A randomised study[74] failed to find significant differences in outcomes (maternal and neonatal) between glyburide and insulin treatment in women with gestational diabetes. It is on this basis, and in the absence of any conflicting evidence, that such a cost minimisation analysis might be justifiable to determine the cost-effectiveness of various gestational diabetes treatments. Of course, no evidence of a difference is not the same as evidence of no difference, but the P values in this study were particularly large and the inference of no difference does not arise as a result of some outcomes being just the wrong side of an arbitrary 5% cut-off point for statistical significance.

Insulin analogue was used in this cost comparison rather than insulin, as this is what would be offered to women with gestational diabetes in the UK. Implicit in this is an assumption that outcomes with an insulin analogue would be equivalent to those with insulin. Metformin was additionally added into this analysis as the ongoing MIG study is assessing its use in women with gestational diabetes and it could potentially be an important treatment option in the UK.

D.7.2 Method

The basic structure of the cost analysis is shown in Figure D.6. It is assumed that a diagnosis of gestational diabetes would be made at a gestational age of 27 weeks. As described in the screening, diagnosis and treatment model, women with gestational diabetes would start with dietary treatment. In women who do not achieve adequate glycaemic control after 10 days, pharmacological therapy would be started and this is the starting point for the cost comparison.

Costs which are common to all treatments, such as those associated with self-monitoring of blood glucose, are not included in the analysis. The costs for a woman taking insulin analogue include the time of a diabetes specialist nurse in providing instruction on how to administer the drug. Women with gestational diabetes are assumed to use a pre-filled disposable injection pen (e.g. Humalog® Mix50) and to be on a daily dose of 20 units administered in twice-daily injections. Therefore, they require two needles per day for their injection pen. The cost of glibenclamide is the drug cost based on a daily dose of 15 mg. Similarly, the cost of metformin is based on a daily dose of 1.5 g.

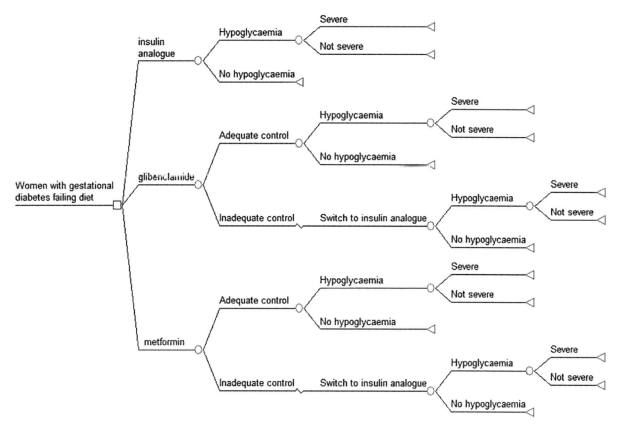

Figure D.6 Gestational diabetes treatment cost model

In addition to the cost of treatment it is important also to consider downstream costs. Overall outcomes are assumed not to differ, but following the Langer study[74] the model addresses a possible differential in the hypoglycaemia risk between the different treatments. It is additionally assumed at baseline that 5% of hypoglycaemic events will be 'severe' and it is these for which there will typically be an NHS resource implication. The cost of a 'severe' hypoglycaemic event is assumed to be the cost of a paramedic ambulance journey and an admission to an accident and emergency department.

The complete list of model parameters is given in Tables D.30 to D.32.

D.7.3   Results

Table D.33 lists the cost per patient of each of the three treatment options. These show the oral hypoglycaemics to be considerably cheaper than analogue insulin. Of the oral hypoglycamics, metformin is the cheapest and, with the assumption of equal clinical effectiveness, the most cost-effective treatment.

D.7.4   Sensitivity analysis

A number of sensitivity analyses were undertaken to determine how robust the conclusion of the baseline result was to changes in model parameters where some uncertainty exists as to their 'true' value. For ease of exposition, most sensitivity analyses focus on a comparison of glibenclamide and insulin analogue on the basis that, apart from a small difference in costs, these are assumed to be identical treatments in terms of both outcomes and downstream costs.

However, threshold analyses were also undertaken which showed that, holding all other factors constant, metformin remained cheapest as long as control on metformin was at least 90.3% (with control on glibenclamide 96%) or control on metformin was at least 72.3% (with control on glibenclamide 77%).

Figure D.7 shows how the incremental cost of insulin analogue varies with different assumptions about the proportion of women with gestational diabetes who achieve adequate glycaemic

Table D.30   Treatment timeframe (days)

Variable	Value (days)	Source	Notes
Treatment duration	80	Diabetes in pregnancy GDG	It is assumed a gestational diabetes diagnosis would be made at 27 weeks of gestation. Women with gestational diabetes would be given approximately 10 days to achieve control with diet and 80 days is a reasonable approximation of the typical time to term at the commencement of pharmacological treatment.
Oral hypoglycaemic trial period	14	ACHOIS[153]	

Table D.31   Costs

Variable	Cost	Source	Notes
Insulin instruction	£47.25	Curtis and Netten (2006)[456] GDG estimate	This is based on an instruction time of 45 minutes with instruction provided by a specialist nurse.
Insulin analogue	£0.57 per day	BNF 52 (2006)[457]	This is based on a dose of 20 units per day. A pre-filled disposable pen has 1500 units and costs £29.46. It is further assumed that injections are twice daily, requiring two needles at £0.09 each.
Glibenclamide	£0.16	BNF 52 (2006)[457]	Based on 15 mg daily. A 5 mg 28 tablet pack costs £1.50.
Metformin	£0.10	BNF 52 (2006)[457]	Based on 1.5 g daily. A 500 mg 84 tablet pack costs £2.85.
Switching cost of oral hypoglycaemia failure	£0.00	GDG estimate	It is assumed there is no additional cost over and above those incurred by all women with gestational diabetes starting insulin analogue treatment.
Treatment of severe hypoglycaemia	£403	Curtis and Netten (2006)[456] NHS Reference Costs 2005–06	Average cost per patient journey for paramedic ambulance: £323. Admission to an accident and emergency department with low-cost investigation: £80.

Table D.32   Probabilities

Variable	Probability	Source	Notes
Control with glibenclamide	0.96	Langer et al. (2000)[74] GDG estimate	A GDG member reported 0.77 for this parameter in his clinical practice.
Control with metformin	0.96	Langer et al. (2000)[74]	Assumed identical to glibenclamide.
Hypoglycaemia on insulin analogue	0.20	Langer et al. (2000)[74]	Assumed to be the same as Langer found for insulin.
Hypoglycaemia on glibenclamide	0.02	Langer et al. (2000)[74]	–
Hypoglycaemia on metformin	0.02	Langer et al. (2000)[74]	Assumed identical to glibenclamide.
Proportion of hypoglycaemia that is 'severe'	0.05	GDG estimate	–

Table D.33   Cost per women with gestational diabetes

Treatment	Average cost per women with gestational diabetes
Insulin analogue	£96.92
Glibenclamide	£16.32
Metformin	£11.68

control with glibenclamide. Although the differential in cost declines with reduced glibenclamide clinical effectiveness, insulin analogue continues to be the more costly option even if only 40% of women achieve adequate glycaemic control with glibenclamide. Figure D.8 shows that the cost analysis is not sensitive to the risk of hypoglycaemia in women taking glibenclamide. Similarly, Figure D.9 shows that the costs of treating hypoglycaemia are not an important determinant of the additional costs of insulin analogue.

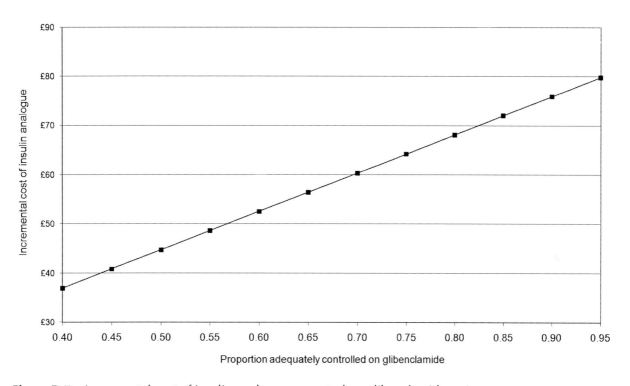

Figure D.7   Incremental cost of insulin analogue as control on glibenclamide varies

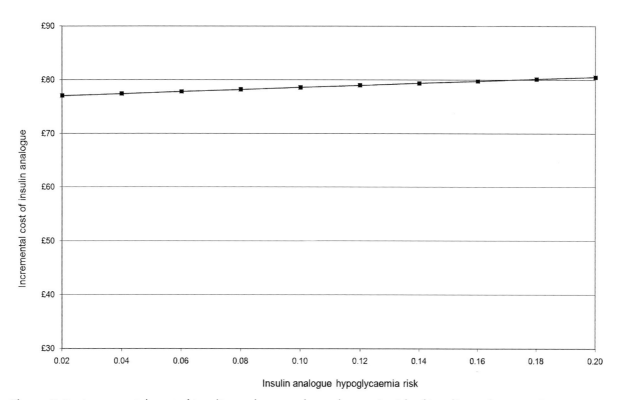

Figure D.8   Incremental cost of insulin analogue as hypoglycaemia risk of insulin analogue varies

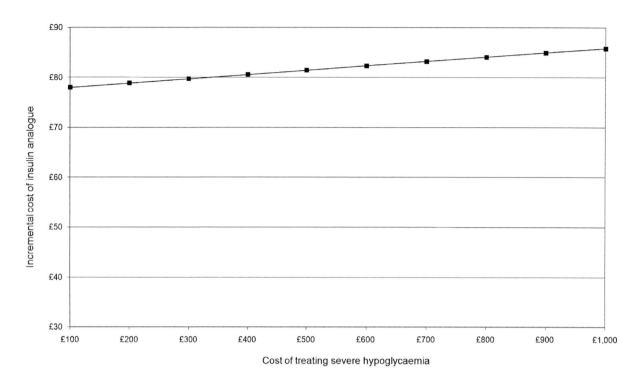

Figure D.9   Incremental cost of insulin analogue as cost of treating severe hypoglycaemia varies

D.7.5   Discussion

Using the data from ACHOIS, this guideline has demonstrated that screening, diagnosis and treatment of gestational diabetes is cost-effective and that this finding is not contingent on the type of pharmacological treatment used (insulin analogue or oral hypoglycaemic agent). However, given that the treatments have different resource implications for the NHS, it does not follow that all treatments are equally cost-effective. One study[74] suggested that 'among women with gestational diabetes, the degree of glycaemic control and the perinatal outcomes were essentially the same for those treated with glyburide (glibenclamide) and those treated with insulin. The lack of differences between the infants born to mothers in the two treatment groups corroborated the results in the mothers'. Therefore, if it is argued on the basis of this study that glibenclamide is equally effective as insulin analogue and would have achieved similar outcomes to those observed with diet and insulin treatment in ACHOIS, then we can say that the results presented here suggest that glibenclamide is a more cost-effective treatment for gestational diabetes than insulin analogue. Sensitivity analysis suggested that this conclusion was robust when model parameters were changed in a one-way fashion. The diabetes in pregnancy GDG has suggested that the proportion of women with gestational diabetes achieving control with glibenclamide may be lower in clinical practice than that observed by Langer et al.[74] However, as the sensitivity analysis shows, glibenclamide continues to be cost-saving compared with insulin analogue even with a much smaller proportion achieving adequate control.

As yet, there is no evidence to justify a cost minimisation approach with metformin. However, if it too was shown to be as effective as insulin analogue then it would be the most cost-effective treatment of all.

One caveat to these findings is the assumption that there is no cost to the NHS in switching from an oral hypoglycaemic agent to insulin analogue, other than those ordinarily incurred for women with gestational diabetes taking insulin analogue. If there were a 'switching cost', then the cost-effectiveness of the oral hypoglycaemic agents would be less than that implied here.

Appendix E

Cost-effectiveness of screening for congenital cardiac malformations

E.1 Introduction

A review of the health economics literature identified a single study addressing the cost-effectiveness of screening for congenital cardiac malformations in pregnant women with diabetes.[413] In the study, a decision-analytic model was used to compare the cost-effectiveness of four screening strategies for congenital cardiac malformations in a healthcare setting in the USA. The strategies were: no screening; selective fetal echocardiography after abnormal detailed anatomical survey (a four chamber view of the heart plus outflow tracts was included as part of the detailed anatomical survey); fetal echocardiography for high HbA_{1c} only; and universal fetal echocardiography. Costs and outcomes were modelled for a hypothetical cohort of 40 000 pregnant women with diabetes and with a 2.1% prevalence of major cardiac malformations. The sensitivities and specificities for each strategy were derived from a literature search and costs included tests, terminations of pregnancy, and the healthcare costs of a major cardiac malformation over and above those needed for a healthy child. Effectiveness was measured using QALYs derived by assigning different utilities to different outcomes (major cardiac defect 0.5, fetal death 0.07, and healthy neonate 1.0) and then multiplying by the life expectancy with each outcome. The utility weights were discounted at a rate of 3% per year. The study reported that selective fetal echocardiogram after abnormal detailed anatomical survey dominated all other strategies with baseline assumptions. However, the study also noted that universal fetal echocardiogram yielded the highest detection rate of cardiac anomalies. As a result of a probabilistic sensitivity analysis, the study reported that the model results were robust when considering parameter uncertainty. However, the scenarios presented did not reflect current UK practice or viable alternatives. In addition, there are concerns about the generalisability of cost-effectiveness results from healthcare settings outside the UK and it was, therefore, decided to develop a model for this guideline to compare the cost-effectiveness of two screening strategies in the UK context.

A decision tree model was developed for the guideline in Microsoft Excel® to assess the cost-effectiveness of second-trimester screening for congenital cardiac malformations in pregnant women with diabetes. Current UK practice is to screen pregnant women using a four chamber ultrasound scan at 20 weeks of gestation, but using a four chamber plus outflow tracts view may allow the detection of some abnormalities, such as TGA and tetralogy of Fallot, which are not usually visible with a four chamber view. Screening for these malformations in pregnant women with diabetes is likely to be relatively more cost-effective than in pregnant women without diabetes because the prevalence of these anomalies is much higher in women with diabetes.[414]

There are two principal reasons why it may be beneficial to screen for congenital cardiac malformations:

- it allows women to consider termination of pregnancy
- improved outcomes for women and/or babies.

There are difficulties in considering the cost-effectiveness of screening using termination as a positive outcome and the evidence that screening produces a survival advantage is limited.[415] Nevertheless, there is some evidence suggesting that an antenatal diagnosis of TGA may reduce mortality. This is important for the health economic analysis because TGA is an anomaly that would not normally be identifiable with a four chamber view, but it would be with the addition of a view of the outflow tracts and, therefore, the model particularly focuses on the cost-effectiveness of antenatal diagnosis of TGA.

The basic decision tree structure is illustrated in Figure E.1. At 20 weeks of gestation women receive either a four chamber view ultrasound scan or four chamber plus outflow tracts view ultrasound scan. Women with a positive result on either scan will then be referred for fetal echocardiography to confirm diagnosis and guide subsequent treatment. If the diagnosis is confirmed then the woman has the option to terminate or continue the pregnancy. If the woman chooses to continue the pregnancy then she will either give birth to a live baby or suffer a pregnancy loss. A proportion of babies born with cardiac malformations will have TGA and they may survive or die.

E.2 Model parameters

The parameter values used in the baseline model are shown in Tables E.1 to E.4.

Table E.1 Population characteristics

Characteristic	Value	Source	Notes
Population	1000		Prevalence data are often given as rates per 1000 head of population and the ICER from the model is not affected by population size.
Prevalence of cardiac malformations at 20 weeks of gestation	0.0032	Wren et al. (2003)[414]	Wren's value of 3.2% is for prevalence at birth.[a]
Proportion of cardiac malformations that are TGA in women with diabetes	0.144	Wren et al. (2003)[414]	
Pregnancy loss after 20 weeks of gestation (no cardiac malformations present)	0.0115	Ritchie et al. (2004)[416]	Derived from survival probability from second trimester to birth.
Pregnancy loss after 20 weeks of gestation (cardiac malformations present)	0.0405	Ritchie et al. (2004)[416]	Derived from survival probability from second trimester to birth.

ICER = incremental cost-effectiveness ratio; TGA = transposition of the great arteries.

[a] The prevalence of cardiac malformations at 20 weeks of gestation may be slightly higher than at birth if terminations and fetal death are higher in affected than non-affected pregnancies. This is likely to represent a small bias in the model against the four chamber plus outflow tracts view, but this is not important if the four chamber plus outflow tracts view is shown to be cost-effective.

Table E.2 Costs

Characteristic	Cost	Source	Notes
Four chamber view ultrasound scan	£34	NHS Reference Costs 2005–06	Mean value for a maternity ultrasound
Four chamber plus outflow tracts view ultrasound scan	£46	GDG estimate	Based on estimate that appointment slots would be 20 minutes compared with 15 minutes for a four chamber view.[a]
Fetal echocardiography	£62	NHS Referemce Costs 2005–06	Mean value for an echocardiogram
Termination of pregnancy	£492	NHS Tariff 2006/07	Cost of a surgical termination
Birth	£3,000	NHS Reference Costs 2003; NHS General Medical Services Revised Fees and Allowances 2003–04	A weighted average including birth, GP fees, other maternity events, outpatient visits, neonatal care, tests

[a] The cost of the four chamber plus outflow tracts view does not take into account the fact that the number of equivocal scans is likely to increase.

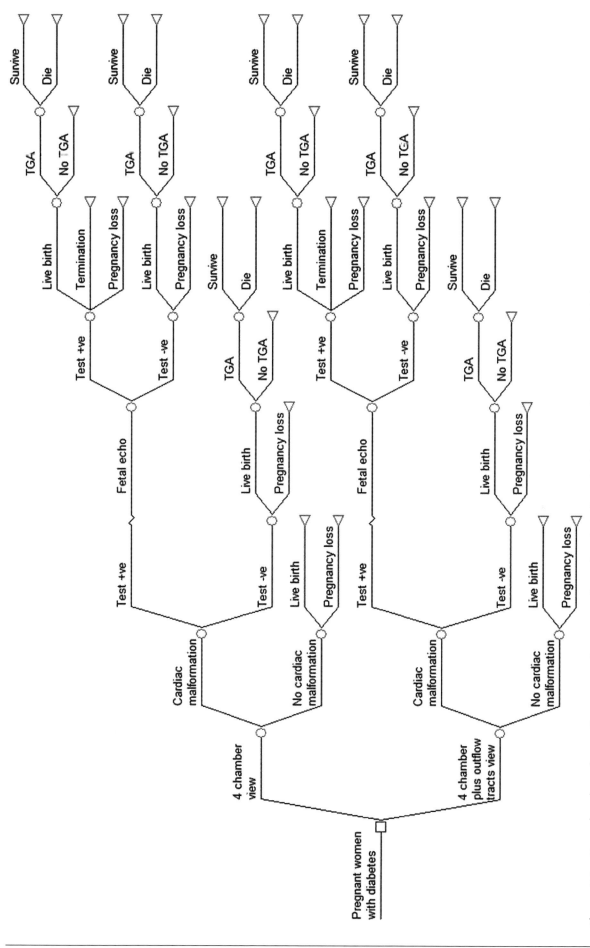

Figure E.1 Four chamber plus outflow tracts view versus four chamber view decision tree for women with diabetes; TGA = transposition of the great arteries

Table E.3 Test characteristics

Characteristic	Value	Source	Notes
Four chamber view sensitivity	0.73	Smith *et al.* (1997)[275] (see www.d4pro.com/IDM/site/idm4cr.pdf)	
Four chamber view specificity	1.00	Smith *et al.* (1997)[275]	
Four chamber plus outflow tracts view sensitivity	0.82	Smith *et al.* (1997)[275]	
Four chamber plus outflow tracts view specificity	1.00	Smith *et al.* (1997)[275]	
TGA proportion of malformations only detectable on four chamber plus outflow tracts view	0.36	Ogge *et al.* (2006)[417]	In 58 cases of congenital cardiac defects, 14 were only usually diagnosable with outflow-tract view. Of these, five were TGA.[a]
Fetal echocardiography sensitivity	0.92	Pan *et al.*[440]	
Fetal echocardiography specificity	0.95	Pan *et al.*[440]	
Termination of pregnancy rate for diagnosis of cardiac malformation	0.25	Ritchie *et al.* (2004)[416]	

TGA = transposition of the great arteries.

[a] Only one TGA was actually detected, giving the four chamber plus outflow tracts view a sensitivity for detecting TGA of only 20%.

Table E.4 Outcomes and quality-adjusted life years

Characteristic	Value	Source	Notes
Life expectancy if TGA treated successfully (years)	76	ONS (2006)	UK life expectancy at birth (2003–05) is 76.6 years for males and 81.0 years for females.
TGA mortality detected antenatally	0.018	Wessex UK (1994–2005), EUROCAT, Bonnet 1988–97,[418] Bonnet 1998–2002,[419] Kumar 1988–96[420]	Results reported in presentation by Wellesley *et al.* (4/226).
TGA mortality detected postnatally	0.166	Wessex UK (1994–2005), EUROCAT, Bonnet 1998–97[418]	Results reported in presentation by Wellesley *et al.* (70/422).
QALY weight successful TGA treatment	1.0		Assumes no long-term morbidity associated with successful TGA treatment.
Annual discount rate	3.5%		Discount rate stipulated by NICE guidelines manual 2007.[23]

QALY = quality-adjusted life year; TGA = transposition of the great arteries.

E.3 Results

With baseline results, the four chamber view is the cheapest strategy for screening for cardiac malformations. As shown in Table E.5, the difference is almost entirely explained by the higher cost of the four chamber plus outflow tracts view ultrasound scan. However, the higher sensitivity of the four chamber plus outflow tracts view results in 1.91 more live births per 1000 pregnancies having detected cardiac malformations antenatally (Table E.6). A proportion of these (36% at baseline) would be TGA and given the baseline assumption about lower mortality for TGA with an antenatal diagnosis this leads to a concomitant 6.86 neonatal deaths averted per 10 000 pregnancies (Table E.7). Following on from these cost and effects the estimated ICER for the four chamber plus outflow tracts view is £3,806 per QALY.

Table E.5 Costs of four chamber and four chamber plus outflow tracts view strategies

Costs	Four chamber view	Four chamber plus outflow tracts view
Cardiac scan	£34,000	£46,000
Fetal echocardiogram	£1,448	£1,627
Termination of pregnancy	£2,643	£2,969
Birth	£2,947,250	£2,945,344
Total cost	£2,985,342	£2,995,940
Cost per woman	£2,985	£2,996

Table E.6 Outcomes of four chamber and four chamber plus outflow tracts view strategies

Outcomes	Four chamber view	Four chamber plus outflow tracts view
Pregnancy loss	12.21	12.18
Termination of pregnancy	5.37	6.04
Healthy live birth	956.87	956.87
Live birth, cardiac malformation detected	15.47	17.37
Live birth, cardiac malformation not detected	10.08	7.54

Table E.7 Incremental cost-effectiveness of four chamber plus outflow tracts view

Incremental values	Four chamber plus outflow tracts view
Costs	£10,598
Antenatal diagnosis of cardiac malformations	1.91
Antenatal diagnosis of TGA	0.686
Neonatal deaths averted	0.102
QALYs	2.784
ICER	£3,806 per QALY

ICER = incremental cost-effectiveness ratio; QALY = quality-adjusted life year; TGA = transposition of the great arteries.

E.4   Sensitivity analysis

A number of one-way sensitivity analyses were undertaken to assess to what extent uncertainty over certain parameter values was likely to be important in interpreting the baseline results. The results of the sensitivity analyses are presented in Figures E.2 to E.7. A £30,000 cost per QALY threshold is indicated in each of the figures.

E.5   Discussion

With baseline values the model suggests that the four chamber plus outflow tracts view is cost-effective for screening for cardiac malformations in pregnant women with diabetes compared with the four chamber view. Although the higher costs of the four chamber plus outflow tracts view make it more expensive than the four chamber view the ICER of £3,806 is substantially below the £20,000 per QALY threshold used by NICE as a willingness to pay for cost-effectiveness. NICE states that interventions with a cost per QALY of less than £20,000 should be considered cost-effective, but there must be 'strong reasons' for considering any intervention to be cost-effective if the cost per QALY is greater than £30,000.[23]

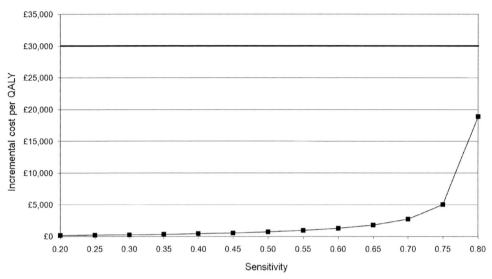

Figure E.2   Incremental cost per QALY, varying sensitivity of the four chamber view

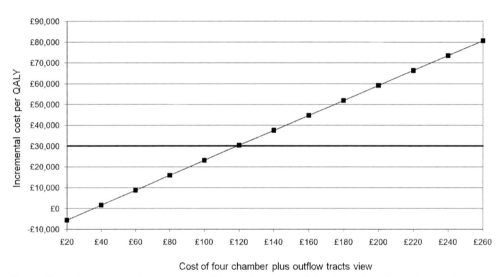

Figure E.3   Incremental cost per QALY, varying cost of the four chamber plus outflow tracts view

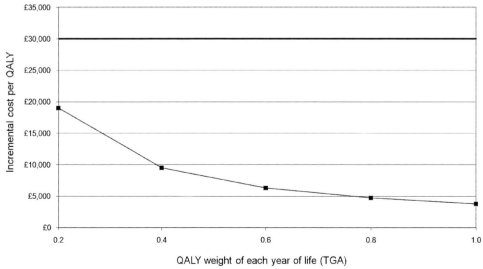

Figure E.4   Incremental cost per QALY, varying QALY weight of each baby treated for transposition of the great arteries (TGA)

The model assumes that TGA is the only cardiac malformation where an antenatal diagnosis confers a benefit in terms of improved health outcomes for the woman and/or the baby. The baseline parameter values give a TGA prevalence of approximately 4.6 per 1000 pregnancies in women with diabetes. With the baseline assumptions for perinatal mortality in relation to TGA detected antenatally or not, one neonatal death would be averted for every seven TGA malformations detected. If a screening strategy involving a four chamber plus outflow tracts view detected all TGA malformations then the number of pregnant women with diabetes needed to screen with the four chamber plus outflow tracts view rather than the four chamber view to avert one neonatal death would be 1466.

The literature does not generally provide test sensitivity and specificity for individual cardiac malformations; instead it gives a value for detecting any cardiac malformation. Hence, the improved sensitivity of the four chamber plus outflow tracts view compared with the four chamber view occurs because the four chamber plus outflow tracts view detects additional malformations that cannot usually be observed with the four chamber view (the sensitivity of detecting TGA with the four chamber view is 0%). The model follows the literature in using overall sensitivities and specificities and it is this which generates the additional 1.91 antenatal diagnoses of cardiac malformations using the four chamber plus outflow tracts view. The model assumption is that these additional diagnoses are for malformations that would not normally be detectable with a four chamber view, but would be detectable with a view of the outflow tracts. However, as TGA is not the only malformation falling into this category, the model does not assume that all additional antenatal diagnoses are TGA. It uses published data[417] to estimate that 36% of the additional diagnoses would be TGA, which leads to the model result that a four chamber plus outflow tracts view would identify 0.686 TGA per 1000 pregnant women with diabetes. It should be noted that, although this is only 15% of the total TGA malformations present in the population, the four chamber plus outflow tracts view still appears cost-effective with such a low detection rate. However, it may be appropriate to assume a relatively low detection rate as published data reported that only one out of five TGA malformations was detected with a four chamber plus outflow tracts view.[417] With the baseline detection rate used in the model it would be necessary to screen approximately 9800 pregnant women with diabetes using a four chamber plus outflow tracts view to avert one neonatal death.

The baseline results suggest that the detection rate threshold for TGA for the four chamber plus outflow tracts view to achieve cost-effectiveness is quite low. The one-way sensitivity analyses indicate thresholds for cost-effectiveness for other parameter values. Figure E.2 suggests that the four chamber plus outflow tracts view would be cost-effective even if the test sensitivity for the four chamber view was within two percentage points of the sensitivity of the four chamber plus outflow tracts view. As the four chamber view sensitivity approaches that of the four chamber plus outflow tracts view there comes a point where there is only very limited added value in terms of detecting cardiac malformations using the four chamber plus outflow tracts view. The key issue here is the difference in test sensitivity between the four chamber view and the four chamber plus outflow tracts view, rather than the absolute values. The one-way sensitivity analysis of the sensitivity of the four chamber view is undertaken holding the sensitivity of the four chamber plus outflow tracts view constant at 82%. The sensitivity analysis suggests that the four chamber plus outflow tracts view requires a sensitivity that is at least four percentage points higher than the sensitivity for the four chamber view in order to achieve cost-effectiveness.

Figure E.3 shows that the cost-effectiveness of the four chamber plus outflow tracts view compared with the four chamber view is quite sensitive to the costs of screening. Again it is the difference between screening costs using the four chamber view and the four chamber plus outflow tracts view that is important, rather than the absolute costs of the screening tests. However, the cost of the four chamber plus outflow tracts view would have to be £120 (for an incremental screening cost of £86) and well above the baseline estimate before the four chamber view would be preferred on cost-effectiveness grounds.

Figures E.4 and E.5 show that the cost-effectiveness of the four chamber plus outflow tracts view is not sensitive to assumptions about QALYs or life expectancy within plausible ranges. Baseline values suggest that the incremental costs of the four chamber plus outflow tracts view are £3,806 in a population of 1000 pregnant women with diabetes. Therefore, only 0.13 incremental QALYs are needed to generate a cost per QALY of £30,000. With baseline values this is approximately 1.3 QALYs per neonatal death averted.

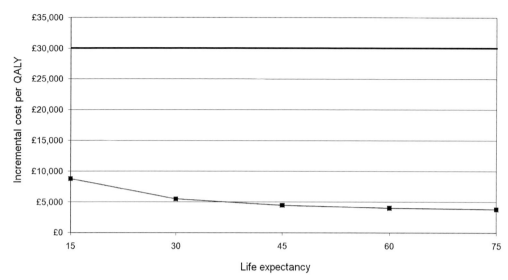

Figure E.5 Incremental cost per QALY, varying life expectancy

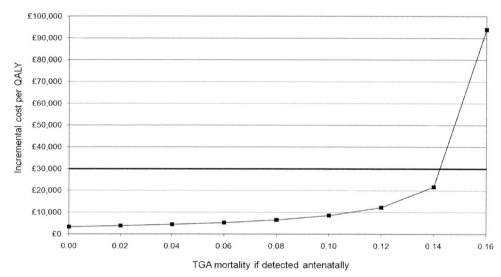

Figure E6 Incremental cost per QALY, varying mortality with diagnosis of transposition of the great arteries (TGA)

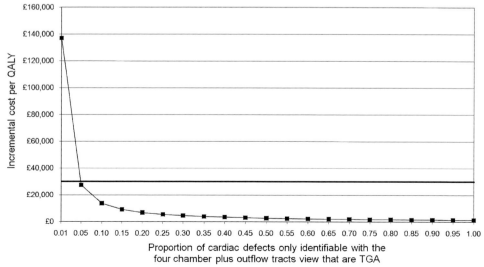

Figure E.7 Incremental cost per QALY, varying the proportion of cardiac malformations only identifiable with four chamber plus outflow tracts view that are transposition of the great arteries (TGA)

Figure E.6 shows that the results of the model are sensitive to the assumptions made in relation to the positive impact that an antenatal diagnosis of TGA has on mortality. However, the 'best' estimate used for baseline mortality for antenatally detected TGA mortality (1.8%) is comfortably below the threshold (14%) needed to yield a cost per QALY of £30,000.

Finally, Figure E.7 shows that cost-effectiveness is sensitive to the proportion of additional cardiac malformations detected with the four chamber plus outflow tracts view that are assumed to be TGA. However, this relates to the earlier discussion about the overall detection rate of TGA. Given the way the model is constructed, a lower proportion of TGA malformations implies a lower detection rate. Here, TGA would have to account for less than 5% of the additional cardiac malformations detected for the ICER for four chamber plus outflow tracts view to exceed £30,000 per QALY.

The results of the sensitivity analyses suggest that the cost-effectiveness of screening for cardiac malformations based on the four chamber plus outflow tracts view is robust and is unaffected by one-way variation of model parameters within plausible ranges.

The model only addresses cost-effectiveness of screening for cardiac malformations in terms of the impact that antenatal diagnosis has on improved health outcomes. It does not address the 'value' or cost-effectiveness of such screening in providing information to inform a decision about termination of pregnancy. Clearly, the cost-effectiveness of termination of pregnancy is problematic ethically and it does not readily fit into a QALY paradigm.

References

1.	Office for National Statistics. *Key Population and Vital Statistics 2005. Local and Health Authority Areas*. No. Series VS, No 32. Basingstoke: Palgrave Macmillan; 2007.

2.	CEMACH. *Confidential Enquiry into Maternal and Child Health: Pregnancy in Women with Type 1 and Type 2 Diabetes in 2002–03, England, Wales and Northern Ireland*. London: CEMACH; 2005.

3.	King H. Epidemiology of glucose intolerance and gestational diabetes in women of childbearing age. *Diabetes Care* 1998;21(Suppl 2): B9–13.

4.	Casson IF. Outcomes of pregnancy in insulin dependent diabetic women: results of a five year population cohort study. *British Medical Journal* 1997;315:275–8.

5.	Hawthorne G. Prospective population based survey of outcome of pregnancy in diabetic women: results of the Northern Diabetic Pregnancy Audit, 1994. *British Medical Journal* 1997;315:279–81.

6.	NHS Executive. *Clinical Guidelines: Using Clinical Guidelines to Improve Patient Care Within the NHS*. London: HMSO; 1996.

7.	National Institute for Clinical Excellence. *Type 1 Diabetes: Diagnosis and Management of Type 1 Diabetes in Children, Young People and Adults*. London: NICE; 2004.

8.	National Institute for Health and Clinical Excellence. *Type 2 Diabetes: the Management of Type 2 Diabetes (Update)*. London: NICE [publication expected April 2008].

9.	National Collaborating Centre for Women's and Children's Health. *Antenatal Care: Routine Care for the Health Pregnant Woman (2008 Update)*. 2nd ed. London: RCOG Press; 2008.

10.	National Collaborating Centre for Women's and Children's Health. *Intrapartum Care: Care of Healthy Women and Their Babies During Childbirth*. London: RCOG Press; 2007.

11.	National Collaborating Centre for Primary Care. *Postnatal Care: Routine Postnatal Care of Women and Their Babies*. London: NICE; 2006.

12.	Royal College of Obstetricians and Gynaecologists. *Induction of Labour*. London: RCOG Press; 1998.

13.	National Collaborating Centre for Women's and Children's Health. *Caesarean Section*. London: RCOG Press; 2004.

14.	National Insitute for Clinical Excellence. *Guidance on the Use of Continuous Subcutaneous Insulin Infusion for Diabetes*. London: NICE; 2003.

15.	National Institute for Clinical Excellence. *Guidance on The Use of Glitazones for the Treatment of Type 2 Diabetes*. London: NICE; 2003.

17.	National Institute for Clinical Excellence. *Guidance on the Use of Long-Acting Insulin Analogues for the Treatment of Diabetes – Insulin Glargine*. London: NICE; 2002.

18.	National Institute for Clinical Excellence. *Guidance on the Use of Patient-Education Models for Diabetes*. London: NICE; 2003.

19.	National Institute for Health and Clinical Excellence. *Improving the Nutrition of Pregnant and Breastfeeding Mothers and Children in Low-Income Households*. NICE public health guidance 11. London: NICE; 2008.

20.	Department of Health. *National Service Framework for Diabetes: Standards*. London: Department of Health; 2002.

21.	National Institute for Clinical Excellence. *Guideline Development Methods: Information for National Collaborating Centres and Guideline Developers*. London: NICE; 2005.

22.	National Institute for Health and Clinical Excellence. *The Guidelines Manual 2006*. London: NICE; 2006.

23.	National Institute for Health and Clinical Excellence. *The Guidelines Manual 2007*. London: NICE; 2007.

24.	Oxman AD, Sackett DL and Guyatt GH. Users' guides to the medical literature. I. How to get started. The Evidence-Based Medicine Working Group. *JAMA: the journal of the American Medical Association* 1993;270(17):2093–5.

25.	Guyatt GH, Sackett DL and Cook DJ. Users' guides to the medical literature. II. How to use an article about therapy or prevention. A. Are the results of the study valid? Evidence-Based Medicine Working Group. *JAMA: the journal of the American Medical Association* 1993;270(21):2598–601.

26.	Guyatt GH, Sackett DL and Cook DJ. Users' guides to the medical literature. II. How to use an article about therapy or prevention. B. What were the results and will they help me in caring for my patients? Evidence-Based Medicine Working Group. *JAMA: the journal of the American Medical Association* 1994;271(1):59–63.

27.	Jaeschke R, Guyatt G and Sackett DL. Users' guides to the medical literature. III. How to use an article about a diagnostic test. A. Are the results of the study valid? Evidence-Based Medicine Working Group. *JAMA: the journal of the American Medical Association* 1994;271(5):389–91.

28.	Jaeschke R, Guyatt GH and Sackett DL. Users' guides to the medical literature. III. How to use an article about a diagnostic test. B. What are the results and will they help me in caring for my patients? The Evidence-Based Medicine Working Group. *JAMA: the journal of the American Medical Association* 1994;271(9):703–7.

29.	Sackett DL, Straus SE, Richardson WS, *et al. Evidence-based medicine. How to practice and teach EBM*. 2nd ed. Edinburgh: Churchill Livingstone; 2000.

30.	Scottish Intercollegiate Guidelines Network. *A guideline developers' handbook*. No. 50. Edinburgh: SIGN; 2001.

31.	World Health Organization and Department of Noncommunicable Disease Surveillance. *Definition, diagnosis and classification of diabetes mellitus and its complications. Report of a WHO consultation. Part 1: diagnosis and classification of diabetes mellitus*. Geneva: World Health Organization; 1999.

32.	CEMACH. *Confidential enquiry into maternal and child health: Maternity services in 2002 for women with type 1 and type 2 diabetes*. London: RCOG Press on behalf of CEMACH; 2004.

33.	Confidential Enquiry into Maternal and Child Health. *Diabetes in pregnancy: are we providing the best care? Findings of a national enquiry: England, Wales and Northern Ireland*. London: CEMACH; 2007.

34.	Drummond MF, Sculpher M, Torrance GW, *et al. Methods for the economic evaluation of health care programmes*. 3rd ed. Oxford: Oxford University Press; 2005.

35. Suhonen L, Hiilesmaa V and Teramo K. Glycaemic control during early pregnancy and fetal malformations in women with type I diabetes mellitus. *Diabetologia* 2000;43(1):79–82.

36. Kitzmiller JL, Gavin LA, Gin GD, *et al.* Preconception care of diabetes. Glycemic control prevents congenital anomalies. *JAMA: the journal of the American Medical Association* 1991;265(6):731–6.

37. Dornhorst A and Frost G. Nutritional management in diabetic pregnancy: a time for reason not dogma. In: Hod M, Jovanovic L, Di Renzo GC, de Leiva A, Langer O, eds. *Diabetes and Pregnancy*. London: Taylor & Francis Group; 2003. p. 340–58.

38. Brand-Miller J, Hayne S, Petocz P, *et al.* Low-glycemic index diets in the management of diabetes: a meta-analysis of randomized controlled trials. *Diabetes Care* 2003;26(8):2261–7.

39. Kaplan JS, Iqbal S, England BG, *et al.* Is pregnancy in diabetic women associated with folate deficiency? *Diabetes Care* 1999;22(7):1017–21.

40. Gillmer MD, Maresh M, Beard RW, *et al.* Low energy diets in the treatment of gestational diabetes. *Acta Endocrinologica, Supplementum* 1986;277:44–9.

41. Ray JG, Vermeulen MJ, Shapiro JL, *et al.* Maternal and neonatal outcomes in pregestational and gestational diabetes mellitus, and the influence of maternal obesity and weight gain: The DEPOSIT study. *QJM: monthly journal of the Association of Physicians* 2001;94(7):347–56.

42. Moore LL, Singer MR, Bradlee ML, *et al.* A prospective study of the risk of congenital defects associated with maternal obesity and diabetes mellitus. *Epidemiology* 2000;11(6):689–94.

43. Kieffer EC, Tabaei BP, Carman WJ, *et al.* The influence of maternal weight and glucose tolerance on infant birthweight in Latino mother-infant pairs. *American Journal of Public Health* 2006;96(12):2201–8.

44. Stotland NE, Cheng YW, Hopkins LM, *et al.* Gestational weight gain and adverse neonatal outcome among term infants. *Obstetrics and Gynecology* 2006;108(3 Pt 1):635–43.

45. Ricart W, Lopez J, Mozas J, *et al.* Body mass index has a greater impact on pregnancy outcomes than gestational hyperglycaemia. *Diabetologia* 2005;48(9):1736–42.

46. Moore H, Summerbell C, Hooper L, *et al.* Dietary advice for the prevention of type 2 diabetes mellitus in adults. (Cochrane Review). In: *Cochrane Database of Systematic Reviews*. Chichester: Wiley Interscience; 2005.

47. Ceysens G, Rouiller D and Boulvain M. Exercise for diabetic pregnant women. (Cochrane Review). In: *Cochrane Database of Systematic Reviews*. Chichester: Wiley Interscience; 2006.

48. Expert Advisory Group. *Folic acid and the prevention of neural tube defects*. Department of Health; Scottish Office, Home and Health Department; Welsh Office; Department of Health and Social Services, Northern Ireland; 1992.

49. The Diabetes Control and Complications Trial Research Group. Pregnancy outcomes in the Diabetes Control and Complications Trial. *American Journal of Obstetrics and Gynecology* 1996;174(4):1343–53.

50. Goldman JA, Dicker D, Feldberg D, *et al.* Pregnancy outcome in patients with insulin-dependent diabetes mellitus with preconceptional diabetic control: a comparative study. *American Journal of Obstetrics and Gynecology* 1986;155(2):293–7.

51. Steel JM, Johnstone FD, Hepburn DA, *et al.* Can prepregnancy care of diabetic women reduce the risk of abnormal babies? *British Medical Journal* 1990;301(6760):1070–4.

52. Fuhrmann K, Reiher H, Semmler K, *et al.* The effect of intensified conventional insulin therapy before and during pregnancy on the malformation rate in offspring of diabetic mothers. *Experimental and Clinical Endocrinology* 1984;83(2):173–7.

53. Fuhrmann K. Treatment of pregnant insulin-dependent diabetic women. *Acta Endocrinologica Supplementum* 1986;277:74–6.

54. Diabetes and Pregnancy Group F. French multicentric survey of outcome of pregnancy in women with pregestational diabetes. *Diabetes Care* 2003;26(11):2990–3.

55. Greene MF, Hare JW, Cloherty JP, *et al.* First-trimester hemoglobin A1 and risk for major malformation and spontaneous abortion in diabetic pregnancy. *Teratology* 1989;39(3):225–31.

56. Ylinen K, Aula P, Stenman UH, *et al.* Risk of minor and major fetal malformations in diabetics with high haemoglobin A1c values in early pregnancy. *British Medical Journal* 1984;289(6441):345–6.

57. Miller E, Hare JW, Cloherty JP, *et al.* Elevated maternal hemoglobin A1c in early pregnancy and major congenital anomalies in infants of diabetic mothers. *New England Journal of Medicine* 1981;304(22):1331–4.

58. Lucas MJ, Leveno KJ, Williams ML, *et al.* Early pregnancy glycosylated hemoglobin, severity of diabetes, and fetal malformations. *American Journal of Obstetrics and Gynecology* 1989;161(2):426–31.

59. Key TC, Giuffrida R and Moore TR. Predictive value of early pregnancy glycohemoglobin in the insulin-treated diabetic patient. [Erratum appears in *Am J Obstet Gynecol* 1987;157(6):1460]. *American Journal of Obstetrics and Gynecology* 1987;156(5):1096–100.

60. Rosenn B, Miodovnik M, Combs CA, *et al.* Glycemic thresholds for spontaneous abortion and congenital malformations in insulin-dependent diabetes mellitus. *Obstetrics and Gynecology* 1994;84(4):515–20.

61. Mills JL, Simpson JL, Driscoll SG, *et al.* Incidence of spontaneous abortion among normal women and insulin-dependent diabetic women whose pregnancies were identified within 21 days of conception. *New England Journal of Medicine* 1988;319(25):1617–23.

62. Rosenn B, Miodovnik M, Combs CA, *et al.* Pre-conception management of insulin-dependent diabetes: improvement of pregnancy outcome. *Obstetrics and Gynecology* 1991;77(6):846–9.

63. Dicker D, Feldberg D, Samuel N, *et al.* Spontaneous abortion in patients with insulin-dependent diabetes mellitus: the effect of preconceptional diabetic control. *American Journal of Obstetrics and Gynecology* 1988;158(5):1161–4.

64. Miodovnik M, Mimouni F, Tsang RC, *et al.* Glycemic control and spontaneous abortion in insulin-dependent diabetic women. *Obstetrics and Gynecology* 1986;68(3):366–9.

65. Miodovnik M, Skillman C, Holroyde JC, *et al.* Elevated maternal glycohemoglobin in early pregnancy and spontaneous abortion among insulin-dependent diabetic women. *American Journal of Obstetrics and Gynecology* 1985;153(4):439–42.

66. Jensen DM, Damm P, Moelsted-Pedersen L, *et al.* Outcomes in type 1 diabetic pregnancies: a nationwide, population-based study. *Diabetes Care* 2004;27(12):2819–23.

67. Gold AE, Reilly R, Little J, *et al.* The effect of glycemic control in the pre-conception period and early pregnancy on birth weight in women with IDDM. *Diabetes Care* 1998;21(4):535–8.

68. Rosenn BM, Miodovnik M, Holcberg G, *et al.* Hypoglycemia: the price of intensive insulin therapy for pregnant women with insulin-dependent diabetes mellitus. *Obstetrics and Gynecology* 1995;85(3):417–22.

69. DAFNE Study Group. Training in flexible, intensive insulin management to enable dietary freedom in people with type 1 diabetes: dose adjustment for normal eating (DAFNE) randomised controlled trial. *British Medical Journal* 2002;325:746–8.

70. Diabetes Control and Complications Trial (DCCT) Research Group. The effect of intensive treatment of diabetes on the development and progression of long-term complications in insulin-dependent diabetes mellitus. *New England Journal of Medicine* 1993;329(14):977–86.

71. Gutzin SJ, Kozer E, Magee LA, *et al.* The safety of oral hypoglycemic agents in the first trimester of pregnancy: A meta-analysis. *Canadian Journal of Clinical Pharmacology* 2003;10(4):179–83.

72. Hawthorne G. Metformin use and diabetic pregnancy – has its time come? *Diabetic Medicine* 2006;23(3):223–7.

73. Gilbert C, Valois M and Koren G. Pregnancy outcome after first-trimester exposure to metformin: a meta-analysis. *Fertility and Sterility* 2006;86(3):658–63.

74. Langer O, Conway DL, Berkus MD, *et al.* A comparison of glyburide and insulin in women with gestational diabetes mellitus. *New England Journal of Medicine* 2000;343(16):1134–8.

75. Elder AT. Contraindications to use of metformin. Age and creatinine clearance need to be taken into consideration. *British Medical Journal* 2003;326(7392):762.

76. Ekpebegh CO, Coetzee EJ, van der ML, *et al.* A 10-year retrospective analysis of pregnancy outcome in pregestational Type 2 diabetes: comparison of insulin and oral glucose-lowering agents. *Diabetic Medicine* 2007;24(3):253–8.

77. Briggs GG, Freeman RK and Yaffe SJ. *Drugs in Pregnancy and Lactation. A Reference Guide to Fetal and Neonatal Risk.* 7th ed. Philadelphia: Lippincott, Williams and Wilkins; 2005.

78. Joint Formulary Committee. *British National Formulary.* 53rd ed. London: British Medical Association and Royal Pharmaceutical Society of Great Britain; 2007.

79. Mathiesen E, Kinsley B, McCance D, *et al.* Maternal hyperglycemia and glycemic control in pregnancy: a randomized trial comparing insulin aspart with human insulin in 322 subjects with type 1 diabetes. *Diabetes* 2006;55(Suppl 1):A40.

80. Jovanovic L, Howard C, Pettitt D, *et al.* Insulin aspart vs. regular human insulin in basal/bolus therapy for patients with gestational diabetes mellitus: safety and efficacy. *Diabetologia* 2005;48(Suppl 1):A317.

81. Kinsley BT, Al-Agha R, Murray S, *et al* R. A comparison of soluble human insulin vs rapid acting insulin analogue in type 1 diabetes mellitus in pregnancy. *Diabetes* 2005;54(Suppl 1):A461 (Abstract).

82. Balaji V and Seshiah V. Insulin aspart – safe during pregnancy. *Diabetes* 2005;54(Suppl 1):A787 (Abstract).

83. Boskovic R, Feig DS, Derewlany L, *et al.* Transfer of insulin lispro across the human placenta: In vitro perfusion studies. *Diabetes Care* 2003;26(5):1390–4.

84. Plank J, Siebenhofer A, Berghold A, *et al.* Systematic review and meta-analysis of short-acting insulin analogues in patients with diabetes mellitus. *Archives of Internal Medicine* 2005;165(12):1337–44.

85. Mecacci F, Carignani L, Cioni R, *et al.* Maternal metabolic control and perinatal outcome in women with gestational diabetes treated with regular or lispro insulin: comparison with non-diabetic pregnant women. *European Journal of Obstetrics, Gynecology and Reproductive Biology* 2003;111(1):19–24.

86. Persson B, Swahn ML, Hjertberg R, *et al.* Insulin lispro therapy in pregnancies complicated by type 1 diabetes mellitus. *Diabetes Research and Clinical Practice* 2002;58(2):115–21.

87. Simmons D. The utility and efficacy of the new insulins in the management of diabetes and pregnancy. *Current Diabetes Reports* 2002;2(4):331–6.

88. Kitzmiller JL and Jovanovic L. Insulin therapy in pregnancy. In: Hod M, Jovanovic L, Di Renzo GC, de Leiva A, Langer O, eds. *Textbook of Diabetes and Pregnancy.* London: Martin Dunitz; 2003. p. 359–78.

89. Garg SK, Frias JP, Anil S, *et al.* Insulin lispro therapy in pregnancies complicated by type 1 diabetes: glycemic control and maternal and fetal outcomes. *Endocrine Practice* 2003;9(3):187–93.

90. Masson EA, Patmore JE, Brash PD, *et al.* Pregnancy outcome in Type 1 diabetes mellitus treated with insulin lispro (Humalog). *Diabetic Medicine* 2003;20(1):46–50.

91. Wyatt JW, Frias JL, Hoyme HE, *et al.* Congenital anomaly rate in offspring of mothers with diabetes treated with insulin lispro during pregnancy. *Diabetic Medicine* 2005;22(6):803–7.

92. Cypryk K, Sobczak M, Pertynska-Marczewska M, *et al.* Pregnancy complications and perinatal outcome in diabetic women treated with Humalog (insulin lispro) or regular human insulin during pregnancy. *Medical Science Monitor* 2004;10(2):PI29–32.

93. Gallen IW and Jaap AJ. Insulin glargine use in pregnancy is not associated with adverse maternal or fetal outcomes. *Diabetes* 2006;55(Suppl 1):A417–1804-P (Abstract).

94. Poyhonen-Alho M, Saltevo J, Ronnemaa T, *et al.* Insulin glargine during pregnancy. *Diabetes* 2006;55(Suppl 1):A417 (Abstract).

95. Price N, Bartlett C and Gillmer MD. Use of insulin glargine during pregnancy: A case–control pilot study. *BJOG: an international journal of obstetrics and gynaecology* 2007;114(4):453–7.

96. Di CG, Volpe L, Lencioni C, *et al.* Use of insulin glargine during the first weeks of pregnancy in five type 1 diabetic women. *Diabetes Care* 2005;28(4):982–3.

97. Woolderink JM, van Loon AJ, Storms F, *et al.* Use of insulin glargine during pregnancy in seven type 1 diabetic women. *Diabetes Care* 2005;28(10):2594–5.

98. Graves DE, White JC and Kirk JK. The use of insulin glargine with gestational diabetes mellitus. *Diabetes Care* 2006;29(2):471–2.

99. Al-Shaikh AA. Pregnant women with type 1 diabetes mellitus treated by glargine insulin. *Saudi Medical Journal* 2006;27(4):563–5.

100. Holstein A, Plaschke A and Egberts EH. Use of insulin glargine during embryogenesis in a pregnant woman with Type 1 diabetes. *Diabetic Medicine* 2003;20(9):779–80.

101. Caronna S, Cioni F, Dall'Aglio E, *et al.* Pregnancy and the long-acting insulin analogue: A case study. *Acta Bio-Medica de l Ateneo Parmense* 2006;77(1):24–6, 62.

102. Conway DL and Longer O. Selecting antihypertensive therapy in the pregnant woman with diabetes mellitus. *Journal of Maternal-Fetal Medicine* 2000;9(1):66–9.

103. Hod M, van Dijk DJ, Karp M, *et al.* Diabetic nephropathy and pregnancy: the effect of ACE inhibitors prior to pregnancy on fetomaternal outcome. *Nephrology Dialysis Transplantation* 1995;10(12):2328–33.

104. Bar J, Chen R, Schoenfeld A, *et al.* Pregnancy outcome in patients with insulin dependent diabetes mellitus and diabetic nephropathy treated with ACE inhibitors before pregnancy. *Journal of Pediatric Endocrinology* 1999;12(5):659–65.

105. Cooper WO, Hernandez-Diaz S, Arbogast PG, *et al.* Major congenital malformations after first-trimester exposure to ACE inhibitors. *New England Journal of Medicine* 2006;354(23):2443–51.

106. Lip GY, Churchill D, Beevers M, *et al.* Angiotensin-converting-enzyme inhibitors in early pregnancy. *Lancet* 1997;350(9089):1446–7.

107. Steffensen FH, Nielsen GL, Sorensen HT, *et al*. Pregnancy outcome with ACE-inhibitor use in early pregnancy. *Lancet* 1998;351(9102):596.

108. Centers for Disease Control and Prevention (CDC). Postmarketing surveillance for angiotensin-converting enzyme inhibitor use during the first trimester of pregnancy--United States, Canada, and Israel, 1987–1995. *MMWR - Morbidity and Mortality Weekly Report* 1997;46(11):240–2.

109. Bar J, Hod M and Merlob P. Angiotensin converting enzyme inhibitors use in the first trimester of pregnancy. *International Journal of Risk and Safety in Medicine* 1997;10(1):23–6.

110. Magee LA, Schick B, Donnenfeld AE, *et al*. The safety of calcium channel blockers in human pregnancy: a prospective, multicenter cohort study. *American Journal of Obstetrics and Gynecology* 1996;174(3):823–8.

111. Belfort MA, Anthony J, Buccimazza A, *et al*. Hemodynamic changes associated with intravenous infusion of the calcium antagonist verapamil in the treatment of severe gestational proteinuric hypertension. *Obstetrics and Gynecology* 1990;75(6):970–4.

112. Holing EV, Beyer CS, Brown ZA, *et al*. Why don't women with diabetes plan their pregnancies? *Diabetes Care* 1998;21(6):889–95.

113. Janz NK, Herman WH, Becker MP, *et al*. Diabetes and pregnancy. Factors associated with seeking pre-conception care. *Diabetes Care* 1995;18(2):157–65.

114. St James PJ, Younger MD, Hamilton BD, *et al*. Unplanned pregnancies in young women with diabetes. An analysis of psychosocial factors. *Diabetes Care* 1993;16(12):1572–8.

115. Casele HL and Laifer SA. Factors influencing preconception control of glycemia in diabetic women. *Archives of Internal Medicine* 1998;158(12):1321–4.

116. Harris K and Campbell E. The plans in unplanned pregnancy: Secondary gain and the partnership. *British Journal of Medical Psychology* 1999;72(1):105–20.

117. Barrett G and Wellings K. What is a 'planned' pregnancy? Empirical data from a British study. *Social Science and Medicine* 2002;55(4):545–57.

118. Charron-Prochownik D, Sereika SM, Falsetti D, *et al*. Knowledge, attitudes and behaviors related to sexuality and family planning in adolescent women with and without diabetes. *Pediatric Diabetes* 2006;7(5):267–73.

119. Charron-Prochownik D, Sereika SM, Wang SL, *et al*. Reproductive health and preconception counseling awareness in adolescents with diabetes: what they don't know can hurt them. *Diabetes Educator* 2006;32(2):235–42.

120. Feig DS, Cleave B and Tomlinson G. Long-term effects of a diabetes and pregnancy program: does the education last? *Diabetes Care* 2006;29(3):526–30.

121. Ray JG, O'Brien TE and Chan WS. Preconception care and the risk of congenital anomalies in the offspring of women with diabetes mellitus: A meta-analysis. *Quarterly Journal of Medicine* 2001;94(8):435–44.

122. Pedersen J. Weight and length at birth of infants of diabetic mothers. *Acta Endocrinologica* 1954;16(4):330–42.

123. Hod M, Rabinerson D and Peled Y. Gestational diabetes mellitus: Is it a clinical entity? *Diabetes Reviews* 1995;3(4):602–13.

124. Scott DA, Loveman E, McIntyre L, *et al*. Screening for gestational diabetes: a systematic review and economic evaluation. *Health Technology Assessment* 2002;6(11):1–172.

125. Dornhorst A, Paterson CM, Nicholls JSD, *et al*. High prevalence of gestational diabetes in women from ethnic minority groups. *Diabetic Medicine* 1992;9:820–5.

126. Ostlund I and Hanson U. Occurrence of gestational diabetes mellitus and the value of different screening indicators for the oral glucose tolerance test. *Acta Obstetricia et Gynecologica Scandinavica* 2003;82(2):103–8.

127. Rayner M, Petersen S, Buckley C, *et al*. *Coronary Heart Disease Statistics: Diabetes Supplement*. London: British Heart Foundation; 2001.

128. Moses R, Griffiths R and Davis W. Gestational diabetes: do all women need to be tested? *Australian and New Zealand Journal of Obstetrics and Gynaecology* 1995;35(4):387–9.

129. Davey RX and Hamblin PS. Selective versus universal screening for gestational diabetes mellitus: an evaluation of predictive risk factors. *Medical Journal of Australia* 2001;174(3):118–21.

130. Doherty DA, Magann EF, Francis J, *et al*. Pre-pregnancy body mass index and pregnancy outcomes. *International Journal of Gynecology and Obstetrics* 2006;95(3):242–7.

131. Keshavarz M, Cheung NW, Babaee GR, *et al*. Gestational diabetes in Iran: incidence, risk factors and pregnancy outcomes. *Diabetes Research and Clinical Practice* 2005;69(3):279–86.

132. Griffin ME, Coffey M, Johnson H, *et al*. Universal vs. risk factor-based screening for gestational diabetes mellitus: detection rates, gestation at diagnosis and outcome. *Diabetic Medicine* 2000;17(1):26–32.

133. Schytte T, Jorgensen LG, Brandslund I, *et al*. The clinical impact of screening for gestational diabetes. *Clinical Chemistry and Laboratory Medicine* 2004;42(9):1036–42.

134. Weijers RN, Bekedam DJ, Goldschmidt HM, *et al*. The clinical usefulness of glucose tolerance testing in gestational diabetes to predict early postpartum diabetes mellitus. *Clinical Chemistry and Laboratory Medicine* 2006;44(1):99–104.

135. Coustan DR, Nelson C, Carpenter MW, *et al*. Maternal age and screening for gestational diabetes: A population-based study. *Obstetrics and Gynecology* 1989;73(4):557–61.

136. Solomon CG, Willett WC, Carey VJ, *et al*. A prospective study of pregravid determinants of gestational diabetes mellitus. *JAMA: the journal of the American Medical Association* 1997;278(13):1078–83.

137. Kim C, Berger DK and Chamany S. Recurrence of gestational diabetes mellitus: a systematic review. *Diabetes Care* 2007;30(5):1314–19.

138. Major CA, DeVeciana M, Weeks J, *et al*. Recurrence of gestational diabetes: who is at risk? *American Journal of Obstetrics and Gynecology* 1998;179(4):1038–42.

139. Spong CY, Guillermo L, Kuboshige J, *et al*. Recurrence of gestational diabetes mellitus: identification of risk factors. *American Journal of Perinatology* 1998;15(1):29–33.

140. Clarke P, Norman P, Coleman MA, *et al*. The introduction of a specific request form for the diagnosis of gestational diabetes (GDM) improves understanding of GDM amongst clinicians but does not increase its detection. *Diabetic Medicine* 2005;22(4):507–8.

141. Agarwal MM, Dhatt GS, Punnose J, *et al*. Gestational diabetes: dilemma caused by multiple international diagnostic criteria. *Diabetic Medicine* 2005;22(12):1731–6.

142. American Diabetes Association. Diagnosis and classification of diabetes mellitus. *Diabetes Care* 2004;27(Suppl 1):S5–10.

143. Tallarigo L, Giampietro O, Penno G, *et al*. Relation of glucose tolerance to complications of pregnancy in nondiabetic women. *New England Journal of Medicine* 1986;315(16):989–92.

144. Weiss PAM, Haeusler M, Tamussino K, *et al.* Can glucose tolerance test predict fetal hyperinsulinism? *BJOG: an international journal of obstetrics and gynaecology* 2000;107(12):1480–5.

145. Sacks DA, Greenspoon JS, bu-Fadil S, *et al.* Toward universal criteria for gestational diabetes: the 75-gram glucose tolerance test in pregnancy. *American Journal of Obstetrics and Gynecology* 1995;172(2 Pt 1):607–14.

146. Mello G, Parretti E, Cioni R, *et al.* The 75-gram glucose load in pregnancy: relation between glucose levels and anthropometric characteristics of infants born to women with normal glucose metabolism. *Diabetes Care* 2003;26(4):1206–10.

147. Sermer M, Naylor CD, Farine D, *et al.* The Toronto Tri-Hospital Gestational Diabetes Project. A preliminary review. *Diabetes Care* 1998;21(Suppl 2):B33–42.

148. Langer O, Brustman L, Anyaegbunam A, *et al.* The significance of one abnormal glucose tolerance test value on adverse outcome in pregnancy. *American Journal of Obstetrics and Gynecology* 1987;157(3):758–63.

149. Jensen DM, Damm P, Sorensen B, *et al.* Proposed diagnostic thresholds for gestational diabetes mellitus according to a 75-g oral glucose tolerance test. Maternal and perinatal outcomes in 3260 Danish women. *Diabetic Medicine* 2003;20(1):51–7.

150. Ostlund I, Hanson U, Bjorklund A, *et al.* Maternal and fetal outcomes if gestational impaired glucose tolerance is not treated. *Diabetes Care* 2003;26(7):2107–11.

151. Saldana TM, Siega-Riz AM, Adair LS, *et al.* The association between impaired glucose tolerance and birth weight among black and white women in central North Carolina. *Diabetes Care* 2003;26(3):656–61.

152. Cheng YW, Esakoff TF, Block-Kurbisch I, *et al.* Screening or diagnostic: markedly elevated glucose loading test and perinatal outcomes. *Journal of Maternal-Fetal and Neonatal Medicine* 2006;19(11):729–34.

153. Crowther CA, Hiller JE, Moss JR, *et al.*; Australian Carbohydrate Intolerance Study in Pregnant Women (ACHOIS) Trial Group. Effect of treatment of gestational diabetes mellitus on pregnancy outcomes. *New England Journal of Medicine* 2005;352(24):2477–86.

154. Dornhorst A and Frost G. The principles of dietary management of gestational diabetes: reflection on current evidence. *Journal of Human Nutrition and Dietetics* 2002;15(2):145–56.

155. de Veciana M, Major CA, Morgan MA, *et al.* Postprandial versus preprandial blood glucose monitoring in women with gestational diabetes mellitus requiring insulin therapy. *New England Journal of Medicine* 1995;333(19):1237–41.

156. Fraser RB. The effect of pregnancy on the normal range of the oral glucose tolerance in Africans. *East African Medical Journal* 1981;58(2):90–4.

157. Fraser RB, Ford FA and Lawrence GF. Insulin sensitivity in third trimester pregnancy. A randomized study of dietary effects. *British Journal of Obstetrics and Gynaecology* 1988;95(3):223–9.

158. Clapp JF 3rd. Effect of dietary carbohydrate on the glucose and insulin response to mixed caloric intake and exercise in both nonpregnant and pregnant women. *Diabetes Care* 1998;21(Suppl 2):B107–12.

159. Clapp JF 3rd. Maternal carbohydrate intake and pregnancy outcome. *Proceedings of the Nutrition Society* 2002;61(1):45–50.

160. Gillen L, Tapsell LC, Martin GS, *et al.* The type and frequency of consumption of carbohydrate-rich foods may play a role in the clinical expression of insulin resistance during pregnancy. *Nutrition and Dietetics: Journal of the Dietitians Association of Australia* 2002;59(2):135–43.

161. Nolan CJ. Improved glucose tolerance in gestational diabetic women on a low fat, high unrefined carbohydrate diet. *Australian and New Zealand Journal of Obstetrics and Gynaecology* 1984;24(3):174–7.

162. Ostman EM, Frid AH, Groop LC, *et al.* A dietary exchange of common bread for tailored bread of low glycaemic index and rich in dietary fibre improved insulin economy in young women with impaired glucose tolerance. *European Journal of Clinical Nutrition* 2006;60(3):334–41.

163. Sacks DA, Chen W, Wolde-Tsadik G, *et al.* When is fasting really fasting? The influence of time of day, interval after a meal, and maternal body mass on maternal glycemia in gestational diabetes. *American Journal of Obstetrics and Gynecology* 1999;181(4):904–11.

164. Dornhorst A, Nicholls JS, Probst F, *et al.* Calorie restriction for treatment of gestational diabetes. *Diabetes* 1991;40(Suppl 2):161–4.

165. Rae A, Bond D, Evans S, *et al.* A randomised controlled trial of dietary energy restriction in the management of obese women with gestational diabetes. *The Australian and New Zealand Journal of Obstetrics and Gynaecology* 2000;40(4):416–22.

166. Algert S, Shragg P and Hollingsworth DR. Moderate caloric restriction in obese women with gestational diabetes. *Obstetrics and Gynecology* 1985;65(4):487–91.

167. Peterson CM and Jovanovic-Peterson L. Randomized crossover study of 40% vs. 55% carbohydrate weight loss strategies in women with previous gestational diabetes mellitus and non-diabetic women of 130–200% ideal body weight. *Journal of the American College of Nutrition* 1995;14(4):369–75.

168. Jovanovic-Peterson L, Durak EP and Peterson CM. Randomized trial of diet versus diet plus cardiovascular conditioning on glucose levels in gestational diabetes. *American Journal of Obstetrics and Gynecology* 1989;161(2):415–19.

169. Brankston GN, Mitchell BF, Ryan EA, *et al.* Resistance exercise decreases the need for insulin in overweight women with gestational diabetes mellitus. *American Journal of Obstetrics and Gynecology* 2004;190(1):188–93.

170. Lesser KB, Gruppuso PA, Terry RB, *et al.* Exercise fails to improve postprandial glycemic excursion in women with gestational diabetes. *Journal of Maternal-Fetal Medicine* 1996;5(4):211–17.

171. Symons DD and Ulbrecht JS. Understanding exercise beliefs and behaviors in women with gestational diabetes mellitus. *Diabetes Care* 2006;29(2):236–40.

172. Persson B, Stangenberg M, Hansson U, *et al.* Gestational diabetes mellitus (GDM). Comparative evaluation of two treatment regimens, diet versus insulin and diet. *Diabetes* 1985;34(Suppl 2):101–4.

173. Thompson DJ, Porter KB, Gunnells DJ, *et al.* Prophylactic insulin in the management of gestational diabetes. *Obstetrics and Gynecology* 1990;75(6):960–4.

174. Wechter DJ, Kaufmann RC, Amankwah KS, *et al.* Prevention of neonatal macrosomia in gestational diabetes by the use of intensive dietary therapy and home glucose monitoring. *American Journal of Perinatology* 1991;8(2):131–4.

175. Botta RM, Di Giovanni BM, Cammilleri F, *et al.* Predictive factors for insulin treatment in women with diagnosis of gestational diabetes. *Annali Dell'Istituto Superiore di Sanita* 1997;33(3):403–6.

176. Bochner CJ, Medearis AL, Williams J 3rd, *et al.* Early third-trimester ultrasound screening in gestational diabetes to determine the risk of macrosomia and labor dystocia at term. *American Journal of Obstetrics and Gynecology* 1987;157(3):703–8.

177. Buchanan TA, Kjos SL, Montoro MN, *et al.* Use of fetal ultrasound to select metabolic therapy for pregnancies complicated by mild gestational diabetes. *Diabetes Care* 1994;17(4):275–83.

178. Kjos SL, Schaefer-Graf U, Sardesi S, *et al.* A randomized controlled trial using glycemic plus fetal ultrasound parameters versus glycemic parameters to determine insulin therapy in gestational diabetes with fasting hyperglycemia. *Diabetes Care* 2001;24(11):1904–10.

179. Schaefer-Graf UM, Kjos SL, Fauzan OH, *et al.* A randomized trial evaluating a predominantly fetal growth-based strategy to guide management of gestational diabetes in Caucasian women. *Diabetes Care* 2004;27(2):297–302.

180. Bonomo M, Cetin I, Pisoni MP, *et al.* Flexible treatment of gestational diabetes modulated on ultrasound evaluation of intrauterine growth: a controlled randomized clinical trial. *Diabetes and Metabolism* 2004;30(3):237–44.

181. Rossi G, Somigliana E, Moschetta M, *et al.* Adequate timing of fetal ultrasound to guide metabolic therapy in mild gestational diabetes mellitus. Results from a randomized study. *Acta Obstetricia et Gynecologica Scandinavica* 2000;79(8):649–54.

182. Bertini AM, Silva JC, Taborda W, *et al.* Perinatal outcomes and the use of oral hypoglycemic agents. *Journal of Perinatal Medicine* 2005;33(6):519–23.

183. Jacobson GF, Ramos GA, Ching JY, *et al.* Comparison of glyburide and insulin for the management of gestational diabetes in a large managed care organization. *American Journal of Obstetrics and Gynecology* 2005;193(1):118–24.

184. Conway DL, Gonzales O and Skiver D. Use of glyburide for the treatment of gestational diabetes: the San Antonio experience. *Journal of Maternal-Fetal and Neonatal Medicine* 2004;15(1):51–5.

185. Kremer CJ and Duff P. Glyburide for the treatment of gestational diabetes. *American Journal of Obstetrics and Gynecology* 2004;190(5):1438–9.

186. Yogev Y, Ben-Haroush A, Chen R, *et al.* Undiagnosed asymptomatic hypoglycemia: diet, insulin, and glyburide for gestational diabetic pregnancy. *Obstetrics and Gynecology* 2004;104(1):88–93.

187. Jovanovic L, Ilic S, Pettitt DJ, *et al.* Metabolic and immunologic effects of insulin lispro in gestational diabetes. *Diabetes Care* 1999;22(9):1422–7.

188. Poyhonen-Alho M, Teramo K and Kaaja R. Treatment of gestational diabetes with short- or long-acting insulin and neonatal outcome: a pilot study. *Acta Obstetricia et Gynecologica Scandinavica* 2002;81(3):258–9.

189. Pettitt DJ, Ospina P, Kolaczynski JW, *et al.* Comparison of an insulin analog, insulin aspart, and regular human insulin with no insulin in gestational diabetes mellitus. *Diabetes Care* 2003;26(1):183–6.

190. Sameshima H, Kamitomo M, Kajiya S, *et al.* Insulin-meal interval and short-term glucose fluctuation in tightly controlled gestational diabetes mellitus. *The Journal of Maternal-Fetal Medicine* 2001;10(4):241–5.

191. Smits MW, Paulk TH and Kee CC. Assessing the impact of an outpatient education program for patients with gestational diabetes. *Diabetes Educator* 1995;21(2):129–34.

192. Mires GJ, Williams FL and Harper V. Screening practices for gestational diabetes mellitus in UK obstetric units. *Diabetic Medicine* 1999;16(2):138–41.

193. Hod M, Jovanovic L, Di Renzo GC, *et al. Textbook of Diabetes and Pregnancy.* London: Martin Dunitz; 2003.

194. Langer O, Rodriguez DA, Xenakis EM, *et al.* Intensified versus conventional management of gestational diabetes. *American Journal of Obstetrics and Gynecology* 1994;170(4):1036–46.

195. Landon MB, Gabbe SG, Piana R, *et al.* Neonatal morbidity in pregnancy complicated by diabetes mellitus: predictive value of maternal glycemic profiles. *American Journal of Obstetrics and Gynecology* 1987;156(5):1089–95.

196. Wyse LJ, Jones M and Mandel F. Relationship of glycosylated hemoglobin, fetal macrosomia, and birthweight macrosomia. *American Journal of Perinatology* 1994;11(4):260–2.

197. Valuk J. Factors influencing birth weight in infants of diabetic mothers. *Diabetes* 1986;35:96A.

198. Jovanovic L, Druzin M and Peterson CM. Effect of euglycemia on the outcome of pregnancy in insulin-dependent diabetic women as compared with normal control subjects. *American Journal of Medicine* 1981;71(6):921–7.

199. Evers IM, De Valk HW, Mol BWJ, *et al.* Macrosomia despite good glycaemic control in Type I diabetic pregnancy; results of a nationwide study in The Netherlands. *Diabetologia* 2002;45(11):1484–9.

200. Jovanovic-Peterson L, Peterson CM, Reed GF, *et al.* Maternal postprandial glucose levels and infant birth weight: the Diabetes in Early Pregnancy Study. The National Institute of Child Health and Human Developmen – Diabetes in Early Pregnancy Study. *American Journal of Obstetrics and Gynecology* 1991;164(1 Pt 1):103–11.

201. Combs CA, Gunderson E, Kitzmiller JL, *et al.* Relationship of fetal macrosomia to maternal postprandial glucose control during pregnancy. *Diabetes Care* 1992;15(10):1251–7.

202. Manderson JG, Patterson CC, Hadden DR, *et al.* Preprandial versus postprandial blood glucose monitoring in type 1 diabetic pregnancy: a randomized controlled clinical trial. *American Journal of Obstetrics and Gynecology* 2003;189(2):507–12.

203. Parretti E, Mecacci F, Papini M, *et al.* Third-trimester maternal glucose levels from diurnal profiles in nondiabetic pregnancies: correlation with sonographic parameters of fetal growth. *Diabetes Care* 2001;24(8):1319–23.

204. Karlsson K and Kjellmer I. The outcome of diabetic pregnancies in relation to the mother's blood sugar level. *American Journal of Obstetrics and Gynecology* 1972;112(2):213–20.

205. Miodovnik M. High spontaneous premature labour rate in insulin-dependent diabetic women: An association with poor glycaemic control. *Scientific abstracts of the seventh Annual Meeting of the Society for Perinatal Obstetrics* Lake Buena Vista, Florida, 5–7 February 1987 (Abstract).

206. Rosenn B. Minor congenital malformations in infants of insulin-diabetic women: association with poor glycaemic control. *Obstetrics and Gynecology* 1990;76:745–9.

207. Nielsen GL, Moller M and Sorensen HT. HbA1c in early diabetic pregnancy and pregnancy outcomes: A Danish population-based cohort study of 573 pregnancies in women with type 1 diabetes. *Diabetes Care* 2006;29(12):2612–16.

208. Fotinos C, Dodson S and French L. Does tight control of blood glucose in pregnant women with diabetes improve neonatal outcomes?. *Journal of Family Practice* 2004;53(10):838–41.

209. Yogev Y, Chen R, Ben-Haroush A, *et al.* Continuous glucose monitoring for the evaluation of gravid women with type 1 diabetes mellitus. *Obstetrics and Gynecology* 2003;101(4):633–8.

210. Kerssen A, De Valk HW and Visser GH. Do HbA(1)c levels and the self-monitoring of blood glucose levels adequately reflect glycaemic control during pregnancy in women with type 1 diabetes mellitus? *Diabetologia* 2006;49(1):25–8.

211. Jovanovic L. The role of continuous glucose monitoring in gestational diabetes mellitus. *Diabetes Technology and Therapeutics* 2000;2(Suppl 1):S67–71.

212. di Biase N, Napoli A, Sabbatini A, *et al.* Telemedicine in the treatment of diabetic pregnancy. *Annali Dell'Istituto Superiore di Sanita* 1997;33(3):347–51.

213. Inkster ME, Fahey TP, Donnan PT, *et al.* Poor glycated haemoglobin control and adverse pregnancy outcomes in type 1 and type 2 diabetes mellitus: Systematic review of observational studies. *BMC Pregnancy and Childbirth* 2006;6:30.

214. Diamond MP, Reece EA, Caprio S, *et al*. Impairment of counterregulatory hormone responses to hypoglycemia in pregnant women with insulin-dependent diabetes mellitus. *American Journal of Obstetrics and Gynecology* 1992;166(1 Pt 1):70–7.

215. Rosenn BM, Miodovnik M, Khoury JC, *et al*. Counterregulatory hormonal responses to hypoglycemia during pregnancy. *Obstetrics and Gynecology* 1996;87(4):568–74.

216. Zarkovic M, Nesovic M, Marisavljevic D, *et al*. Short term parenteral nutrition in a pregnant diabetic woman with hyperemesis gravidarum. *Archives of Gastroenterohepatology* 1995;14(1–2):33–5.

217. Brimacombe J. Midazolam and parenteral nutrition in the management of life-threatening hyperemesis gravidarum in a diabetic patient. *Anaesthesia and Intensive Care* 1995;23(2):228–30.

218. Carroll MA and Yeomans ER. Diabetic ketoacidosis in pregnancy. *Critical Care Medicine* 2005;33(10 Suppl):S347–53.

219. Rodgers BD and Rodgers DE. Clinical variables associated with diabetic ketoacidosis during pregnancy. *Journal of Reproductive Medicine* 1991;36(11):797–800.

220. Levetan CS, Passaro MD, Jablonski KA, *et al*. Effect of physician specialty on outcomes in diabetic ketoacidosis. *Diabetes Care* 1999;22(11):1790–5.

221. National Collaborating Centre for Chronic Conditions. *Type 1 diabetes in adults - national clinical guideline for diagnosis and management in primary and secondary care*. London: Royal College of Physicians; 2004.

222. Nachum Z, Ben Shlomo I, Weiner E, *et al*. Twice daily versus four times daily insulin dose regimens for diabetes in pregnancy: randomised controlled trial. *British Medical Journal* 1999;319(7219):1223–7.

223. Gonzalez C, Santoro S, Salzberg S, *et al*. Insulin analogue therapy in pregnancies complicated by diabetes mellitus. *Expert Opinion on Pharmacotherapy* 2005;6(5):735–42.

224. Farrar D, Tuffnell DJ and West J. Continuous subcutaneous insulin infusion versus multiple daily injections of insulin for pregnant women with diabetes. *Cochrane Database of Systematic Reviews* 2007;(3).

225. Coustan DR, Reece EA, Sherwin RS, *et al*. A randomized clinical trial of the insulin pump vs intensive conventional therapy in diabetic pregnancies. *JAMA : the journal of the American Medical Association* 1986;255(5):631–6.

226. Laatikainen L, Teramo K and Hieta-Heikurainen H. A controlled study of the influence of continuous subcutaneous insulin infusion treatment on diabetic retinopathy during pregnancy. *Acta Medica Scandinavica* 1987;221(4):367–76.

227. Burkart W, Hanker JP and Schneider HP. Complications and fetal outcome in diabetic pregnancy. Intensified conventional versus insulin pump therapy. *Gynecologic and Obstetric Investigation* 1988;26(2):104–12.

228. Lapolla A, Dalfra MG, Masin M, *et al*. Analysis of outcome of pregnancy in type 1 diabetics treated with insulin pump or conventional insulin therapy. *Acta Diabetologica* 2003;40(3):143–9.

229. Simmons D, Thompson CF, Conroy C, *et al*. Use of insulin pumps in pregnancies complicated by type 2 diabetes and gestational diabetes in a multiethnic community. *Diabetes Care* 2001;24(12):2078–82.

230. Gabbe SG, Holing E, Temple P, *et al*. Benefits, risks, costs, and patient satisfaction associated with insulin pump therapy for the pregnancy complicated by type 1 diabetes mellitus. *American Journal of Obstetrics and Gynecology* 2000;182(6):1283–91.

231. Klein R, Klein BE, Moss SE, *et al*. The Wisconsin epidemiologic study of diabetic retinopathy. II. Prevalence and risk of diabetic retinopathy when age at diagnosis is less than 30 years. *Archives of Ophthalmology* 1984;102(4):520–6.

232. Diabetes Prevention Program Research Group., Nathan DM, Chew E, *et al*. The prevalence of retinopathy in impaired glucose tolerance and recent-onset diabetes in the diabetes prevention program. *Diabetic Medicine* 2007;24(2):137–44.

233. The Diabetes Control and Complications Trial Research Group. Effect of pregnancy on microvascular complications in the diabetes control and complications trial the diabetes control and complications trial research group. *Diabetes Care* 2000;23(8):1084–91.

234. Maayah J, Shammas A and Haddadin A. Effect of pregnancy on diabetic retinopathy. *Bahrain Medical Bulletin* 2001;23(4):163–5.

235. Klein BE, Moss SE and Klein R. Effect of pregnancy on progression of diabetic retinopathy. *Diabetes Care* 1990;13(1):34–40.

236. Chew EY, Mills JL, Metzger BE, *et al*. Metabolic control and progression of retinopathy: The Diabetes in Early Pregnancy Study. *Diabetes Care* 1995;18(5):631–7.

237. Phelps RL, Sakol P and Metzger BE. Changes in diabetes retinopathy during pregnancy. Correlations with regulation of hyperglycemia. *Archives of Ophthalmology* 1986;104(12):1806–10.

238. Axer-Siegel R, Hod M, Fink-Cohen S, *et al*. Diabetic retinopathy during pregnancy. *Ophthalmology* 1996;103(11):1815–19.

239. Rosenn B, Miodovnik M, Kranias G, *et al*. Progression of diabetic retinopathy in pregnancy: Association with hypertension in pregnancy. *American Journal of Obstetrics and Gynecology* 1992;166(4):1214–18.

240. Dibble CM, Kochenour NK and Worley RJ. Effect of pregnancy on diabetic retinopathy. *Obstetrics and Gynecology* 1982;59(6):699–704.

241. Temple RC, Aldridge VA, Sampson MJ, *et al*. Impact of pregnancy on the progression of diabetic retinopathy in Type 1 diabetes. *Diabetic Medicine* 2001;18(7):573–7.

242. Lauszus F, Klebe JG and Bek T. Diabetic retinopathy in pregnancy during tight metabolic control. *Acta Obstetricia et Gynecologica Scandinavica* 2000;79(5):367–70.

243. Diabetes Control and Complications Trial (DCCT) Research Group. Early worsening of diabetic retinopathy in the DCCT. *Archives of Ophthalmology* 1998;116:874–86.

244. Kroc Collaborative Study Group. Diabetic retinopathy after two years of intensified insulin treatment. Follow-up of the Kroc Collaborative Study. *JAMA: the journal of the American Medical Association* 1988;260(1):37–41.

245. Dahl-Jorgensen K, Brinchmann-Hansen O, Hanssen KF, *et al*. Rapid tightening of blood glucose control leads to transient deterioration of retinopathy in insulin dependent diabetes mellitus: the Oslo study. *British Medical Journal* 1985;290(6471):811–15.

246. Lauritzen T, Frost-Larsen K, Larsen HW, *et al*. Effect of 1 year of near-normal blood glucose levels on retinopathy in insulin-dependent diabetics. *Lancet* 1983;1(8318):200–4.

247. Early Treatment Diabetic Retinopathy Study Research Group. Photocoagulation for diabetic macular edema. Early treatment diabetic retinopathy study report number 1. *Archives of Ophthalmology* 1985;103:1796–806.

248. Early Treatment Diabetic Retinopathy Study Research Group. Treatment techniques and clinical guidelines for photocoagulation of diabetic macular edema. Early Treatment Diabetic Retinopathy Study Report Number 2. *Ophthalmology* 1987;94(7):761–74.

249. Early Treatment Diabetic Retinopathy Study Research Group. Early photocoagulation for diabetic retinopathy. ETDRS report number 9. *Ophthalmology* 1991;98(5 Suppl):766–85.

250. Bailey CC, Sparrow JM, Grey RH, *et al*. The National Diabetic Retinopathy Laser Treatment Audit. I. Maculopathy. *Eye* 1998;12(Pt 1):69–76.

251. Bailey CC, Sparrow JM, Grey RH, *et al.* The National Diabetic Retinopathy Laser Treatment Audit. III. Clinical outcomes. *Eye* 1999;13(Pt 2):151–9.

252. The Diabetic Retinopathy Study Research Group. Four risk factors for severe visual loss in diabetic retinopathy. The third report from the Diabetic Retinopathy Study. *Archives of Ophthalmology* 1979;97(4):654–5.

253. Diabetic Retinopathy Study Research Group. Photocoagulation treatment of proliferative diabetic retinopathy: clinical application of Diabetic Retinopathy Study (DRS) findings, DRS report Number 8. *Ophthalmology* 1981;88(7):583–600.

254. Chase HP, Garg SK, Jackson WE, *et al.* Blood pressure and retinopathy in type I diabetes. *Ophthalmology* 1990;97(2):155–9.

255. Joner G, Brinchmann-Hansen O, Torres CG, *et al.* A nationwide cross-sectional study of retinopathy and microalbuminuria in young Norwegian type 1 (insulin-dependent) diabetic patients. *Diabetologia* 1992;35(11):1049–54.

256. Klein R, Klein BE, Moss SE, *et al.* The Wisconsin Epidemiologic Study of Diabetic Retinopathy: XVII. The 14-year incidence and progression of diabetic retinopathy and associated risk factors in type 1 diabetes. *Ophthalmology* 1998;105(10):1801–15.

257. UK Prospective Diabetes Study Group. Tight blood pressure control and risk of macrovascular and microvascular complications in type 2 diabetes: UKPDS 38. [Erratum appears in *BMJ* 1999;318(7175):29]. *British Medical Journal* 1998;317(7160):703–13.

258. Stratton IM, Kohner EM, Aldington SJ, *et al.* UKPDS 50: risk factors for incidence and progression of retinopathy in Type II diabetes over 6 years from diagnosis. *Diabetologia* 2001;44(2):156–63.

259. Estacio RO, Jeffers BW, Gifford N, *et al.* Effect of blood pressure control on diabetic microvascular complications in patients with hypertension and type 2 diabetes. *Diabetes Care* 2000;23(Suppl 2):B54–64.

260. Matthews DR, Stratton IM, Aldington SJ, *et al.* Risks of progression of retinopathy and vision loss related to tight blood pressure control in type 2 diabetes mellitus: UKPDS 69. *Archives of Ophthalmology* 2004;122(11):1631–40.

261. Mogensen CE, Christensen CK and Vittinghus E. The stages in diabetic renal disease. With emphasis on the stage of incipient diabetic nephropathy. *Diabetes* 1983;32(Suppl 2):64–78.

262. Rosenn BM and Miodovnik M. Diabetic vascular complications in pregnancy: nephropathy. In: Hod M, Jovanovic L, Di Renzo GC, de Leiva A, Langer O, eds. *Diabetes and Pregnancy*. London: Taylor & Francis Group; 2003. p. 486–94.

263. Ekbom P, Damm P, Feldt-Rasmussen B, *et al.* Pregnancy outcome in type 1 diabetic women with microalbuminuria. *Diabetes Care* 2001;24(10):1739–44.

264. Nielsen LR, Muller C, Damm P, *et al.* Reduced prevalence of early preterm delivery in women with Type 1 diabetes and microalbuminuria – Possible effect of early antihypertensive treatment during pregnancy. *Diabetic Medicine* 2006;23(4):426–31.

265. McLeod L and Ray JG. Prevention and detection of diabetic embryopathy. *Community Genetics* 2002;5(1):33–9.

266. Macintosh MC, Fleming KM, Bailey JA, *et al.* Perinatal mortality and congenital anomalies in babies of women with type 1 or type 2 diabetes in England, Wales and Northern Ireland: population based study. *British Medical Journal* 2006;333(7560):177.

267. EUROCAT Central Registry. *European Registration of Congenital Anomalities: report 8: surveillance of congenital anomallies in Europe 1980–1999*. Newtownabbey: University of Ulster; 2002.

268. Huttly W, Rudnicka A and Wald NJ. Second-trimester prenatal screening markers for Down syndrome in women with insulin-dependent diabetes mellitus. *Prenatal Diagnosis* 2004;24(10):804–7.

269. Spencer K, Cicero S, Atzei A, *et al.* The influence of maternal insulin-dependent diabetes on fetal nuchal translucency thickness and first-trimester maternal serum biochemical markers of aneuploidy. *Prenatal Diagnosis* 2005;25(10):927–9.

270. Pedersen JF, Sorensen S and Molsted-Pedersen L. Serum levels of human placental lactogen, pregnancy-associated plasma protein A and endometrial secretory protein PP14 in first trimester of diabetic pregnancy. *Acta Obstetricia et Gynecologica Scandinavica* 1998;77(2):155–8.

271. Wong SF, Chan FY, Cincotta RB, *et al.* Routine ultrasound screening in diabetic pregnancies. *Ultrasound in Obstetrics and Gynecology* 2002;19(2):171–6.

272. Greene MF and Benacerraf BR. Prenatal diagnosis in diabetic gravidas: utility of ultrasound and maternal serum alpha-fetoprotein screening. *Obstetrics and Gynecology* 1991;77(4):520–4.

273. Albert TJ, Landon MB, Wheller JJ, *et al.* Prenatal detection of fetal anomalies in pregnancies complicated by insulin-dependent diabetes mellitus. *American Journal of Obstetrics and Gynecology* 1996;174(5):1424–8.

274. Giancotti A, Ferrero A, Marceca M, *et al.* Mid-second trimester fetal echocardiographic examination for detecting cardiac malformations in pregnancies complicated by pregestational diabetes. *Italian Journal of Gynaecology and Obstetrics* 1995;7(2):79–82.

275. Smith RS, Comstock CH, Lorenz RP, *et al.* Maternal diabetes mellitus: which views are essential for fetal echocardiography? *Obstetrics and Gynecology* 1997;90(4 Pt 1):575–9.

276. Muller PR, James A, Feldman K, *et al.* Utility of fetal echocardiogram in high-risk patients. *Australian and New Zealand Journal of Obstetrics and Gynaecology* 2005;45(2):117–21.

277. Stratton JF, Scanaill SN, Stuart B, *et al.* Are babies of normal birth weight who fail to reach their growth potential as diagnosed by ultrasound at increased risk? *Ultrasound in Obstetrics and Gynecology* 1995;5(2):114–18.

278. Coomarasamy A, Connock M, Thornton J, *et al.* Accuracy of ultrasound biometry in the prediction of macrosomia: a systematic quantitative review. *BJOG: an international journal of obstetrics and gynaecology* 2005;112(11):1461–6.

279. Hadlock FP, Harrist RB, Fearneyhough TC, *et al.* Use of femur length/abdominal circumference ratio in detecting the macrosomic fetus. *Radiology* 1985;154(2):503–5.

280. Parry S, Severs CP, Sehdev HM, *et al.* Ultrasonographic prediction of fetal macrosomia. Association with cesarean delivery. *Journal of Reproductive Medicine* 2000;45(1):17–22.

281. Levine AB, Lockwood CJ, Brown B, *et al.* Sonographic diagnosis of the large for gestational age fetus at term: does it make a difference? *Obstetrics and Gynecology* 1992;79(1):55–8.

282. Wong SF, Chan FY, Cincotta RB, *et al.* Sonographic estimation of fetal weight in macrosomic fetuses: diabetic versus non-diabetic pregnancies. *Australian and New Zealand Journal of Obstetrics and Gynaecology* 2001;41(4):429–32.

283. Bancerraf BR. Songraphically estimated fetal weights: accuracy and limitations. *American Journal of Obstetrics and Gynecology* 1988;159:118–21.

284. Kehl RJ, Krew MA, Thomas A, *et al.* Fetal growth and body composition in infants of women with diabetes mellitus during pregnancy. *Journal of Maternal-Fetal Medicine* 1996;5(5):273–80.

285. Combs CA, Rosenn B, Miodovnik M, *et al.* Sonographic EFW and macrosomia: is there an optimum formula to predict diabetic fetal macrosomia? *Journal of Maternal-Fetal Medicine* 2000;9(1):55–61.

286. Colman A, Maharaj D, Hutton J, et al. Reliability of ultrasound estimation of fetal weight in term singleton pregnancies. *New Zealand Medical Journal* 2006;119(1241):U2146.

287. Farrell T, Owen P, Kernaghan D, et al. Can ultrasound fetal biometry predict fetal hyperinsulinaemia at delivery in pregnancy complicated by maternal diabetes? *European Journal of Obstetrics, Gynecology, and Reproductive Biology* 2007;131(2):146–50.

288. Kernaghan D, Ola B, Fraser RB, et al. Fetal size and growth velocity in the prediction of the large for gestational age (LGA) infant in a glucose impaired population. *European Journal of Obstetrics and Gynecology* 2007;132(2):189–92.

289. Johnstone FD, Prescott RJ, Steel JM, et al. Clinical and ultrasound prediction of macrosomia in diabetic pregnancy. *British Journal of Obstetrics and Gynaecology* 1996;103(8):747–54.

290. Williams KP, Farquharson DF, Bebbington M, et al. Screening for fetal well-being in a high-risk pregnant population comparing the nonstress test with umbilical artery Doppler velocimetry: a randomized controlled clinical trial. *American Journal of Obstetrics and Gynecology* 2003;188(5):1366–71.

291. Neilson JP and Alfirevic Z. Doppler ultrasound for fetal assessment in high risk pregnancies. (Cochrane Review). In: *Cochrane Database of Systematic Reviews*. Chichester: Wiley Interscience; 2000.

292. Bricker L and Neilson JP. Routine doppler ultrasound in pregnancy. (Cochrane Review). In: *Cochrane Database of Systematic Reviews*. Chichester: Wiley Interscience; 2001.

293. Salvesen K. Routine ultrasound scanning in pregnancy. *British Medical Journal* 1993;307(6911):1064.

294. Wong SF, Chan FY, Cincotta RB, et al. Use of umbilical artery Doppler velocimetry in the monitoring of pregnancy in women with pre-existing diabetes. *Australian and New Zealand Journal of Obstetrics and Gynaecology* 2003;43(4):302–6.

295. Leung WC, Lam H, Lee CP, et al. Doppler study of the umbilical and fetal middle cerebral arteries in women with gestational diabetes mellitus. *Ultrasound in Obstetrics and Gynecology* 2004;24(5):534–7.

296. Zimmermann P, Kujansuu E and Tuimala R. Doppler velocimetry of the umbilical artery in pregnancies complicated by insulin-dependent diabetes mellitus. *European Journal of Obstetrics, Gynecology, and Reproductive Biology* 1992;47(2):85–93.

297. Johnstone FD, Steel JM, Haddad NG, et al. Doppler umbilical artery flow velocity waveforms in diabetic pregnancy. *British Journal of Obstetrics and Gynaecology* 1992;99(2):135–40.

298. Bracero LA, Figueroa R, Byrne DW, et al. Comparison of umbilical Doppler velocimetry, nonstress testing, and biophysical profile in pregnancies complicated by diabetes. *Journal of Ultrasound in Medicine* 1996;15(4):301–8.

299. Ben-Ami M, Battino S, Geslevich Y, et al. A random single Doppler study of the umbilical artery in the evaluation of pregnancies complicated by diabetes. *American Journal of Perinatology* 1995;12(6):437–8.

300. Kofinas AD, Penry M and Swain M. Uteroplacental Doppler flow velocity waveform analysis correlates poorly with glycemic control in diabetic pregnant women. *American Journal of Perinatology* 1991;8(4):273–7.

301. Reece EA, Hagay Z, Assimakopoulos E, et al. Diabetes mellitus in pregnancy and the assessment of umbilical artery waveforms using pulsed Doppler ultrasonography. *Journal of Ultrasound in Medicine* 1994;13(2):73–80.

302. Reece EA, Hagay Z, Moroder W, et al. Is there a correlation between aortic Doppler velocimetric findings in diabetic pregnant women and fetal outcome? *Journal of Ultrasound in Medicine* 1996;15(6):437–40.

303. Lauszus FF, Fuglsang J, Flyvbjerg A, et al. Preterm delivery in normoalbuminuric, diabetic women without preeclampsia: The role of metabolic control. *European Journal of Obstetrics, Gynecology, and Reproductive Biology* 2006;124(2):144–9.

304. Mathiesen ER, Christensen AB, Hellmuth E, et al. Insulin dose during glucocorticoid treatment for fetal lung maturation in diabetic pregnancy: test of an algorithm [correction of an algorithm]. *Acta Obstetricia et Gynecologica Scandinavica* 2002;81(9):835–9.

305. Kaushal K, Gibson J and Railton A. A protocol for improved glycaemic control following corticosteroid therapy in diabetic pregnancies. *Diabetic Medicine* 2003;20(1):73–5.

306. Royal College of Obstetricians and Gynaecologists. Tocolytic drugs for women in preterm labour. London, RCOG Press; 2002.

307. Giugliano D, Passariello N, Torella R, et al. Effects of acetylsalicylic acid on plasma glucose, free fatty acid, betahydroxybutyrate, glucagon and C-peptide responses to salbutamol in insulin-dependent diabetic subjects. *Acta Diabetologica Latina* 1981;18(1):27–36.

308. Fredholm BB, Lunell NO, Persson B, et al. Actions of salbutamol in late pregnancy: plasma cyclic AMP, insulin and C-peptide, carbohydrate and lipid metabolites in diabetic and non-diabetic women. *Diabetologia* 1978;14(4):235–42.

309. Lenz S, Kuhl C, Wang P, et al. The effect of ritodrine on carbohydrate and lipid metabolism in normal and diabetic pregnant women. *Acta Endocrinologica* 1979;92(4):669–79.

310. Tibaldi JM, Lorber DL and Nerenberg A. Diabetic ketoacidosis and insulin resistance with subcutaneous terbutaline infusion: a case report. *American Journal of Obstetrics and Gynecology* 1990;163(2):509–10.

311. Halpren EW, Soifer NE, Haenel LC, et al. Ketoacidosis secondary to oral ritodrine use in a gestational diabetic patient: Report of a case. *Journal of the American Osteopathic Association* 1988;88(2):241–4.

312. Richards SR and Klingelberger CE. Intravenous ritodrine as a possibly provocative predictive test in gestational diabetes. A case report. *Journal of Reproductive Medicine* 1987;32(10):798–800.

313. Mordes D, Kreutner K, Metzger W, et al. Dangers of intravenous ritodrine in diabetic patients. *JAMA: the journal of the American Medical Association* 1982;248(8):973–5.

314. Schilthuis MS and Aarnoudse JG. Fetal death associated with severe ritodrine induced ketoacidosis. *Lancet* 1980;1(8178):1145.

315. Feig DS, Razzaq A, Sykora K, et al. Trends in deliveries, prenatal care, and obstetrical complications in women with pregestational diabetes: a population-based study in Ontario, Canada, 1996–2001. *Diabetes Care* 2006;29(2):232–5.

316. Ehrenberg HM, Durnwald CP, Catalano P, et al. The influence of obesity and diabetes on the risk of cesarean delivery. *American Journal of Obstetrics and Gynecology* 2004;191(3):969–74.

317. Bernstein IM and Catalano PM. Examination of factors contributing to the risk of cesarean delivery in women with gestational diabetes. *Obstetrics and Gynecology* 1994;83(3):462–5.

318. Naylor CD, Sermer M, Chen E, et al. Cesarean delivery in relation to birth weight and gestational glucose tolerance. Pathophysiology or practice style? *JAMA: the journal of the American Medical Association* 1996;275(15):1165–70.

319. Kolderup LB, Laros RK, Jr. and Musci TJ. Incidence of persistent birth injury in macrosomic infants: association with mode of delivery. *American Journal of Obstetrics and Gynecology* 1997;177(1):37–41.

320. Naeye RL. The outcome of diabetic pregnancies: a prospective study. *Ciba Foundation symposium* 1978;(63)227–41.

321. Patel RR, Peters TJ and Murphy DJ. Prenatal risk factors for Caesarean section. Analyses of the ALSPAC cohort of 12 944 women in England. *International Journal of Epidemiology* 2005;34(2):353–67.

322. Modanlou H and Dorchester W. Maternal, fetal and immediate neonatal morbidity and operative delivery. *Neonatal Epidemiology & Follow-up* 1987;400A.

323. Kjos SL, Henry OA, Montoro M, *et al.* Insulin-requiring diabetes in pregnancy: a randomized trial of active induction of labor and expectant management. *American Journal of Obstetrics and Gynecology* 1993;169(3):611–15.

324. Hod M, Bar J, Peled Y, *et al.* Antepartum management protocol. Timing and mode of delivery in gestational diabetes. *Diabetes Care* 1998;21(Suppl 2):B113–17.

325. Conway DL and Langer O. Elective delivery of infants with macrosomia in diabetic women: reduced shoulder dystocia versus increased cesarean deliveries. *American Journal of Obstetrics and Gynecology* 1998;178(5):922–5.

326. Levy AL, Gonzalez JL, Rappaport VJ, *et al.* Effect of labor induction on cesarean section rates in diabetic pregnancies. *Journal of Reproductive Medicine* 2002;47(11):931–2.

327. Gonen O, Rosen DJ, Dolfin Z, *et al.* Induction of labor versus expectant management in macrosomia: a randomized study. *Obstetrics and Gynecology* 1997;89(6):913–17.

328. Incerpi MH, Fassett MJ, Kjos SL, *et al.* Vaginally administered misoprostol for outpatient cervical ripening in pregnancies complicated by diabetes mellitus. *American Journal of Obstetrics and Gynecology* 2001;185(4):916–19.

329. Khonjandi M, Tsai M and Tyson JE. Gestational diabetes: the dilemma of delivery. *Obstetrics and Gynecology* 1974;43(1):1–6.

330. Takoudes TC, Weitzen S, Slocum J, *et al.* Risk of cesarean wound complications in diabetic gestations. *American Journal of Obstetrics and Gynecology* 2004;191(3):958–63.

331. Lurie S, Insler V and Hagay ZJ. Induction of labor at 38 to 39 weeks of gestation reduces the incidence of shoulder dystocia in gestational diabetic patients class A2. *American Journal of Perinatology* 1996;13(5):293–6.

332. Coleman TL, Randall H, Graves W, *et al.* Vaginal birth after cesarean among women with gestational diabetes. *American Journal of Obstetrics and Gynecology* 2001;184(6):1104–7.

333. Holt VL and Mueller BA. Attempt and success rates for vaginal birth after caesarean section in relation to complications of the previous pregnancy. *Paediatric and Perinatal Epidemiology* 1997;11(Suppl 1):63–72.

334. Marchiano D, Elkousy M, Stevens E, *et al.* Diet-controlled gestational diabetes mellitus does not influence the success rates for vaginal birth after cesarean delivery. *American Journal of Obstetrics and Gynecology* 2004;190(3):790–6.

335. Rees GA, Hayes TM and Pearson JF. Diabetes, pregnancy and anaesthesia. *Clinics in Obstetrics and Gynaecology* 1982;9(2):311–32.

336. Lattermann R, Carli F, Wykes L, *et al.* Epidural blockade modifies perioperative glucose production without affecting protein catabolism. *Anesthesiology* 2002;97(2):374–81.

337. Tsen LC. Anesthetic management of the parturient with cardiac and diabetic diseases. *Clinical Obstetrics and Gynecology* 2003;46(3):700–10.

338. Ramanathan S, Khoo P and Arismendy J. Perioperative maternal and neonatal acid-base status and glucose metabolism in patients with insulin-dependent diabetes mellitus. *Anesthesia and Analgesia* 1991;73(2):105–11.

339. Hebl JR, Kopp SL, Schroeder DR, *et al.* Neurologic complications after neuraxial anesthesia or analgesia in patients with preexisting peripheral sensorimotor neuropathy or diabetic polyneuropathy. *Anesthesia and Analgesia* 2006;103(5):1294–9.

340. Saravanakumar K, Rao SG and Cooper GM. Obesity and obstetric anaesthesia. *Anaesthesia* 2006;61(1):36–48.

341. Datta S, Kitzmiller JL, Naulty JS, *et al.* Acid-base status of diabetic mothers and their infants following spinal anesthesia for cesarean section. *Anesthesia and Analgesia* 1982;61(8):662–5.

342. Andersen O, Hertel J, Schmolker L, *et al.* Influence of the maternal plasma glucose concentration at delivery on the risk of hypoglycaemia in infants of insulin-dependent diabetic mothers. *Acta Paediatrica Scandinavica* 1985;74(2):268–73.

343. Miodovnik M, Mimouni F and Tsang RC. Management of the insulin-dependent diabetic during labor and delivery. Influences on neonatal outcome. *American Journal of Perinatology* 1987;4(2):106–14.

344. Curet LB, Izquierdo LA, Gilson GJ, *et al.* Relative effects of antepartum and intrapartum maternal blood glucose levels on incidence of neonatal hypoglycemia. *Journal of Perinatology* 1997;17(2):113–15.

345. Lean ME, Pearson DW and Sutherland HW. Insulin management during labour and delivery in mothers with diabetes. *Diabetic Medicine* 1990;7(2):162–4.

346. Feldberg D, Dicker D, Samuel N, *et al.* Intrapartum management of insulin-dependent diabetes mellitus (IDDM) gestants. A comparative study of constant intravenous insulin infusion and continuous subcutaneous insulin infusion pump (CSIIP). *Acta Obstetricia et Gynecologica Scandinavica* 1988;67(4):333–8.

347. Balsells M, Corcoy R, Adelantado JM, *et al.* Gestational diabetes mellitus: Metabolic control during labour. *Diabetes, Nutrition and Metabolism - Clinical and Experimental* 2000;13(5):257–62.

348. Carron Brown S, Kyne-Grzebalski D, Mwangi B, *et al.* Effect of management policy upon 120 Type 1 diabetic pregnancies: policy decisions in practice. *Diabetic Medicine* 1999;16(7):573–8.

349. Taylor R, Lee C, Kyne-Grzebalski D, *et al.* Clinical outcomes of pregnancy in women with type 1 diabetes. *Obstetrics and Gynecology* 2002;99(4):537–41.

350. Mimouni F. Perinatal asphyxia in infants of diabetic mothers is associated with maternal vasclopathy and hyperglycaemia in labour. *Neonatal Epidemiology & Follow-up* 1987;400A.

351. Rosenberg VA, Eglinton GS, Rauch ER, *et al.* Intrapartum maternal glycemic control in women with insulin requiring diabetes: a randomized clinical trial of rotating fluids versus insulin drip. *American Journal of Obstetrics and Gynecology* 2006;195(4):1095–9.

352. Fuloria M and Kreiter S. The newborn examination: Part I. Emergencies and common abnormalities involving the skin, head, neck, check, and respiratory and cardiovascular systems. *American Family Physician* 2002;65(1):61–8.

353. Edstrom CS and Christensen RD. Evaluation and treatment of thrombosis in the neonatal intensive care unit. *Clinics in Perinatology* 2000;27(3):623–41.

354. Akera C and Ro S. Medical concerns in the neonatal period. *Clinics in Family Practice* 2003;5(2):265–92.

355. Aucott SW, Williams TG, Hertz RH, *et al.* Rigorous management of insulin-dependent diabetes mellitus during pregnancy. *Acta Diabetologica* 1994;31(3):126–9.

356. Haworth JC, Dilling LA and Vidyasagar D. Hypoglycemia in infants of diabetic mothers: effect of epinephrine therapy. *The Journal of Pediatrics* 1973;82(1):94–7.

357. Van Howe RS and Storms MR. Hypoglycemia in infants of diabetic mothers: experience in a rural hospital. *American Journal of Perinatology* 2006;23(2):105–10.

358. Alam M, Raza SJ, Sherali AR, *et al*. Neonatal complications in infants born to diabetic mothers. [Erratum appears in *J Coll Physicians Surg Pak* 2006;16(8):566 Note: Akhtar, SM [corrected to Akhtar, ASM]. *Journal of the College of Physicians and Surgeons – Pakistan: JCPSP* 2006;16(3):212–15.

359. Jones CW. Gestational diabetes and its impact on the neonate. *Neonatal Network - Journal of Neonatal Nursing* 2001;20(6):17–23.

360. Teramo K, Kari MA, Eronen M, *et al*. High amniotic fluid erythropoietin levels are associated with an increased frequency of fetal and neonatal morbidity in type 1 diabetic pregnancies. *Diabetologia* 2004;47(10):1695–703.

361. Dalgic N, Ergenekon E, Soysal S, *et al*. Transient neonatal hypoglycemia--long-term effects on neurodevelopmental outcome. *Journal of Pediatric Endocrinology* 2002;15(3):319–24.

362. Cordero L, Treuer SH, Landon MB, *et al*. Management of infants of diabetic mothers. *Archives of Pediatrics and Adolescent Medicine* 1998;152(3):249–54.

363. Halliday HL. Hypertrophic cardiomyopathy in infants of poorly-controlled diabetic mothers. *Archives of Disease in Childhood* 1981;56(4):258–63.

364. Watson D, Rowan J, Neale L, *et al*. Admissions to neonatal intensive care unit following pregnancies complicated by gestational or type 2 diabetes. *Australian and New Zealand Journal of Obstetrics and Gynaecology* 2003;43(6):429–32.

365. Scottish Intercollegiate Guidelines Network. *Management of diabetes. A national clinical guideline*. Edinburgh: SIGN; 2001.

366. Williams AF. Hypoglycaemia of the newborn: a review. *Bulletin of the World Health Organization* 1997;75(3):261–90.

367. Lucas A, Morley R and Cole TJ. Adverse neurodevelopmental outcome of moderate neonatal hypoglycaemia. *British Medical Journal* 1988;297(6659):1304–8.

368. Cornblath M, Hawdon JM, Williams AF, *et al*. Controversies regarding definition of neonatal hypoglycemia: suggested operational thresholds. *Pediatrics* 2000;105(5):1141–5.

369. Beard AG, Panos TC, Marasigan BV, *et al*. Perinatal stress and the premature neonate. II. Effect of fluid and calorie deprivation on blood glucose. *The Journal of Pediatrics* 1966;68(3):329–43.

370. Wharton BA and Bower BD. Immediate or later feeding for premature babies? *A controlled trial*. Lancet 1965;2(7420):769–72.

371. Hawdon JM, Ward Platt MP and Aynsley-Green A. Patterns of metabolic adaptation for preterm and term infants in the first neonatal week. *Archives of Disease in Childhood* 1992;67(4 Spec No):357–65.

372. Lucas A, Boyes S, Bloom SR, *et al*. Metabolic and endocrine responses to a milk feed in six-day-old term infants: differences between breast and cow's milk formula feeding. *Acta Paediatrica Scandinavica* 1981;70(2):195–200.

373. Ratzmann KP, Steindel E, Hildebrandt R, *et al*. Is there a relationship between metabolic control and glucose concentration in breast milk of type 1 (insulin-dependent) diabetic mothers? *Experimental and Clinical Endocrinology* 1988;92(1):32–6.

374. Plagemann A, Harder T, Franke K, *et al*. Long-term impact of neonatal breast-feeding on body weight and glucose tolerance in children of diabetic mothers. *Diabetes Care* 2002;25(1):16–22.

375. Rodekamp E, Harder T, Kohlhoff R, *et al*. Long-term impact of breast-feeding on body weight and glucose tolerance in children of diabetic mothers: role of the late neonatal period and early infancy. *Diabetes Care* 2005;28(6):1457–62.

376. Rodekamp E, Harder T, Kohlhoff R, *et al*. Impact of breast-feeding on psychomotor and neuropsychological development in children of diabetic mothers: role of the late neonatal period. *Journal of Perinatal Medicine* 2006;34(6):490–6.

377. Plagemann A, Harder T, Kohlhoff R, *et al*. Impact of early neonatal breast-feeding on psychomotor and neuropsychological development in children of diabetic mothers. *Diabetes Care* 2005;28(3):573–8.

378. Gerstein HC. Cow's milk exposure and type I diabetes mellitus. A critical overview of the clinical literature. *Diabetes Care* 1994;17(1):13–19.

379. Norris JM and Scott FW. A meta-analysis of infant diet and insulin-dependent diabetes mellitus: do biases play a role? *Epidemiology* 1996;7(1):87–92.

380. Meloni T, Marinaro AM, Mannazzu MC, *et al*. IDDM and early infant feeding. Sardinian case–control study. *Diabetes Care* 1997;20(3):340–2.

381. Ferris AM, Neubauer SH, Bendel RB, *et al*. Perinatal lactation protocol and outcome in mothers with and without insulin-dependent diabetes mellitus. *American Journal of Clinical Nutrition* 1993;58(1):43–8.

382. Gagne MP, Leff EW and Jefferis SC. The breast-feeding experience of women with type I diabetes. *Health Care for Women International* 1992;13(3):249–60.

383. van Beusekom CM, Zeegers TA, Martini IA, *et al*. Milk of patients with tightly controlled insulin-dependent diabetes mellitus has normal macronutrient and fatty acid composition. *American Journal of Clinical Nutrition* 1993;57(6):938–43.

384. Cox SG. Expressing and storing colostrum antenatally for use in the newborn periods. *Breastfeeding Review* 2006;14(3):16.

386. Screening guidelines for newborns at risk for low blood glucose. *Paediatrics and Child Health* 2004;9(10):723–40.

387. CREST. *Management of Diabetes in Pregnancy*. Belfast: CREST; 2001. p. 1–74.

388. Rennie JM. *Robertson's Textbook of Neonatology*. Edinburgh: Churchill Livingstone; 2005.

389. Saez-de-Ibarra L, Gaspar R, Obesso A, *et al*. Glycaemic behaviour during lactation: postpartum practical guidelines for women with type 1 diabetes. *Practical Diabetes International* 2003;20(8):271–5.

390. Ferris AM, Dalidowitz CK, Ingardia CM, *et al*. Lactation outcome in insulin-dependent diabetic women. *Journal of the American Dietetic Association* 1988;88(3):317–22.

391. Davies HA, Clark JD, Dalton KJ, *et al*. Insulin requirements of diabetic women who breast feed. *British Medical Journal* 1989;298(6684):1357–8.

392. Briggs GG, Ambrose PJ, Nageotte MP, *et al*. Excretion of metformin into breast milk and the effect on nursing infants. *Obstetrics and Gynecology* 2005;105(6):1437–41.

393. Feig DS, Briggs GG, Kraemer JM, *et al*. Transfer of glyburide and glipizide into breast milk. *Diabetes Care* 2005;28(8):1851–5.

394. Kim C, Newton KM and Knopp RH. Gestational diabetes and the incidence of type 2 diabetes: a systematic review. *Diabetes Care* 2002;25(10):1862–8.

395. Lauenborg J, Hansen T, Jensen DM, *et al*. Increasing incidence of diabetes after gestational diabetes: a long-term follow-up in a Danish population. *Diabetes Care* 2004;27(5):1194–9.

396. Lobner K, Knopff A, Baumgarten A, *et al*. Predictors of postpartum diabetes in women with gestational diabetes mellitus. *Diabetes* 2006;55(3):792–7.

397. Wein P, Beischer NA and Sheedy MT. Studies of postnatal diabetes mellitus in women who had gestational diabetes. Part 2. Prevalence and predictors of diabetes mellitus after delivery. *Australian and New Zealand Journal of Obstetrics and Gynaecology* 1997;37(4):420–3.

398. Lee CP, Wong HS, Chan FY, *et al*. Long-term prognosis of women with abnormal glucose tolerance in pregnancy. *Australian and New Zealand Journal of Obstetrics and Gynaecology* 1994;34(5):507–10.

399. Linne Y, Barkeling B and Rossner S. Natural course of gestational diabetes mellitus: Long term follow up of women in the SPAWN study. *BJOG: an international journal of obstetrics and gynaecology* 2002;109(11):1227–31.

400. Aberg AE, Jonsson EK, Eskilsson I, *et al*. Predictive factors of developing diabetes mellitus in women with gestational diabetes. *Acta Obstetricia et Gynecologica Scandinavica* 2002;81(1):11–16.

401. Jarvela IY, Juutinen J, Koskela P, *et al*. Gestational diabetes identifies women at risk for permanent type 1 and type 2 diabetes in fertile age: predictive role of autoantibodies. *Diabetes Care* 2006;29(3):607–12.

402. Pettitt DJ, Narayan KM, Hanson RL, *et al*. Incidence of diabetes mellitus in women following impaired glucose tolerance in pregnancy is lower than following impaired glucose tolerance in the non-pregnant state. *Diabetologia* 1996;39(11):1334–7.

403. Stage E, Ronneby H and Damm P. Lifestyle change after gestational diabetes. *Diabetes Research and Clinical Practice* 2004;63(1):67–72.

404. Knowler WC, Barrett-Connor E, Fowler SE, *et al*. Reduction in the incidence of type 2 diabetes with lifestyle intervention or metformin. *New England Journal of Medicine* 2002;346(6):393–403.

405. Tuomilehto J, Lindstrom J, Eriksson JG, *et al*. Prevention of type 2 diabetes mellitus by changes in lifestyle among subjects with impaired glucose tolerance. *New England Journal of Medicine* 2001;344(18):1343–50.

406. Smith BJ, Cheung NW, Bauman AE, *et al*. Postpartum physical activity and related psychosocial factors among women with recent gestational diabetes mellitus. *Diabetes Care* 2005;28(11):2650–4.

407. Gillies CL, Abrams KR, Lambert PC, *et al*. Pharmacological and lifestyle interventions to prevent or delay type 2 diabetes in people with impaired glucose tolerance: systematic review and meta-analysis. *British Medical Journal* 2007;334(7588):299–302.

408. Holt RI, Goddard JR, Clarke P, *et al*. A postnatal fasting plasma glucose is useful in determining which women with gestational diabetes should undergo a postnatal oral glucose tolerance test. *Diabetic Medicine* 2003;20(7):594–8.

409. Tan YY, Yeo SH and Liauw PC. Is postnatal oral glucose tolerance testing necessary in all women with gestational diabetes. *Singapore Medical Journal* 1996;37(4):384–8.

410. Elixhauser A, Weschler JM, Kitzmiller JL, *et al*. Cost-benefit analysis of preconception care for women with established diabetes mellitus. *Diabetes Care* 1993;16(8):1146–57.

411. Shearer A, Bagust A, Sanderson D, *et al*. Cost-effectiveness of flexible intensive insulin management to enable dietary freedom in people with Type 1 diabetes in the UK. *Diabetic Medicine* 2004;21(5):460–7.

412. Gregory R and Tattersall RB. Are diabetic pre-pregnancy clinics worth while? *Lancet* 1992;340(8820):656–8.

413. Odibo AO, Coassolo KM, Stamilio DM, *et al*. Should all pregnant diabetic women undergo a fetal echocardiography? A cost-effectiveness analysis comparing four screening strategies. *Prenatal Diagnosis* 2006;26(1):39–44.

414. Wren C, Birrell G and Hawthorne G. Cardiovascular malformations in infants of diabetic mothers. *Heart* 2003;89(10):1217–20.

415. Sullivan ID. Prenatal diagnosis of structural heart disease: does it make a difference to survival? *Heart* 2002;87(5):405–6.

416. Ritchie K, Boynton J, Bradbury I, *et al*. *Routine Ultrasound Scanning Before 24 Weeks of Pregnancy*. Consultation report. NHS Quality Improvement; 2003 [www.nhshealthquality.org/nhsqis/files/Ultrasound%20CAR.pdf].

417. Ogge G, Gaglioti P, Maccanti S, *et al*. Prenatal screening for congenital heart disease with four-chamber and outflow-tract views: A multicenter study. *Ultrasound in Obstetrics and Gynecology* 2006;28(6):779–84.

418. Bonnet D, Coltri A, Butera G, *et al*. Detection of transposition of the great arteries in fetuses reduces neonatal morbidity and mortality. *Circulation* 1999;99(7):916–18.

419. Bonnet D, Jouannic JM and Fermont L. Impact of prenatal diagnosis on perinatal care of transposition of the great arteries. *Ultrasound in Obstetrics and Gynecology* 2003;22(S1):66–7.

420. Kumar RK, Newburger JW, Gauvreau K, *et al*. Comparison of outcome when hypoplastic left heart syndrome and transposition of the great arteries are diagnosed prenatally versus when diagnosis of these two conditions is made only postnatally. *American Journal of Cardiology* 1999;83(12):1649–53.

421. Schaefer-Graf UM, Buchanan TA, Xiang A, *et al*. Patterns of congenital anomalies and relationship to initial maternal fasting glucose levels in pregnancies complicated by type 2 and gestational diabetes. *American Journal of Obstetrics and Gynecology* 2000;182(2):313–20.

422. Checa MA, Requena A, Salvador C, *et al*. Insulin-sensitizing agents: Use in pregnancy and as therapy in polycystic ovary syndrome. *Human Reproduction Update* 2005;11(4):375–90.

423. Hod M, Visser GHA, Damm P, *et al*. Safety and perinatal outcome in pregnancy: a randomized trial comparing insulin aspart with human insulin in 322 subjects with type 1 diabetes. *Diabetes* 2006;55(Suppl 1):A 417.

424. Halaska M, Martan A, Voigt R, *et al*. Tolerance and effectiveness of propiverine hydrochloride in 752 patients with symptoms of hyperactivity of the detruser, increased sensitivity and irritability of the urinary bladder: Results of an investigation of the use of a drug. *Ceska Gynekologie* 1997;62(5):259–64.

425. Glueck CJ, Goldenberg N, Wang P, *et al*. Metformin during pregnancy reduces insulin, insulin resistance, insulin secretion, weight, testosterone and development of gestational diabetes: Prospective longitudinal assessment of women with polycystic ovary syndrome from preconception throughout pregnancy. *Human Reproduction* 2004;19(3):510–21.

426. Langer O, Yogev Y, Most O, *et al*. Gestational diabetes: the consequences of not treating. *American Journal of Obstetrics and Gynecology* 2005;192(4):989–97.

427. Wang Y, Storlien LH, Jenkins AB, *et al*. Dietary variables and glucose tolerance in pregnancy. *Diabetes Care* 2000;23(4):460–4.

428. Catalano PM, Thomas A, Huston-Presley L, *et al*. Increased fetal adiposity: a very sensitive marker of abnormal in utero development. *American Journal of Obstetrics and Gynecology* 2003;189(6):1698–704.

429. Simmons D and Robertson S. Influence of maternal insulin treatment on the infants of women with gestational diabetes. *Diabetic Medicine* 1997;14(9):762–5.

430. Drexel H, Bichler A, Sailer S, *et al*. Prevention of perinatal morbidity by tight metabolic control in gestational diabetes mellitus. *Diabetes Care* 1988;11(10):761–8.

431. Stainton MC, Lohan M, Fethney J, *et al*. Women's responses to two models of antepartum high-risk care: Day stay and hospital stay. *Women and Birth* 2006;19(4):89–95.

432. Carta Q, Meriggi E, Trossarelli GF, *et al*. Continuous subcutaneous insulin infusion versus intensive conventional insulin therapy in type I and type II diabetic pregnancy. *Diabète & Métabolisme* 1986;12(3):121–9.

433. Nosari I, Maglio ML, Lepore G, et al. Is continuous subcutaneous insulin infusion more effective than intensive conventional insulin therapy in the treatment of pregnant diabetic women? *Diabetes, Nutrition and Metabolism - Clinical and Experimental* 1993;6(1):33–7.

434. Abramowicz JS, Rana S and Abramowicz S. Fetal cheek-to-cheek diameter in the prediction of mode of delivery. *American Journal of Obstetrics and Gynecology* 2005;192(4):1205–11.

435. Best G and Pressman EK. Ultrasonographic prediction of birth weight in diabetic pregnancies. *Obstetrics and Gynecology* 2002;99(5 Pt 1):740–4.

436. Bracero LA, Haberman S and Byrne DW. Maternal glycemic control and umbilical artery Doppler velocimetry. *Journal of Maternal-Fetal and Neonatal Medicine* 2002;12(5):342–8.

437. Chauhan SP, Parker D, Shields D, et al. Sonographic estimate of birth weight among high-risk patients: feasibility and factors influencing accuracy. *American Journal of Obstetrics and Gynecology* 2006;195(2):601–6.

438. de la Vega A and Verdiales M. Failure of intensive fetal monitoring and ultrasound in reducing the stillbirth rate. *Puerto Rico Health Sciences Journal* 2002;21(2):123–5.

439. Smith MC, Moran P, Ward MK, et al. Assessment of glomerular filtration rate during pregnancy using the MDRD formula. *BJOG: an International Journal of Obstetrics and Gynaecology* 2008;115(1):109–12.

440. Pan W, Wu GP, Li YF, et al. The experience of diagnosis the abnormal fetal heart by fetal echocardiography to 900 fetuses. Guangzhou, China: Guangdong Cardiovascular Institute; undated [available from www.unepsa.org/china/ab/1327.HTM; accessed 30 August 2006].

441. Poncet B, Touzet S, Rocher L, et al. Cost-effectiveness analysis of gestational diabetes mellitus screening in France. *European Journal of Obstetrics, Gynecology and Reproductive Biology* 2002;103(2):122–9.

442. Di CG, Volpe L, Casadidio I et al. Universal screening and intensive metabolic management of gestational diabetes: cost-effectiveness in Italy. *Acta Diabetologica* 2002;39(2):69–73.

443. Nicholson WK, Fleisher LA, Fox HE et al. Screening for gestational diabetes mellitus: a decision and cost-effectiveness analysis of four screening strategies. *Diabetes Care* 2005;28(6):1482–4.

444. Reed BD. Screening for gestational diabetes--analysis by screening criteria. *Journal of Family Practice* 1984;19(6):751–5.

445. Massion C, O'Connor PJ, Gorab R et al. Screening for gestational diabetes in a high-risk population. *Journal of Family Practice* 1987;25(6):569–75.

446. Lavin JP, Barden TP and Miodovnik M. Clinical experience with a screening program for gestational diabetes. *American Journal of Obstetrics and Gynecology* 1981;141(5):491–4.

447. Larijani B, Hossein-nezhad A and Vassigh A-R. Effect of varying threshold and selective versus universal strategies on the cost in gestational diabetes mellitus. *Archives of Iranian Medicine* 2004;7(4):267–71.

448. National Collaborating Centre for Women's and Children's Health. *Fertility: Assessment and Management for People with Fertility Problems.* London: RCOG Press; 2004.

449. Reichelt AJ, Spichler ER, Branchtein L, Nucci LB, Franco LJ, Schmidt MI. Fasting plasma glucose is a useful test for the detection of gestational diabetes. Brazilian Study of Gestational Diabetes (EBDG) Working Group. *Diabetes Care* 1998;21:1246–9.

450. Ostlund I and Hanson U. Repeated random blood glucose measurements as universal screening test for gestational diabetes mellitus. *Acta Obstetricia et Gynecologica Scandinavica* 2004;83(1):46–51.

451. Seshiah V, Balaji V, Balaji MS, et al. Gestational diabetes mellitus in India. *Journal of the Association of Physicians of India.* 2004;52:707–11.

452. Coustan DR. Methods of screening for and diagnosing of gestational diabetes. *Clinics in Perinatology* 1993;20(3):593–602.

453. Weeks JW, Major CA, de Veciana M et al. Gestational diabetes: Does the presence of risk factors influence perinatal outcome? *American Journal of Obstetrics and Gynecology* 1994; 171:1003–7.

454. Danilenko-Dixon D, Van Winter J, Nelson R, Ogburn P. Universal versus selective gestational diabetes screening: application of 1997 American Diabetes Association recommendations. *American Journal of Obstetrics and Gynecology* 1999;181:798–802.

455. Williams CB, Iqbal S, Zawacki CM, Yu D, Brown MB, Herman WH. Effect of selective screening for gestational diabetes. *Diabetes Care* 1999;22:418–21.

456. Curtis L, Netten A. *Unit Costs of Health and Social Care.* Canterbury: Personal and Social Services Research Unit University of Kent at Canterbury; 2006.

457. Joint Formulary Committee. *British National Formulary.* 52nd ed. London: British Medical Association and Royal Pharmaceutical Society of Great Britain; 2006.

458. Davies L and Drummond M. Management of labour: consumer choice and cost implications. *Journal of Obstetrics and Gynaecology* 1991;11(Suppl 1):s28–s33.

459. Davies L and Drummond M. *The Costs of Induction of Labour by Prostaglandin E_2 or Oxytocin: Refining the Estimates.* York: University of York; 1993.

460. Briggs A, Claxton K, Sculpher M. *Decision Modelling for Health Economic Evaluation.* Oxford: Oxford University Press; 2006.

461. Goetzl L and Wilkins I. Glyburide compared to insulin for the treatment of gestational diabetes mellitus: A cost analysis. *Journal of Perinatology* 2002;22(5):403–6.

462. Williams CB, Iqbal S, Zawacki CM, et al. Effect of selective screening for gestational diabetes. *Diabetes Care* 1999;22:418–21.

Index